T0313228

Bayesian Analysis with R for Drug Development

Concepts, Algorithms, and Case Studies

Chapman and Hall/CRC
Biostatistics Series

Shein-Chung Chow, Duke University School of Medicine
Byron Jones, Novartis Pharma AG
Jen-pei Liu, National Taiwan University
Karl E. Peace, Georgia Southern University
Bruce W. Turnbull, Cornell University

Recently Published Titles

Self-Controlled Case Series Studies: A Modelling Guide with R
Paddy Farrington, Heather Whitaker, Yonas Ghebremichael Weldeselassie

Bayesian Methods for Repeated Measures
Lyle D. Broemeling

Modern Adaptive Randomized Clinical Trials: Statistical and Practical Aspects
Oleksandr Sverdlov

Medical Product Safety Evaluation: Biological Models and Statistical Methods
Jie Chen, Joseph Heyse, Tze Leung Lai

Statistical Methods for Survival Trial Design: With Applications to Cancer Clinical Trials Using R
Jianrong Wu

Bayesian Applications in Pharmaceutical Development
Satrajit Roychoudhury, Soumi Lahiri

Platform Trials in Drug Development: Umbrella Trials and Basket Trials
Zoran Antonjevic and Robert Beckman

Innovative Strategies, Statistical Solutions and Simulations for Modern Clinical Trials
Mark Chang, John Balser, Robin Bliss, Jim Roach

Bayesian Cost-Effectiveness Analysis of Medical Treatments
Elias Moreno, Francisco Jose Vazquez-Polo, Miguel Angel Negrin-Hernandez

Analysis of Incidence Rates
Peter Cummings

Mixture Modelling for Medical and Health Sciences
Shu-Kay Ng, Liming Xiang, Kelvin Kai Wing Yau

Economic Evaluation of Cancer Drugs: Using Clinical Trial and Real-World Data
Iftekhar Khan, Ralph Crott, Zahid Bashir

Bayesian Analysis with R for Drug Development: Concepts, Algorithms, and Case Studies
Harry Yang and Steven J. Novick

For more information about this series, please visit: https://www.crcpress.com/go/biostats

Bayesian Analysis with R for Drug Development

Concepts, Algorithms, and Case Studies

Harry Yang and Steven J. Novick
AstraZeneca, Gaithersburg, Maryland

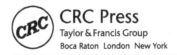

CRC Press
Taylor & Francis Group
Boca Raton London New York

CRC Press is an imprint of the
Taylor & Francis Group, an **informa** business

A CHAPMAN & HALL BOOK

CRC Press
Taylor & Francis Group
6000 Broken Sound Parkway NW, Suite 300
Boca Raton, FL 33487-2742

© 2019 by Taylor & Francis Group, LLC
CRC Press is an imprint of Taylor & Francis Group, an Informa business

No claim to original U.S. Government works

Printed on acid-free paper

International Standard Book Number-13: 978-1-1382-9587-2 (Hardback)

Library of Congress Cataloging-in-Publication Data

Names: Yang, Harry, author. | Novick, Steven, author.
Title: Bayesian analysis with R for biopharmaceuticals / Harry Yang, Steven Novick.
Description: Boca Raton : CRC Press, Taylor & Francis Group, 2019. | Includes bibliographical references and index.
Identifiers: LCCN 2019005802 | ISBN 9781138295872 (hardback : alk. paper)
Subjects: LCSH: Drug development. | Biopharmaceutics. | Clinical trials. | Bayesian statistical decision theory. | R (Computer program language)
Classification: LCC RM301.25 .Y36 2019 | DDC 615.1/9--dc23
LC record available at https://lccn.loc.gov/2019005802

Visit the Taylor & Francis Web site at
http://www.taylorandfrancis.com

and the CRC Press Web site at
http://www.crcpress.com

Contents

Section III   Chemistry, Manufacturing, and Control

Preface

Drug development is an empirical problem-solving process, characterized by trial and error. Knowledge gleaned from the previous study is often used to guide the next experiment. The sequential learning nature of experimentation and reliance on knowledge from various drug development stages calls for statistical methods that enable synthesis of information from disparate sources to aid better decision-making.

Bayesian statistics provide a flexible framework for continuous update of learning based on new information. In addition, Bayesian analysis allows for the incorporation of prior knowledge, in terms of either expert opinion or historical data, in its statistical inferences. This not only helps ease the reliance on large sample approximations that are often required for frequentist methods but also often results in greater efficiency in study design. Furthermore, many practitioners in drug development find it difficult to interpret the frequentist interval estimates and p-values, consequently creating a challenging and confusing situation for decision-makers. In contrast, the results of Bayesian analysis are typically presented through probabilistic statements. For example, after analyzing data from a two-arm comparative study, in which a test drug is assessed against the standard of care (SOC) therapy, both the frequentist and Bayesian conclude that the experimental drug is more effective than the SOC. The Bayesian directly concludes that the experimental drug is 20% more effective than the SOC with 95% probability. In contrast, the frequentist deduces that, conditioned on the data, the effectiveness of the experimental drug cannot be equal to that of the SOC (and thus, the experimental drug must be the better treatment). The straightforward feature of the Bayesian inference is extremely desirable as it brings a risk-based approach to bear for decision-making in drug development, as recommended by the current regulatory guidelines.

In the past two decades, the advances in Bayesian computations such as Markov chain Monte Carlo (MCMC) simulation have made it possible to implement sophisticated Bayesian analysis. The release of regulatory guidance on the potential use of Bayesian statistics in medical device development and regulatory endorsement of the Bayesian methods for early clinical development has further fueled the enthusiasm for Bayesian applications to drug development issues, including those previously considered intractable.

Although several Bayesian books have been published to address a broad array of drug development problems, they are primarily focused on clinical trial design, safety analysis, observational studies, and cost-effectiveness assessment. Bayesian methodologies remain unfamiliar to the majority of statistical practitioners in the non-clinical areas. Suffice to say, the lack of adoption of Bayesian methods in those non-clinical areas, including drug discovery, analytical method development, process optimization, and manufacturing control has resulted in many missed opportunities for statisticians to make meaningful differences. Neither is this in keeping with the recent regulatory initiatives of quality by design (QbD), which achieves product quality through greater understanding of the product and manufacturing process, based on knowledge and data collected throughout the lifecycle of the product development.

It is the desire to fill the aforesaid gap that motivates us to write this book. The aim of this book is to provide Bayesian applications to a wide range of clinical and non-clinical issues in drug development. Each Bayesian method in the book is used to address a specific scientific question and illustrated through a case study. The R code used for implementing the method is discussed and included. It is our belief that the publication of this book will promote the use of Bayesian approaches in pharmaceutical practices.

The book consists of three parts, totaling 11 chapters. Since the primary aim of this book is to use case studies, examples, and easy-to-follow R code to demonstrate Bayesian applications in the entire spectrum of drug development, it is, by no means, meant to be comprehensive in literature review, nor is it intended to be exhaustive in expounding each application. Below is a brief description of each chapter:

Part I (Chapters 1–3) provides backgrounds of drug research and development, and basics of Bayesian statistics.

In Chapter 1, after a brief overview of drug research and development centered on drug discovery, pre-clinical and clinical programs, and CMC development, we discuss the opportunities and challenges of Bayesian applications. Chapter 2 is concerned with the basic theory of Bayesian inference and computational tools. Chapter 3 uses three examples, one regarding lot release and the other two concerning Bayesian study designs, to illustrate how sample size is determined for the purpose of hypothesis testing.

Part II (Chapters 4–7) discuss various Bayesian applications in pre-clinical animal studies and clinical development, notably with focus on Phase I and II clinical trials. In Chapter 4, novel Bayesian methods are explained, which utilize historical data to compensate for the usual lack of large sample size and, thus, the inferential power of statistical tests in animal efficacy assessment. Chapter 5 is concentrated on model-based Phase I dose-finding study design and analysis. Two examples are presented to illustrate the use of Bayesian continuous reassessment methods. Chapter 6 describes the use of the Bayesian method in dose-ranging studies. Chapter 7 discusses Bayesian Phase II studies, consisting of an example of a single-arm Phase IIa study with continuous monitoring to show the early efficacy of an experimental therapy, and another case study of Phase IIb to determine an optimum dose regimen for future Phase III trials.

Part III (Chapters 8–11) focuses on selected topics of Bayesian methods used for CMC development. Chapter 8 shows how to validate the performance of an analytical method regarding precision, accuracy, and linearity using Bayesian inferences. Chapter 9 deals with the construction of a Bayesian design space for process development. Chapters 10 and 11 are concentrated on the discussion of stability analysis and process control.

Throughout the above chapters, some of the computer code calls upon external *.csv files. These files are available for download at the following site: https://www.crcpress.com/9781138295872 under "Additional Resources". In addition, various applications are carried out using R code written in JAGS. For readers who are more familiar with Stan, we include R code in Stan in the appendix.

We thank John Kimmel, executive editor, Chapman & Hall/CRC Press, for providing us with the opportunity to write this book. We express our gratitude to Lorin Roskos for reviewing the entire book, and four anonymous reviewers for their review and comments on the book proposal. We also thank Jianchun Zhang for helping resolve an R-coding issue with one of the examples in Chapter 8.

Lastly, the views expressed in this book are those of the authors and not necessarily those of AstraZeneca.

Harry Yang and Steven Novick
Gaithersburg, Maryland

Authors

Harry Yang is senior director and head of Statistical Sciences at AstraZeneca. He has 24 years of experience across all aspects of drug research and development and extensive global regulatory experiences. He has published six statistical books, 15 book chapters, and over 90 peer-reviewed papers on diverse scientific and statistical subjects, including 15 joint statistical works with Dr. Novick. Dr. Yang is a frequently invited speaker at national and international conferences. He also developed statistical courses and conducted training at the FDA and USP, as well as in Peking University, China.

Steven Novick is director of Statistical Sciences at AstraZeneca. He has extensively contributed statistical methods to the biopharmaceutical literature. Dr. Novick is a skilled Bayesian computer programmer and is frequently invited to speak at conferences, having developed and taught courses in several areas, including drug combination analysis and Bayesian methods in clinical areas. He served on IPAC-RS and has chaired several national statistical conferences.

Section I

Background

1

Bayesian Statistics in Drug Development

1.1 Introduction

Drug research and development is a long, costly, and arduous process. Despite advances and breakthroughs in science and technologies, the attrition rate of new drugs remains high. According to a recent report, bringing a novel drug to the market may cost as much as 1.8 billion dollars and take 13 years. Adding to pharmaceutical-industry woes, an increasing number of drug recalls due to manufacturing issues have caused product safety concerns. In recent years, a growing emphasis has been placed on better prediction of clinical outcomes and control of manufacturing risk, using all available data. Bayesian statistics, a well-known framework for synthesizing information from disparate sources, provides such an opportunity. In this chapter, we begin with a brief overview of the drug development process. Subsequently, we discuss the opportunities and challenges of applying Bayesian statistics in drug development.

1.2 Overview of Drug Development

The overarching aim of drug development is to bring safe and effective drugs to the market to meet the unmet medical needs. Drug development is a complex, lengthy, and resource-intensive process. It involves drug discovery, formulation development, pre-clinical animal studies, clinical trials, and regulatory filings. As reported by Bunnage (2011), it takes as much as 1.8 billion US dollars and approximately 13 years to develop an effective drug. Furthermore, drug development is strictly regulated by laws and governmental policies. Ever since the Kefauver–Harris Amendments, a drug must be shown to be both safe and efficacious before marketing approval (Peltzman 1973; FDA 2012). To this end, scientifically well-designed and controlled studies in both animal and human populations are required. In addition, regulations, such as the US current Good Manufacturing Practice (cGMP), require that modern standards and technologies be adopted in the design, monitoring, and control of manufacturing processes and facilities to ensure a consistent supply of high-quality drug products to the consumer or public (FDA 1995). In 2004, the FDA launched a significant initiative entitled "Pharmaceutical cGMPs for the 21st Century: A Risk-Based Approach" (FDA 2004a). The initiative was driven by a vision to achieve a desired state of the pharmaceutical industry as "a maximally efficient, agile, flexible manufacturing sector that reliably produces high-quality drug products without extensive regulatory oversight" (Woodcock 2012). The subsequent publications of several regulatory documents (ICH 2006, 2007a, 2007b, 2011a) further stress the importance of manufacturing process development based on systematic product and process understanding, control of risk, and implementation of quality management systems. Increasingly regulatory guidelines stipulate the use of statistics and good statistical practice in study design and analysis (ICH 1998; FDA 2001, 2004a, 2011a, 2016a). The reliance on statistics has been further intensified as the industry becomes more focused on use of "big data" such as genomics, proteomics, transcriptomics, and real-world evidence to develop precision medicine.

Figure 1.1 presents a diagram of drug development. An outline of each stage is provided in the following sections.

1.2.1 Basic Research

Drug development begins with research on the inner working of a disease at the molecular level. Specifically, various studies are conducted to gain insights on causes of gene mutations, effect of proteins they encode, interaction among those proteins in living cells and their host tissues, and ultimately the patient (Petrova 2012). For example, for years, researchers have

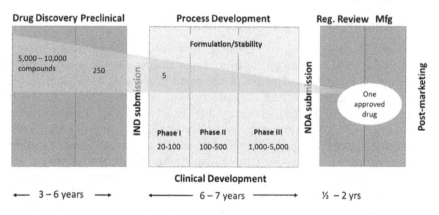

FIGURE 1.1
Drug development process.

noted that some cancers grow quickly and spread rapidly while others do not; however, the cause of the phenomenon has been elusive. It was not until the discovery of the mutated gene called HER2 in breast cancer that scientists understood that the excessive growth of cancer cells in patients with breast cancer was likely caused by high expression of HER2. This critical discovery sparked researchers to look for ways to block HER2 genes in order to slow the growth of HER2-positive breast cancer. The effort finally led to the successful development of trastuzumab (Herceptin®). Advances in genomics, proteomics, and computational capacity have presented unprecedented opportunities for scientists to understand the underlying causes of a disease. The desire to bring innovative medicines to the market has also inspired broad collaborations among researchers from industry, academia, and government. These collective efforts have contributed greatly to the development of innovative drugs.

1.2.2 Drug Discovery

Understanding the causes of a disease often leads to the identification of a biological target. A biological target is any component in a living organism that influences the disease. Examples of common biological targets include genes and proteins. As previously noted (PhRMA 2015), even at this early stage of drug discovery, it is critical to choose a target that can potentially interact with and be affected by a drug molecule. After a target is identified, its association with the disease must be validated through *in vitro* and *in vivo* experiments. Drawing from the understanding of underpinnings of the disease and the potential target, scientists begin to find a drug molecule that can interact with the target and change the course of the disease. Most notable among various methods used for this purpose are 1) screening chemical libraries of synthetic small molecules, natural products, or extracts using *in vitro* assays (usually low-to-medium throughput) to look for compounds of desired therapeutic effect (https://en.wikipedia.org/wiki/Drug_discovery); 2) high-throughput screening of large compound libraries in search of disease-altering molecules; and 3) genetically engineering of molecules that have high affinity to the target. These lead compounds advance to the next stage of testing in which their toxic-kinetic properties are evaluated in cell and animal models. Those compounds that meet the selection criteria are further optimized to increase affinity, selectivity, efficacy, and stability.

1.2.3 Formulation

Drugs must be properly formulated in certain dosage forms to ease production and delivery and maximize therapeutic benefits. The objective of formulation development is to design and establish both a formulation composition and its manufacturing process to meet the above requirements. The development of an acceptable dosage form can be extremely challenging particularly for biological products (Ng and Rajagopalan 2009). The difficulties stem from the fact that biological products are inherently complex and heterogeneous. This makes it formidable to characterize the product and establish the links between the product attributes and process parameters as well as clinical performance (Singh et al. 2009). Formulation development is a continuous endeavor throughout drug development. At the early stage, only a small amount of the drug is produced in a laboratory setting for early phase clinical studies. As the drug program advances to late-stage clinical trials, large quantities of the drug are needed. Since techniques for small-scale production of the drug often do not translate easily to large scales, additional efforts are needed to enhance and optimize the formulation. In recent years, manufacturers began to embrace the Quality by Design principles for formulation development.

1.2.4 Laboratory Test Methods

Analytical testing is an integral part of drug research and development. Analytical methods are developed to determine identity, strength, quality, purity, and potency of the drug. According to regulatory guidance (FDA 2015; USP 1989, 2013), an analytical method should be validated for its intended use. In the early stage of drug development, analytical results are used to guide the selection of lead compound. For pre-clinical and clinical programs, analytical methods aid optimal dose selection and assessment of study endpoints. They are also widely used for formulation and process development and ultimately manufacturing control to ensure the quality of the drug substance and finished product. Additionally, the development of clinical testing methods such as immunogenicity assays also plays a very important role in the overall drug development. For example, immunogenicity assays are used to detect, quantify, and characterize anti-drug antibodies, which may have profound impact on drug safety and efficacy. The development and validation of such assays are also strictly regulated (FDA 2007 and WHO 2009) and pose a host of unique challenges, requiring extra care in both study design and data analysis (Yang et al. 2016).

1.2.5 Pre-Clinical Studies

Before testing an investigational drug in human subjects, animal studies are carried out with the primary aims of selecting a safe dose for human trials and determining the safety profile of the studied drug. Pre-clinical testing can be performed both *in vitro* and *in vivo*. Although different types of pre-clinical studies may be required, in most cases, toxicity pharmacodynamics, pharmacokinetics, and absorption, distribution, metabolism, and excretion (ADME) studies are carried out to determine a safe dose for human testing. It is also important to note that all pre-clinical studies must be conducted in accordance with Good Laboratory Practice (GLP) (FDA 2007).

1.2.6 Clinical Development

Upon completion of pre-clinical development, the drug is ready to be studied in human subjects. The sponsor must submit an Investigational New Drug Application (IND) with the FDA or Investigational Medicinal Product Dossier (IMPD) with the EMA if a clinical trial is to be conducted in one or more European Union member states. IND and IMPD are requests for FDA and EMA authorization to administer the investigational drug to humans. Both filings contain data from non-clinical studies, quality, manufacture, and control of the investigational drug as well as comparator(s) if applicable. In addition to the regulatory approval, the intended clinical study must also be endorsed by the Institutional Review Board (IRB) at the sites where the trial is conducted.

1.2.6.1 Phase I Clinical Trial

The primary objective of a Phase I study is to determine the safety profile and to study the pharmacokinetic property of the drug. For drugs with moderate toxicity, the trial is normally carried out using healthy male volunteers. However, for cytotoxic agents, Phase I trials are usually conducted in the target patient populations to minimize unnecessary exposures of the drugs in healthy volunteers. Dose-escalation designs may be used (see Chapter 5). They typically begin with a low dose of the drug predicted from the animal studies and progressively escalate to higher doses if the drug is well tolerated. A range of doses is explored, and the maximum tolerated dose is determined. The study also collects pharmacodynamic and pharmacokinetic data to address important questions such as side effects, therapeutic effects, and ADME. The knowledge garnered from this stage of development, including the safe dosing range, is used to guide the next phase of clinical development.

1.2.6.2 Phase II Clinical Trial

After a maximum tolerated dose is identified from Phase I trials, Phase II studies are carried out with the primary focus on demonstrating the efficacy of the drug and finding an optimum dosing regimen. The studies are usually conducted in patients who have an illness or condition that the drug is intended to treat. These are relatively larger trials with several hundreds of patients. Phase II trials can be further divided into Phase IIa and Phase IIb studies. The former are typically single-arm trials to screen out inefficacious drugs. The latter usually contain treatment arms of the drug at different dose levels and dosing schedules and a control arm. They are often randomized trials to allow for accurate assessment of treatment effects. At the conclusion of the Phase II trials, researchers expect either to have identified the effective dose, route of administration, and dosing range for Phase III trials, or to decide to terminate the clinical development of the drug.

1.2.6.3 Phase III Clinical Trial

Phase III trials, also known as pivotal or confirmatory trials, are conducted on a much larger number of patients to substantiate safety and efficacy findings from the previous studies in support of market approval of the drug. These studies are often lengthy, multi-center, possibly global, and are consequently very costly to complete. Most Phase III trials are randomized, double-blind, and multi-armed with a comparator. To gain marketing approval by regulatory approval, typically two Phase III trials are required.

1.2.6.4 Phase IV Clinical Trial

For a new drug, Phase IV trials are conducted for various purposes. They may be used to assess the long-term effect of the drug. They may also be carried out to determine risk and benefit in specific subgroups of patients. Further, a Phase IV trial may be conducted to support market authorizations in different regions or countries and expand product label.

1.2.7 Translational Research

In recent years, a great deal of emphasis has been placed on translational research to expedite and shorten the time of "bench-to-bedside" of a new medicine, by harnessing knowledge of both basic science and clinical research. Translational research leverages data generated from advanced technologies, such as next-generation gene sequencing, proteomics, bioinformatics, and robotics, to identify drug candidates that have greater potential to be developed into novel drugs. In addition, it also promotes incorporation of learnings from the clinical setting in drug discovery. For instance, the analysis of patient samples might help identify a subgroup that responds better to the treatment. Thus, a companion diagnostic tool based on genomic or proteomic markers may ensure more targeted therapy development and enhance the probability of success. It is for these reasons that translational research techniques have been widely utilized to advance new drug development.

1.2.8 Chemistry, Manufacturing, and Controls

Chemistry, manufacturing, and controls (CMC) is an integral part of the overall drug development and is required in marketing approval. It consists of several important components, including manufacturing of bulk drug substance and final drug product, setting specifications, release criteria, stability testing, comparability studies after process changes, and analytical method development and validation. CMC issues become increasingly complex as a candidate drug is being advanced to late-stage development. Often statistical methods such as modeling simulation and design of experiments (DOE) are used to develop, optimize, and validate CMC processes so that they are fit for their intended purposes. To ensure drug safety, efficacy, and quality, manufacturing processes are strictly controlled according to GMP (FDA 2004a). Many regulatory guidelines have been established, governing the process control, product characterization, and release. In recent years, pharmaceutical companies have been encouraged to embrace the advances in manufacturing technologies to modernize their production system and meet regulatory standards.

1.2.9 Regulatory Registration

Although the regulatory requirements for premarketing approval of a new drug and review vary, there are common elements in new drug applications (NDA) and biologics license applications (BLA). In the United States, the FDA requires that an NDA/BLA include integrated summaries of pre-clinical and clinical study results. In addition, the application should also contain information on CMC and proposed labeling (FDA 1999). The NDA/BLA is reviewed by the FDA. After comprehensive review, the FDA may approve the drug product or request additional data or studies. For marketing authorization application in Europe and other regions, similar requirements are mandated by regulatory authorities. While the regulatory agencies have the ultimate authority to approve or disapprove the applications, they may solicit the opinion of an independent advisory committee, consisting of experts in the field.

1.3 Statistics in Drug Research and Development

Statistics has been broadly used in virtually all aspects of drug research and development. There are several drivers behind the statistical applications. Firstly, there is growing governmental control over the content and claim of medicinal products. For example, ever since 1906, the United States has passed several laws such as the Federal Food, Drug, and Cosmetics Act in Kefauver–Harris Drug Amendment in 1962, and the NDA Rewrite in 1990, which require drug manufacturers to demonstrate drug safety and effectiveness through well-controlled and designed studies. These regulatory requirements entail the needs of statistics in pre-clinical and clinical testing (ICH 1998). The recent advances in regulatory policies have brought statistics to the forefront of other areas of drug development including formulation, analytical method, and manufacturing control (ICH 2006, 2007a, 2007b, 2011). In both the FDA's PAT (process analytical technologies) and process validation guidance (FDA 2004a, 2011a), the use of multivariate tools for design, data acquisition, and analysis is specifically recommended. In addition, the advances in platforms in areas such as genomics and proteomics enable scientists to generate large quantities of data in a very short time period. The need to make sense out of the data to drive key decision-making necessitates the use of statistics. Moreover, innovations in statistics such as adaptive design have brought flexibility and economy into clinical development (Chow and Chang 2007; Chang 2008).

In drug development, two commonly used statistical approaches are the frequentist and Bayesian methods. The former addresses a scientific question solely based on data collected from an experiment designed to answer the question; whereas the latter reaches an answer using not only the data from the current experiment but also prior knowledge of the question. Consider a two-arm clinical study intended to demonstrate that an innovative drug improves the rate of a disease by 40% over a comparator drug. In the frequentist paradigm, the rates of responses of the two drugs are deemed to be fixed as is the hypothesized difference of 40%. The question is answered by testing the null hypothesis, H_0: there is no difference in response rate between the two drugs, against the alternative hypothesis, H_a: the rates differ by at least 40%. Upon completion of the study, the rate difference δ based on the trial data is estimated. Under the null hypothesis, the probability for the future rate difference from a repeated experiment to exceed the observed difference δ is calculated. This probability, often called the p-value, depends on the statistical model or distribution assumed for the data, the observed results from the current experiment, and the fixed difference in rate. The null hypothesis is rejected and a significant difference claim is made if the p-value is small; otherwise, a lack of difference conclusion is reached. By contrast, the Bayesian approach blends data from the current study with prior beliefs/knowledge about the treatment effect. In addition, under the Bayesian setting, the unknown treatment effect is viewed as a variable that varies according to a distribution. The prior knowledge is updated in light of the trial results and expressed as a posterior distribution. From this distribution, the probability of the rate difference $\geq 40\%$ is calculated. If this probability is high, say, exceeding 90%, one may conclude that there is a significant difference between the two drugs. The idea is illustrated in Figure 1.2.

The derivation of the posterior distribution is obtained through Bayes' Theorem, which is briefly discussed below. Elucidation of the prior distribution and inference based on the posterior distribution is discussed in Chapter 2. Bayes' Theorem also makes it possible to make inference about the future observations from repeated experiment(s) through predictive probability. Central to this inference is the derivation of the probability distribution of the future observations conditional on the data from the current study.

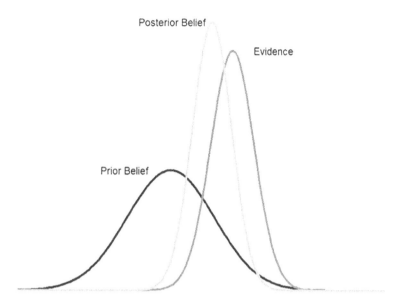

FIGURE 1.2
Posterior distribution incorporates new evidence from the current study into the prior distribution.

1.4 Bayesian Statistics

As previously discussed, there are two types of statistical methodologies, namely, frequentist and Bayesian, that are applicable for study design and analysis in drug development. Traditionally the frequentist methods were predominantly used for drug experimental design and analysis. In recent years, the advances in both Bayesian methodologies and computations have propelled Bayesian methods to the forefront of drug research and development. An important fundamental difference between frequentist and Bayesian methodologies is the use of prior information. Although frequentists use prior beliefs at the study design stage, they do not use it in formal analysis. In contrast, the Bayesian system provides a formal framework to combine prior information with current data to make inferences about a quantity of interest. In addition, the Bayesian approach provides great flexibility to update inferences each time new data become available. Bayesian analysis also affords the advantages of straightforward predictive model-building and lack of reliance on large sample approximations (Natanegara et al. 2014). Furthermore, Bayesian inference can greatly facilitate decision-making as results are typically expressed in terms of probabilistic statements that directly correspond with scientific questions and hypotheses of interest.

1.5 Opportunities of the Bayesian Approach

In the past decades, Bayesian statistics has made significant inroads in drug development, notably in clinical trial design and analysis. More recently, thanks to the regulatory initiatives regarding Quality by Design and risk-based lifecycle principles for pharmaceutical development, there is a significant increase in Bayesian applications to CMC areas. In the following sections, the opportunities of the Bayesian approach are highlighted.

1.5.1 Pre-Clinical Development

Pre-clinical studies in animals are known for small sample sizes due to ethical concerns. The sample size is often large enough to detect a meaningful treatment effect relative to a control group, but too small to differentiate several promising treatments. One way to address this issue is to combine data from different studies, in which the studied drug was tested at different dose levels. Due to differences in study design, however, data may be difficult to directly combine and analyze; e.g., data points are collected at different time points. This makes traditional analyses such as ANOVA or Repeated Measurement Analysis challenging. When good prior information exists (Novick et al. 2018), the utilization of the Bayesian approach has the potential to circumvent the issues of small sample size and observations collected at different time points. In addition, it is also straightforward to carry out Bayesian inference based on complex models such as hierarchical models even when useful prior information is not available.

1.5.2 CMC Development

As previously discussed, the launch of the FDA initiative, "Pharmaceutical Current Good Manufacturing Practices (cGMPs) for the 21st Century", and subsequent publications of other regulatory guidance including ICH Q8-Q11 regarding Quality by Design and quality risk management ushered in a risk-based and lifecycle approach to CMC development, and also stimulated the use of statistics. It is now well understood that the assurance of the robustness of manufacturing processes and quality products is often stated in probabilistic terms. Such assurance is achieved through understanding, quantifying, and controlling the variability of CMC processes. Bayesian analysis provides useful tools for identifying design space, which is a constrained region of manufacturing process parameters providing greater probability for the product to be within its specifications (Peterson 2008, 2009; Peterson and Lief 2010; Peterson and Yahyah 2009). Various Bayesian methods were developed for assay validation (Sondag et al. 2016; USP 2018), formulation development (LeBrun et al. 2018), process monitoring (Colosimo and del Castillo 2007), and general QC troubleshooting (see Chapter 11). These applications, powered by the advances in Bayesian computation techniques such as the Markov Chain Monte Carlo simulation method, render ready solutions to many problems related to drug research, which were long thought to be intractable (Colosimo and del Castillo 2007).

1.5.3 Clinical Trials

Clinical trials are experiments conducted in human subjects in strictly controlled settings to address specific questions regarding the safety and efficacy of a medical intervention. Depending on the questions at hand, different study designs may be used. Early studies are small in size, and progressively large comparative studies are run as confidence in the drug safety and efficacy is gained. In general, clinical trials are carried out in a sequential fashion in which the learning from the previous experiment is used to guide the design of the next. Despite their controlled nature, clinical trials encounter many uncertainties such as varying medical practice at different sites and unknown patient or disease characteristics which are unaccounted for in the trial inclusion or exclusion criteria. Robust evaluation of drug safety and efficacy lies in the researcher's ability to synthesize information from various sources, including different stages of clinical development, and incorporate known variability in the inference of the clinical research questions. It also requires the statistical method to be adaptive in the sense that inference can be updated based on new information. Bayesian approaches are most suitable for this purpose.

In the past two decades, significant advances in Bayesian applications in clinical trial and analysis have been made. There has also been greater regulatory acceptance of Bayesian approaches to study design and analysis, as evidenced by the publication of the FDA guidance on the use of Bayesian statistics in medical device clinical trials (FDA 2010a) and acceptance by regulatory agencies of Bayesian methods for early and exploratory phases of drug development. Bayesian adaptive study design and analysis have been widely used for Phase I dose-finding studies (Chevret 2006) and Phase II efficacy assessment (Berry and Stangl 1996a,b; Spiegelhalter et al. 2004; Berry et al. 2011).

1.6 Challenges of the Bayesian Approach

1.6.1 Objection to Bayesian

Despite its potentially wide-ranging application in drug research and development, Bayesian inference remains one of the most controversial methods (Gelman 2008). Central to the objection to the Bayesian method is its requirement of a prior distribution, which is based on expert opinions and historical data. Inevitably, potential biases may be introduced in prior selection; e.g., expert opinions often vary. Two Bayesian statisticians who analyze the same data may reach different conclusions based solely on the priors they choose. Although sensitivity analysis based on various choices of prior beliefs may alleviate some of the concern of subjectivity, it is not favored by practitioners who look for straightforward answers (Little 2006). Therefore, the application of the Bayesian approach to drug development requires deeper vetting of relevant sources of information and scientific expertise, greater level of engagement among stakeholders, and the ability to synthesize information from different sources and build realistic complex Bayesian models (Ohlssen 2016).

1.6.2 Regulatory Hurdles

Although there have been growing applications of the Bayesian approach in drug development in the past two years, by and large, they are intended to assist internal decision-making. The preponderance of statistical methods used for data analysis in support of regulatory filings are from traditional frequentist approaches. The ICH E9 Statistical Principles for Clinical Trials state "Because the predominant approaches to the design and analysis of clinical trials have been based on frequentist statistical methods, the guidance largely refers to the use of frequentist methods [...] when discussing hypothesis testing and/or confidence intervals. This should not be taken to imply that other approaches are not appropriate: the use of Bayesian [...] and other approaches may be considered when the reasons for their use are clear and when the resulting conclusions are sufficiently robust." Although the guidance presents opportunities for clinical trials, there is no clear regulatory pathway on how exactly the Bayesian methods can contribute to the totality of evidence in support of regulatory filings. In addition, regulators have concerns about Bayesian treatment of multiple testing (Kay 2015). For example, under a frequentist sequential design, the Type I error is allocated across tests at the interim looks to ensure the overall Type I error remains as planned, say, 5%. However, with the Bayesian approach, the posterior distribution at each interim is updated with new data by treating the previous posterior as the prior. The resulting updated posterior distribution levies no additional costs regardless of how many interim looks of the data are carried out. Although several remedies have been suggested in the published literature that imbues the Bayesian sequential testing procedures with the frequentist property in controlling the overall Type I error (Spiegelhalter et al. 2004), there is no precedent that these methods are acceptable to the regulators.

1.7 Concluding Remarks

In the past decades, the advances in Bayesian computations have broadened the use of Bayesian approaches in various industries. Despite progress, applications of Bayesian methods in drug development has been modest (Winkler 2001; Moyé 2008; Chevret 2006; Rogatko et al. 2007; Natanegara 2014). Except clinical trials of medical devices, there is a clear lack of regulatory guidance on Bayesian-driven design and analysis of clinical trials for new drugs. In addition, general regulatory acceptance of Bayesian methods for late-stage studies in support of regulatory submissions is low. An important factor that may have contributed to this issue is the unfamiliarity of Bayesian methods and computational tools for practitioners who are involved in late-stage drug development. The pharmaceutical industry has been facing unprecedented challenges of high attribution rate and unsustainable level of R&D costs. Such challenges argue for quantitative methods that synthesize information from diverse sources to aid robust decision-making and that bring both flexibility and economy into study designs. The Bayesian approach provides this opportunity. To fully capitalize on the benefits of the Bayesian approach, however, it is essential to develop best practices of Bayesian statistics, gain consensus among sponsors and regulators, and continue demonstration of the utilities of Bayesian in all aspects of drug development.

2

Basics of Bayesian Statistics

2.1 Introduction

Bayesian statistics is a branch of statistics founded upon Bayesian probability theory. Reverend Thomas Bayes, a Presbyterian minister in England, developed a specific form of Bayes' Theorem for making inference about the parameter of a binomial distribution. His work, published posthumously, was independently formulated by French mathematician Pierre-Simon Laplace. Although both frequentist and Bayesian inferences rely on probability theories, the interpretation of probability is very different for the two schools of thought. Frequentist practitioners view probability as the limit of the relative frequency of an event after a large number of trials (Stigler 1986). By contrast, from the Bayesian perspective, probability is a measure of the uncertainty of an event based on the current knowledge of the event. As such, the probability can change as new information becomes available. In this sense, Bayesian probability is a subjective measure of likelihood as opposed to the frequentist notion of probability as a fixed quantity. Bayes' Theorem provides a framework to update this probability, combining prior beliefs with the current data. The results of Bayesian analysis are often provided in statements quantified through probabilities. For these reasons, Bayesian inference is intellectually attractive; however, the adoption of Bayesian methods has been slow due to practical considerations. In recent years owing to the rapid advances in the field of Bayesian computation, increasing interest has arisen in Bayesian applications in various areas of drug research and development. This chapter provides an overview of Bayesian statistics after briefly highlighting the differences between the frequentist and Bayesian methods. Topics covered include Bayes' Theorem, prior and posterior distributions, predictive probability, and Bayesian computation.

2.2 Statistical Inferences

2.2.1 Research Questions

Researchers in drug development use scientifically designed experiments to collect data and address research questions such as (1) Is the new drug more effective than the standard care therapy? (2) Does a newly produced product lot meet its specifications for quality? (3) What conditions of a cell culture system render the maximum yield? Answers to these questions can be obtained through applications of statistical methods.

2.2.2 Probability Distribution

A probability distribution of a random variable is a theoretical structure of the variable. For a continuous random variable, the distribution describes the characteristics of a variable, such as its prespecified range. Data generated from a study also follow a distribution. In the Bayesian framework, the data distribution is defined by parameters, some of which are related to the question at hand. Consider the example in which an investigator is interested in the effect of an experimental drug in a single-arm study. Suppose that the response is binary. The drug effect, p, often characterized by response rate, is an unknown parameter. Let Y denote the number of patients (out of n) who responded to the treatment. Under the assumptions that the patients' responses to the drug are assessed independently and each patient responds to the drug with the same probability p, Y follows a binomial distribution binomial(n, p). That is, the probability for Y to be equal to the value k (= 0, 1, ..., n) is given by

$$\Pr[Y = k] = \binom{n}{k} p^y (1-p)^{n-k}. \tag{2.1}$$

The above distribution can be used to make inferences about the response rate p.

2.2.3 Frequentist Methods

In the frequentist paradigm, inference is made strictly based on data from the current study. For the above example, the parameter p can be estimated by $\hat{p} = Y/n$. For example, if 55 out of 100 patients respond, then an estimate of p is given by $55/100 = 0.55$. The performance of the estimation method can be characterized through a $(1-\alpha) \times 100\%$ confidence interval, $\left[A(Y), B(Y) \right]$ such that

$$\Pr\left[A(Y) < p < B(Y) \right] = 1 - \alpha. \tag{2.2}$$

$A(Y)$ and $B(Y)$ are calculated solely based on the current data Y. One of these intervals was derived by Clopper and Pearson (1934):

$$\frac{1}{1+\dfrac{n-y+1}{y}F_{2(n-y+1),2y,\frac{\alpha}{2}}} < p < \frac{\dfrac{y+1}{n-y}F_{2(y+1),2(n-y),\alpha/2}}{1+\dfrac{y+1}{n-y}F_{2(y+1),2(n-y),\alpha/2}} \tag{2.3}$$

where y is the observed value of the random variable Y and $F_{n_1,n_2,\alpha/2}$ is the $(1-\alpha/2)\times 100$ percentile of an F distribution with degrees of freedom of n_1 and n_2.

Frequentists view probability as the limit of the relative long-run frequency at which an event occurs. According to this notion of probability, the $(1-\alpha)$ confidence level can be interpreted as the probability for the interval $[A(Y), B(Y)]$ to contain the true value of the unknown parameter. In other words, if the same experiment were to be repeated an infinite number of times, $100(1-\alpha)\%$ of the resulting intervals would contain the true parameter of p. In practice, however, the above $(1-\alpha)$ confidence interval is often misinterpreted as a probability statement regarding likely values of the unknown parameter p on the basis of the observed data.

In general, in the frequentist paradigm, parameters are considered fixed and statistical inference is made based on the sampling distribution of the data. The performance of a statistical procedure is characterized through repeated sampling under the same conditions.

2.2.4 Bayesian Inference

In contrast with frequentist methods, Bayesians do not view unknown parameters as fixed. Parameters are imbued with uncertainties that can be described through probability distributions. In addition, while frequentists make inferences based solely on the current experimental data, Bayesian methods utilize data from the current experiment as well as information from other sources. In such a context, probability is defined as the plausibility of a random event, representing degrees of belief. Unlike the frequentist definition, it does not rely on the concept of infinitely repeating an experiment of interest. Instead, it starts with a prior belief in the plausibility of the event and then updates the information when data from the current experiment become available. This is made possible by Bayes' rule, which is briefly described below.

2.2.4.1 Bayes' Theorem and Posterior Distribution

Let θ, y, and $\tilde{y}$ denote the parameter of interest, observable data, and future data, respectively. Bayesian methods begin by describing θ and y through a prior distribution for the parameters $\pi(\theta)$ and a conditional probability function for the data $\pi(y|\theta)$. The latter is also called the likelihood function after y is observed and is often depicted as $L(\theta|y)$. The frequentist believes that all information concerning the unknown parameter θ is contained in the likelihood $\pi(y|\theta)$ after the experiment is complete and consequently bases all statistical inference about θ solely upon $\pi(y|\theta)$. In the Bayesian approach, the prior information is updated through Bayes' Theorem to give rise to a posterior distribution:

$$\pi(\theta|y) = \frac{\pi(\theta)\pi(y|\theta)}{\pi(y)}, \tag{2.4}$$

where $\pi(y) = \int \pi(\theta)\pi(y|\theta)d\theta$.

The posterior distribution has two key components, $\pi(\theta)$ and $\pi(y|\theta)$. The former, which is referred to as the prior distribution of θ, represents the information of the parameters before the current data are observed. The latter is the likelihood to observe the current data, conditioned on θ. Together, they represent the totality of knowledge of the parameter up to the current data. Bayes' Theorem also provides a means for updating the posterior distribution as new data become available, using the current posterior as the prior for the future posterior distribution. This is very useful for studies, such as dose-finding trials (see Chapter 5), in which observations are sequentially obtained and estimates are continuously updated based on new information.

2.2.4.2 Inference about Parameters

Inferences regarding θ can be made based on the posterior distribution. For example, either the mode, mean, or median of the distribution may be used as an estimate of the parameter. Moreover, an interval estimator (a, b) can also be constructed for a univariate parameter θ such that

$$\Pr[a \le \theta \le b \,|\, y] = 1 - \alpha. \tag{2.5}$$

The interval (a, b) is often referred to as a $(1-\alpha) \times 100\%$ Bayesian credible interval. Unlike the frequentist confidence interval, the interval in Equation (2.5) has a probabilistic interpretation; it covers the parameter with a probability of $1-\alpha$. Multivariate intervals may be constructed for parameter vectors θ.

Consider the previous example. It is assumed that the response rate p has a beta prior distribution of $\text{Beta}(\alpha_1, \alpha_2)$. That is,

$$\pi(p) \propto p^{(\alpha_1 - 1)}(1-p)^{\alpha_2 - 1}. \tag{2.6}$$

where the symbol "$\propto$" means "proportional to".

From Equations (2.1), (2.4), and (2.6), it follows that the posterior is also a beta distribution

$$\pi(p\,|\,y) \propto p^y (1-p)^{n-y} \times p^{(\alpha_1-1)}(1-p)^{\alpha_2-1} = p^{\alpha_1+y-1}(1-p)^{\alpha_2+n-y-1}. \quad (2.7)$$

From Equation (2.7), it can be shown that

$$p\,|\,y \sim \text{Beta}(\alpha_1 + y, \alpha_2 + n - y).$$

The limits of the $(1-\alpha)\times 100\%$ Bayesian credible interval, $a(y)$ and $b(y)$, can be chosen to be $((\alpha/2)\times 100)^{th}$ and $[(1-\alpha/2)\times 100]^{th}$ percentiles of Beta$(\alpha_1 + y, \alpha_2 + n - y)$, respectively. There are many ways to construct Bayesian credible intervals. Notable is the highest posterior density (HPD) interval, which is determined by finding the shortest width interval among all $(1-\alpha)\times 100\%$ credible intervals. That is, it satisfies

$$b_{\text{HPD}}(y) - a_{\text{HPD}}(y) = \min\left\{ b(y) - a(y) : \int_{a(y)}^{b(y)} \pi(\theta\,|\,y)d\theta = 1 - \alpha \right\}.$$

2.2.4.3 Inference of Future Observations

One of the frequently encountered investigational questions focuses on the likely distribution of future observations. Thus, it is of interest to predict future observation, $\tilde{y}$, based on the current data y. This can be accomplished relatively easily within the Bayesian framework. Specifically, the posterior predictive distribution is obtained by

$$\pi(\tilde{y}\,|\,y) = \int \pi(\tilde{y}\,|\,\theta)\pi(\theta\,|\,y)d\theta. \quad (2.8)$$

In essence, $\pi(\tilde{y}\,|\,y)$ is the sampling distribution of the future observations $\tilde{y}$ weighted over the updated distribution of the parameter θ. Based on this distribution, prediction regarding the behavior of $\tilde{y}$ can be readily made. For example, both point and interval estimates of $\tilde{y}$ can be obtained from the distribution in Equation (2.8). It is worth noting that inference based on this distribution is different from that of the classical frequentist using the condition distribution $\pi(\tilde{y}\,|\,\hat{\theta})$, where $\hat{\theta}$ is an estimate of the parameter. As noted by Colosimo and del Castillo (2007), the classical prediction interval often does not take into account the uncertainty in the parameter θ. There are many applications of the predictive distribution. It is particularly useful for multi-stage clinical trials in defining stopping rules (Lee and Liu 2008; Qian et al. 1996), power calculation (Spiegelhalter et al. 2004), and model validation and diagnosis (Berry and Stangl 1996a).

2.2.5 Selection of Priors

The key component of Bayesian inference is in the selection of prior distributions. Since the prior reflects expert opinion and depends on personal judgment, it can be subjective in nature. Because most controversies surrounding Bayesian analysis are centered on the selection of priors, care should be given in prior selection. Before data collection, one must assess the relative accuracy and weight of the prior information (Schoot et al. 2013).

Three major categories of prior distributions are conjugate priors, non-conjugate priors, and non-informative priors. A conjugate prior yields a posterior that belongs to the same family of the prior distribution. There are two important advantages in the use of a conjugate prior. First, it is mathematically and computationally simple, particularly in sequential studies (Colosimo and del Castillo 2007). Second, in many cases, the prior may directly be viewed as additional data. For example, a $\text{Beta}(\alpha, \beta)$ prior for an experiment with binary response discussed previously can be considered as data from an early experiment which had α successes and β failures. In a similar vein, Morita et al. (2008) formulated the effective sample size that is contributed by any prior distribution, whether it is conjugate or not. Unfortunately, conjugate priors can sometimes be too restrictive to reflect the expert knowledge and other prior beliefs (Irwin 2005).

In contrast, a non-conjugate prior can vary in complexity and so one may always find a non-conjugate prior that possesses the flexibility to characterize historical knowledge. The extra complexity often comes at the price of no closed form for Equation (2.4). Although the use of non-conjugate priors previously posed significant computational challenges, with the advances in MCMC methods, the issue has been attenuated.

A key subtype of prior distributions is the non-informative priors, which are well suited for cases in which little knowledge about the parameters is available. For example, a flat prior that is uniform over the entire real line is non-informative in the sense that the parameter value is believed to be equally likely to assume any value. Over the past decades, a variety of methods for deriving non-informative priors have been suggested (Yang and Berger 1998). Jeffreys (1961) proposed a general method that constructs non-informative priors based on the so-called invariant principle, which states that posterior inferences based on either the original prior $\pi(\theta)$ or the prior $\pi(g(\theta))$, with $g(\theta)$ being a one-to-one transformation, results in the same conclusion. Under such constraint, Jeffreys showed that a prior $\pi(\theta)$ meeting the invariant principle satisfies

$$\pi(\theta) \propto \sqrt{\det[I(\theta)]}$$

where "det" stands for determinant and $I(\theta)$ is the Fisher information matrix given by

$$I(\theta) = -E_\theta \left[\frac{d^2 \log\left[\pi(y \mid \theta) \right]}{d^2\theta} \right].$$

As an example, when the response $Y \sim N(\mu, \sigma^2)$, the Jeffreys non-informative prior of $\theta = (\mu, \sigma^2)$ is given by

$$\pi(\theta) \propto \frac{1}{\sigma^3}.$$

2.3 Bayesian Computation

As noted by Robert (2013), it has long been a bane of the Bayesian approach that the solutions it proposes are intellectually attractive but inapplicable in practice. The difficulty in implementing Bayesian solutions had long hindered the adoption of these methods; however, the advances of Bayesian computational methods in the past two decades have spurred the interest in Bayesian applications in various areas including drug research and development. In this section, we discuss two computational methods, namely, Monte Carlo simulation and MCMC.

2.3.1 Monte Carlo Simulation

The posterior distribution is given by Equation (2.4). The denominator $\pi(y) = \int \pi(\theta) \pi(y \mid \theta) d\theta$ is called the normalizing constant. Making statistical inference about θ can be a mathematically difficult problem depending on many factors, including the dimensionality of θ, the complexity of the likelihood function/prior distribution, and the ability to calculate the normalizing constant. Even with complete knowledge of the posterior probability density function (PDF), calculating posterior probabilities may require multiple integrations of a complicated function. In place of analytically (or numerically) calculating the integral, Monte Carlo integration (Robert and Casella 2004) may be performed. By sampling random variables x_b ($b = 1, 2, \ldots, B$) from a PDF $f(x)$, the integral $\Pr(X \in A) = \iint_{x \in A} f(x) dx$ is approximated by its Monte Carlo counterpart $(1/B) \sum 1[x_b \in A]$. By the central limit theorem, the Monte Carlo integral converges to the true probability as B goes to infinity. Luckily, widely available software solutions exist to provide Bayesian practitioners with the ability to explore the posterior distribution via Monte

Carlo methods (see Section 2.4). Before delving into the pre-packaged software, a primer on Monte Carlo sampling methods is offered in this section to furnish the user with background on sampling methods and Monte Carlo integration.

Monte Carlo integration may also be used to obtain the marginal posterior density of parameters. Suppose $X = (X_1, X_2)$ is a random variable with PDF $f(x_1, x_2)$. The marginal density of X_1 is $\int f(x_1, x_2) dx_2$. By sampling random variables $(x_{b,1}, x_{b,2})$ from $f(x_1, x_2)$, $b = 1, 2, \ldots, B$, the marginal density of X_1 is given by $\{x_{b,1} : x_2 = x_{b,2}\}$. In other words, the marginal distribution of X_1 is generated by ignoring the values of $x_{b,2}$ (assuming that they represent the true distribution of x_2) and examining only the set of $\{x_{b,1}\}$.

2.3.2 Example

To illustrate Monte Carlo integration, we examine a "simple" problem with a known solution. Consider directly calculating a joint posterior probability for parameters $\theta = (\mu, \sigma)$ from independent, identically distributed data

$$y_i \mid \mu, \sigma^2 \sim N\left(\mu, \sigma^2\right), \quad i = 1, 2, \ldots, n,$$

with conjugate prior

$$\mu \mid \sigma^2 \sim N\left(\mu_0, \frac{\sigma^2}{k_0}\right)$$

$$\tau = \frac{1}{\sigma^2} \sim Ga\left(\frac{v_0}{2}, \frac{v_0 \sigma_0^2}{2}\right).$$

Eight ($n = 8$) normally distributed values were generated in R (R Core Team 2018) with mean 98 and standard deviation 5 and given as $y = (87.3, 89.8, 91.8, 96.7, 97, 97.7, 98.2, 99.7)$ so that the sample mean and sample variance are $\bar{y} = 94.775$ and $s^2 = 20.382$. The joint posterior probability $\Pr(95 < \mu < 105, \sigma < 5 \mid y)$ is calculated with prior hyperparameters $\mu_0 = 100$, $k_0 = 1.5$, $v_0 = 2$, and $\sigma_0^2 = 64$. In addition, the marginal posterior distribution of μ is examined through the posterior 5%, 50%, and 95% quantiles.

The joint posterior distribution $\pi(\mu, \tau \mid y)$ is known to be normal-gamma (NG) distributed $\left(\mu_n, k_n, \frac{v_n}{2}, \frac{v_n \sigma_n^2}{2}\right)$, with PDF

$$\pi(\mu, \tau \mid y) = \frac{\left(\frac{v_n \sigma_n^2}{2}\right)^{\frac{v_n}{2}} \sqrt{k_n}}{\Gamma\left(\frac{v_n}{2}\right) \sqrt{2\pi}} \tau^{\frac{v_n - 1}{2}} \exp\left(-\tau \frac{v_n \sigma_n^2 + k_n \left(\mu - \mu_n\right)^2}{2}\right) \qquad (2.9)$$

where, borrowing notation from Gelman et al. (2013, Chapter 3),

$$\mu_n = \left(\frac{k_0}{k_0 + n} \right) \mu_0 + \left(\frac{n}{k_0 + n} \right) \bar{y},$$

$$k_n = k_0 + n, \quad \nu_n = \nu_0 + n, \text{ and}$$

$$\sigma_n^2 = \left(\frac{1}{\nu_n} \right) \left\{ \nu_0 \sigma_0^2 + (n-1)s^2 + \frac{k_0 n}{k_0 + n} (\bar{y} - \mu_0)^2 \right\},$$

so that posterior hyperparameters are $\mu_n = 95.6$, $k_n = 9.5$, $\nu_n = 10$, and $\sigma_n^2 = 30.516$. In R, the PDF in Equation (2.9) is written as

```
## Posterior hyperparameters
mu.n = 95.6
k.n = 9.5
nu.n = 10
sigSq.n = 30.516



## Normal-gamma pdf
dNG = function(mu, tau)
{
  ldens = 0.5*nu.n*log( 0.5*nu.n*sigSq.n ) +
  0.5*log(k.n) -
          lgamma(0.5*nu.n) - 0.5*log(2*pi) +
          0.5*(nu.n-1)*log(tau) -
          0.5*(nu.n*sigSq.n)*tau -
          0.5*k.n*tau*(mu-mu.n)^2
  out = exp(ldens)
  return(out)
}
```

The posterior probability of interest is a double integral

$$\Pr\left(95 < \mu < 105, \sigma < 5 \mid y\right)$$

$$= \Pr\left(95 < \mu < 105, \tau > \frac{1}{5^2} \mid y\right)$$

$$= \int_{0.04}^{\infty} \int_{95}^{105} \pi(\mu, \tau \mid y) d\mu d\tau$$

The marginal posterior $100 \times p$ percentile of μ may be determined by finding the value M that satisfies

$$\int\limits_{0}^{\infty}\int\limits_{-\infty}^{M} \pi(\mu,\tau\,|\,y)\,d\mu\,d\tau = p.$$

Though there are more sophisticated algorithms, the double integral may be numerically approximated in R with two calls to the *integrate()* function as follows.

```
## Pr( 95 < mu < 105, tau > 0.04 | y ) = double
integral
InnerFunc = function(mu, tau){ dNG(mu, tau) }
    InnerIntegral = Vectorize(function(tau.inner) {
      integrate(InnerFunc, lower=95, upper=105, tau=tau.
              inner)$value})
pr = integrate(InnerIntegral, lower=0.04, upper=Inf)
print(pr)
> 0.1797854 with absolute error < 5.3e-05

## Determine marginal posterior 5%, 50%, and 95%-iles
    for mu
InnerIntegral = Vectorize(function(tau.inner, M) {
      integrate(InnerFunc, lower=-Inf, upper=M, tau=tau.
      inner)$value})
mu.quantile = function(m0, p=0.5)
{
  ( integrate(InnerIntegral, lower=0, upper=Inf, M=m0)
            $value - p )^2
}
  ## Find m0 such that Pr( mu < m0 | y ) = 2.5%, 50%,
      97.5%.
  ## Integrate over tau.
sapply( c(0.025, 0.5, 0.975), function(p){
      optimize( mu.quantile, interval=c(90, 110), p=p )
              $minimum } )
> 91.60657 95.60000 99.59342
```

The posterior probability $\Pr(95 < \mu < 105, \sigma < 5\,|\,y) = 0.18$ and the marginal posterior 2.5%-, 50%-, and 97.5%-iles for μ are respectively given as 91.61, 95.60, and 99.59.

While the double-integration method works well for this problem, as the dimensionality of the parameter space increases, direct numerical integration becomes less feasible. In its place, Monte Carlo integration may be used.

By drawing samples $\{(\mu_b, \sigma_b^2)\}$ from Equation (2.9), $b = 1, 2, \ldots, B$, the Monte Carlo integral for the probability is

$$\Pr(95 < \mu < 105, \sigma < 5 \mid y) \approx \left(\frac{1}{B}\right) \Sigma \, 1[95 < \mu_b < 105, \sigma_b < 5].$$

The marginal posterior quantiles for μ may be determined by Monte Carlo integration simply by looking at the quantiles of $\{\mu_b\}$.

The simplest Monte Carlo integration method involves direct sampling from the posterior distribution. Several authors (e.g., Gelman et al. 2013, Chapter 3) derive the NG sampling distribution directly by noting that

$$\pi(\mu, \tau \mid y) = \pi(\mu \mid y, \tau) \times \pi(\tau \mid y).$$

It can be shown that

$$\tau \mid y \sim \text{Ga}\left(\frac{v_n}{2}, \frac{v_n \sigma_n^2}{2}\right) \text{ and}$$

$$\mu \mid y, \sigma^2 \sim N\left(\mu_n, \frac{\sigma^2}{k_n}\right),$$

where $\tau = (1/\sigma^2)$.

In R, the computer code to calculate the Monte Carlo probability is given below.

```
set.seed(089)
tau.ng = rgamma( 10000, shape=0.5*nu.n,
                 rate=0.5*nu.n*sigSq.n ) # tau|y
sigSq.ng = 1/tau.ng
mu.ng = rnorm(10000, mean=mu.n, sd=sqrt(sigSq.ng/k.n))
             # mu|tau, y


 ## Calculate Monte Carlo probability
mean(mu.ng > 95 & mu.ng < 105 & sigSq.ng < 25)
> 0.1797

quantile( mu.ng, p=c(0.025, 0.5, 0.975) )
>       5%          50%                95%
>    91.59147  95.58921   99.62328
```

The Monte Carlo posterior probability (with $B = 10,000$) of 0.1797 (Monte Carlo error < 0.01) is remarkably close to the numerical integrated value of 0.1798. In addition, the Monte Carlo marginal posterior quantiles for μ are also quite close to the true values. The Monte Carlo marginal quantiles will be set aside for now and revisited in Section 2.4.

2.3.3 Rejection Sampling

For situations in which the PDF is known but the sampling distribution is not, rejection sampling (Robert and Casella 2004) may be used. Instead of sampling from $\pi(\theta|\mathbf{y})$, random variables are generated from a proposal distribution $q(\theta)$, where the distribution of $q(\theta)$ must envelop $\pi(\theta|\mathbf{y})$. Let $m > 1$ be a constant and let $u \sim U(0, 1)$. A sample θ^* from $q(\theta)$ is accepted if $(\theta^*|\mathbf{y})/mq(\theta^*) > u$. Otherwise, the sample is rejected and a new pair (θ^*, u) are generated and tested. Ordinarily, $q(.)$ is a multivariate normal or multivariate T distribution. For better sampling properties, we reparameterize the PDF in Equation (2.9) with $\lambda = \ln(\sigma^2) = -\ln(\tau)$ so that the joint posterior density of (μ, λ) is $\pi(\mu, \exp(-\lambda)|y)\exp(-\lambda)$. We set $m = 100$ and $q(.)$ to be a bivariate normal distribution with mean (100, 4) and variance–covariance matrix $\begin{pmatrix} 10^2 & 0 \\ 0 & 10^2 \end{pmatrix}$. Though a simple procedure, rejection sampling can be costly. A sample of size B requires approximately $m \times B$ random variables to be generated. For example, with $m = 100$, about 1 million random variables are needed to generate 10,000 draws. Note that choosing m and $q(.)$ are beyond the scope of this chapter. In R, the rejection sampling algorithm and Monte Carlo integration are coded as follows.

```
reject.sampling = function(m)
{

x.out = rep(NA, 2)
while(TRUE)
{
  ## theta.star = proposal
  theta.star = c( rnorm(1, mean=100, sd=10),rnorm(1,
                  mean=4, sd=10) )
  u = runif(1, 0, 1)
  p.x = dNG(mu=theta.star[1], tau=exp(-theta.star[2]))*
              exp(-theta.star[2])
  q.x = dnorm(theta.star[1], mean=100, sd=10)*
           dnorm(theta.star[2], mean=4, sd=10)
  ratio = p.x/(m*q.x)
  if ( ratio > u )  ## Accept the sample
  {
   x.out = theta.star
```

```
    break
  }
  ## Otherwise, reject the sample
  }
  return(x.out)
}
## Generate 10,000 posterior draws with rejection
    sampling using m=100
set.seed(822)
th.post.reject = t( sapply(1:10000, function(i){
                              reject.sampling(m=100) }))
colnames(th.post.reject) = c("mu", "lambda")

 ## Calculate Monte Carlo probability
mean(th.post.reject[,"mu"] > 95 & th.post.reject
      [,"mu"] < 105 &
                          th.post.reject[,"lambda"]
                          < log(25))
> 0.1747
```

The rejection sampling Monte Carlo posterior probability (with B=10,000) of 0.1747 (Monte Carlo error < 0.01) is a good estimate for the true value of 0.180.

2.3.4 Markov Chain Monte Carlo

While rejection sampling bestows its user with independent random numbers, it requires knowledge of the normalizing constant $\pi(y)$ in Equation (2.4). For most statistical modeling situations, calculation of the normalizing constant is a complex, sometimes intractable mathematical problem. MCMC sampling, however, only requires knowledge of $h(\theta) = \pi(\theta)\pi(y|\theta)$, a function proportional to the posterior distribution, up to the normalizing constant. Two important algorithms for MCMC sampling are discussed, namely Gibbs (Casella and George 1992) and Metropolis–Hastings (Robert and Casella 2004).

2.3.4.1 Gibbs Sampling

Gibbs sampling breaks up the parameter space into two (or more) blocks $\theta = (\theta_1, \theta_2)$. The unconditional joint distribution of $\pi(\theta|y)$ may be sampled by iteratively generating random numbers from $\pi(\theta_1^{(k+1)}|y, \theta_2^{(k)})$ and $\pi(\theta_2^{(k1)}|y, \theta_1^{(k+1)})$, $k = 1, \ldots, K$, given a starting value for $\theta_2^{(1)}$. According to Gibbs sampling theory (Casella and George 1992), the iteratively sampled distribution eventually converges to the true distribution. The resulting set of samples are referred to as an MCMC *chain* (Robert and Casella 2004).

Because Gibbs sampling requires time to converge, a poorly chosen start-ing value $\theta_2^{(1)}$ can yield unlikely samples at the beginning of the chain. As a rule, the first B samples, called the *burn in*, are thrown away to allow the algo-rithm to steer the chain into a more desirable sampling space. Also, because the generation of the $(k+1)$st parameter depends on the value of the kth parameter, Gibbs sampling can suffer from autocorrelation. Autocorrelated samples may possess a smaller-than-expected *effective sample size* (ESS) of MCMC posterior draws. ESS is the approximate number of samples that would have been generated from the posterior distribution if draws were made independently. The "coda" package in R calculates ESS automatically for objects of class "mcmc" with the function *effectiveSize()*. An ESS of 10,000 or more for all parameters is usually sufficient for most statistical inference.

In some cases, such as in our example problem, one or both of $\pi(\theta_1|y,\theta_2)$ and $\pi(\theta_2|y,\theta_1)$ may be exactly identified. Setting $\theta_1=\mu$ and $\theta_2=\tau$, it can be shown that

$$\mu\,|\,y,\sigma^2 \sim N\left(\mu_n, \frac{\sigma^2}{k_n}\right) \text{ and}$$

$$\tau\,|\,y,\mu \sim Ga\left(\frac{n+v_0+1}{2}, \left(\frac{1}{2}\right)\left\{(n-1)s^2 + n(\bar{y}-\mu)^2 + k_0\left(\mu-\mu_0\right)^2 + v_0\sigma_0^2\right\}\right).$$

The R code for Gibbs sampling used to calculate $\Pr\left(95 < \mu < 105, \sigma < 5|\,y\right)$ is shown below.

```
set.seed(121)
th.post.gibbs = matrix(NA, 10000, 2)
sigSq.lag = sSq  ## Starting value for posterior
                    distribution of sigSq
for ( b in 1:5000 )  ## Burn-in period of 5,000
{
 mu.lag = rnorm(1, mean=mu.n, sd=sqrt(sigSq.lag/
             (n+k0)))
 rate = 0.5*( (n-1)*sSq + n*(ybar-mu.lag)^2 +
                 k0*(mu.lag-mu0)^2 + nu0*sigSq0 )
 tau.lag = rgamma(1, shape=0.5*(n+nu0+1), rate=rate)
 sigSq.lag = 1/tau.lag
}
for ( b in 1:10000 ) ## Collect 10,000 posterior samples
{
 mu.lag = rnorm(1, mean=mu.n, sd=sqrt(sigSq.lag/(n+k0)))
 rate = 0.5*( (n-1)*sSq + n*(ybar-mu.lag)^2 +
                 k0*(mu.lag-mu0)^2 + nu0*sigSq0 )
 tau.lag = rgamma(1, shape=0.5*(n+nu0+1), rate=rate)
 sigSq.lag = 1/tau.lag
```

```
th.post.gibbs[b,1:2] = c(mu.lag, log(sigSq.lag))
}
colnames(th.post.gibbs) = c("mu", "lambda")
mean(th.post.gibbs[,"mu"] > 95 & th.post.gibbs
[,"mu"] < 105 & th.post.gibbs[,"lambda"] < log(25))
>   0.1771
```

The Gibbs sampling Monte Carlo posterior probability of 0.1771 is in good agreement with the other methods. Using the coda library function effectiveSize(as.mcmc(th.post.gibbs)), the ESS for μ is about 10,000 and the ESS for σ^2 is about 8,100. Though adequate for this exercise, it may be a good idea to increase the number of posterior draws until the ESS for both parameters is larger than 10,000.

2.3.4.2 Metropolis–Hastings

The Metropolis–Hastings (M–H) algorithm (Robert and Casella 2004) is a form of MCMC rejection sampling that also only requires knowledge of $h(\theta) = \pi(y|\theta)\pi(\theta)$. This algorithm requires a starting value $\theta^{(1)}$. In the kth step of M–H, a sample θ^* is drawn from a proposal distribution $q(\theta)$. If $\alpha = h(\theta^*)/h(\theta^{(k-1)}) \geq 1$ (i.e., the candidate θ^* is more likely than $\theta^{(k-1)}$), the candidate is accepted and $\theta^{(k)}$ is set to θ^*. Otherwise, the candidate is accepted with probability α or else rejected. If rejected, set $\theta^{(k)} = \theta^{(k-1)}$. The proposal distribution $q(.)$ must be symmetric and is often a multivariate normal or multivariate T distribution. As with Gibbs sampling, the M–H procedure can also suffer from a poorly chosen initial value and so a burn-in period is recommended. M–H also induces autocorrelation by sometimes setting the current posterior draw to its immediate predecessor. Autocorrelation may be overcome by increasing the sample size until a sufficient ESS is established. For sample sizes that strain computer storage capacity, *thinning* is recommended. Thinning the sample by m, for example, means that every mth sample is saved and the other $(m–1)$ samples are discarded. Though the draws from a thinned sample may be nearly independent (low or negligible autocorrelation), throwing away draws after the burn-in period results in a less efficient sample set.

For our example with posterior Equation (2.9),

$$\pi(\mu,\tau|y) \propto h(\mu,\tau|y) = \prod \left\{ N\left(y_i;\mu,\sigma^2\right)\right\} \times N\left(\mu;\mu_0,\frac{\sigma_0^2}{k_0}\right) \times \text{Ga}\left(\tau;\frac{v_0}{2},\frac{v_0\sigma_0^2}{2}\right).$$

In R, using $\lambda = \ln(\sigma^2) = -\ln(\tau)$, the M–H algorithm and Monte Carlo integration of the posterior probability of interest are written as follows. As before, the proposal distribution is bivariate normal with mean (100, 4) and variance–covariance matrix

$$\begin{pmatrix} 10^2 & 0 \\ 0 & 10^2 \end{pmatrix}.$$

```r
h.theta = function(mu, lambda)
{
## Likelihood x Prior. Proportional to posterior
density
  sigma = exp(0.5*lambda)
  ldens = sum( dnorm( y, mean=mu, sd=sigma, log=TRUE )) +
      dnorm( mu, mean=mu0, sd=sigma/sqrt(k0), log=TRUE ) +
      dgamma( exp(-lambda), shape=0.5*nu0,
          rate=0.5*nu0*sigSq0, log=TRUE) - lambda

  out = exp(ldens)
  return(out)
}
mh.sampling = function(mu0, lambda0)
{
## (mu0, lambda0) = (k-1)st draw

  x.out = c(mu0, lambda0)
  ## theta.star = proposal
  theta.star = c( rnorm(1, mean=100, sd=10), rnorm(1,
              mean=4, sd=10) )
  u = runif(1, 0, 1)

  ratio = h.theta(mu=theta.star[1], lambda=theta.
              star[2]) / h.theta(mu=mu0,
              lambda=lambda0)
  alpha = min(1, ratio)
  if ( u < alpha ) ## accept new proposal
    x.out = theta.star
  return(x.out)
}


## Generate 10,000 MCMC samples with M-H
set.seed(663)
th.post.mh = matrix(NA, 10000, 2)
theta.lag = c( mean(y), log(sSq) )
for ( b in 1:10000 )
{
  th.post.mh[b,] = mh.sampling(mu0=theta.lag[1],
          lambda0=theta.lag[2])
  theta.lag = as.vector(th.post.mh[b,])
}

colnames(th.post.mh) = c("mu", "lambda")
```

```
mean(th.post.mh[,"mu"] > 95 & th.post.mh[,"mu"] < 105 &
                     th.post.mh[,"lambda"] < log(25))
>  0.141
```

Considering that 10,000 samples were drawn, the estimated posterior probability of 0.141 from M–H is quite far from the numerical integrated value of 0.180. The inadequate result stems from the small ESS of the MCMC posterior draws. The output of *effectiveSize(th.post.mh)* is 136 for μ and 156 for σ^2, a far cry from the desired 10,000 independent draws.

To obtain an ESS of about 10,000, we set a burn-in period of 20,000 draws and increased the number of collected samples to 15,000 with thinning by 100. Computer code follows.

```
set.seed(303)
th.post.mh2 = matrix(NA, 15000, 2)

theta.lag = c( ybar+100, log(sSq)+2 ) ## A poorly chosen
            initial value
print(theta.lag)
>       194.775000  5.014659
for ( burnin in 1:20000 ) ## Burn-in: Discard the
first 20,000 draws
{
 theta.new = mh.sampling(mu0=theta.lag[1],
                         lambda0=theta.lag[2])
 theta.lag = theta.new
}
print(theta.lag)  ## The initial value improves after
a burn-in period
>  92.992802 3.709665

for ( mcmc in 1:15000 )  ## Save 15,000 posterior draws
{
 for ( thin in 1:100 )  ## Thin by 100
 {
  theta.new = mh.sampling(mu0=theta.lag[1], lambda0
  =theta.lag[2])
  theta.lag = theta.new
 }
 th.post.mh2[mcmc,] = theta.new
}
colnames(th.post.mh2) = c("mu", "lambda")

mean(th.post.mh2[,"mu"] > 95 & th.post.mh2[,"mu"]
< 105 & th.post.mh2[,"lambda"] < log(25))
```

```
> 0.1840667

effectiveSize(as.mcmc(th.post.mh2))
>          mu        lambda
> 10978.75    10300.98
```

With an ESS of about 10,000, the M–H Monte Carlo estimate 0.184 agrees with all other methods.

In all, 1,520,000 samples were drawn by M–H in order to achieve an ESS of about 10,000, putting M–H on a par with the rejection sampling algorithm.

Luckily, Bayesian practitioners need not write sophisticated sampling procedures. For nearly all statistical modeling problems, pre-packaged computer code with far superior algorithms written by expert statisticians, mathematicians, and computer scientists are available. These are explored in Section 2.4.

2.4 Computational Tools

2.4.1 BUGS and JAGS

Though not yet in a golden age for Bayesian statistical software, mature computer algorithms for sampling from the posterior distribution have been developed. Started in 1989, the Bayesian inference Using Gibbs Sampling (BUGS) language (Lunn et al. 2009) was among the first to provide a generic interface to MCMC sampling. BUGS, written in 32-bit Component Pascal, performs a combination of M–H and Gibbs sampling, breaking up parameters into correlated groups. For those running Microsoft Windows operating systems, WinBUGS provided a graphical user interface until development was discontinued in 2007 in favor of OpenBUGS.

As computers grew faster with multiple CPU cores and moved from 32-bit to 64-bit, there was a desire to port BUGS to other platforms (e.g., Linux, MacIntosh). The community threw its support behind Just Another Gibbs Sampler (JAGS) (Plummer 2003). JAGS is written in C++, supports 32-bit and 64-bit computing systems, and may be compiled for a variety of computer platforms. In addition, JAGS provides a similar user interface to the BUGS language so that nearly all BUGS code can be run in JAGS and vice versa with little editing. Though it appears that BUGS is no longer actively developed, JAGS was last updated in August 2017.

Both BUGS and JAGS are powered with expert software programming tricks and techniques to perform Metropolis–Hastings with a random-walk updater, Gibbs, and slice sampling. The latest general MCMC software system, called Stan (Carpenter et al. 2017), implements the "No-U-Turn sampler" (NUTS), a variant of Hamiltonian Monte Carlo. Relative to the random walk, the NUTS algorithm performs a more thorough search of the parameter space of the posterior distribution. Like JAGS, Stan is based on C++ for 32-bit and 64-bit systems and has been ported to various computing platforms.

Various interfaces are available for all three MCMC software engines. Most prominently, OpenBugs may be called from R using one of the many available R libraries. In addition, macros were written to call OpenBugs from Excel, SAS, Matlab, and Stata. JAGS may be accessed from R, Python, or Matlab. The Stan website lists interfaces with R, Python, Matlab, Julia, Stata, and Mathematica. Thus, MCMC may be approached from many popular mathematical/statistical computing platforms. Taking advantage of multiple CPUs, many of the interfaces can perform parallel computing with BUGS, JAGS, or Stan.

2.4.2 SAS PROC MCMC

The list is incomplete without SAS Proc MCMC (SAS 2016). Originally released in SAS 9.2 with an experimental set of MCMC functions, Proc MCMC in SAS 9.4 has matured into a feature-complete MCMC system, rivaling JAGS and Stan, with the ability to perform various MCMC sampling, including random walk and NUTS. We note that, while BUGS, JAGS, and Stan may be downloaded as "freeware", SAS is a for-profit company and Proc MCMC is part of its commercial software. Currently, SAS permits free use of its procedures for non-profit research.

2.4.3 Utility of JAGS

We are not endorsing one MCMC platform over another; however, to maintain consistency throughout the book, most of the examples will be given using JAGS via an R interface. In this manner, historical BUGS and JAGS code that may be freely downloaded by the reader will be easily understood. In addition, relative to Stan, JAGS programming statements tend to be more compact. For the reader's benefit, computer code written in JAGS will be analogously provided in Stan in the appendix of this book. As an example, consider the competing "model" statements in JAGS and Stan for the univariate normal random variable example given in Section 2.3. JAGS and Stan code are given in Table 2.1. Stan uses explicit data and parameter declarations, whereas such statements are implicit in JAGS, allowing JAGS scripts to generally be written with far fewer lines of code. Also note that Stan and JAGS often parameterize distributions differently. In the example below, JAGS uses the mean-precision parameterization and Stan uses the mean-standard deviation parameterization for the normal distribution.

Our favorite JAGS interface is through the run.jags() function in the *runjags* R library, which depends on the *rjags* library. We illustrate the run.jags() function, noting that the model statement must be given either with the contents of Table 2.1 in a separate text file or by placing the model statement in quotes.

TABLE 2.1

JAGS and Stan Statements for Univariate Normal Distribution

JAGS	Stan
```model{ ## Prior mu ~ dnorm(mu0, k0*tau) tau ~ dgamma(0.5*nu0, 0.5*nu0*sigSq0) sigmaSq <- 1/tau lambda <- log(sigmaSq) ## Likelihood for (i in 1:n) { y[i] ~ dnorm(mu, tau) } }```	```data{ int<lower=0> n; real y[n]; // hyperparameters real mu0; real k0; real nu0; real sigSq0; } parameters{ real mu; real tau; } transformed parameters{ real sigma; sigma = 1/sqrt(tau); } model{ // Prior mu ~ normal(mu0, sigma/sqrt(k0)); tau ~ gamma(0.5*nu0, 0.5*nu0*sigSq0); // Likelihood for (i in 1:n) { y[i] ~ normal(mu, sigma); } }```

```
require(rjags); require(runjags)

## Prepare the model for JAGS by placing it in quotes.
model.txt = "
model{

  ## Prior
  mu ~ dnorm( mu0, k0*tau )
  tau ~ dgamma( 0.5*nu0, 0.5*nu0*sigSq0 )

  sigmaSq <- 1/tau
  sigma <- 1/sqrt(tau)
  lambda <- log(sigmaSq)

  ## Likelihood
```

```
for ( i in 1:n )
{
 y[i] ~ dnorm( mu, tau )
}

}"

## Prepare the data for JAGS
data = list(n=length(y), y=y, mu0=100, k0=1.5, nu0=2,
sigSq0=64 )

## Call JAGS via run.jags() using 3 CPUs
set.seed(777)
fitb = run.jags( model=model.txt, monitor=c("mu",
                 "sigma", "lambda"), data=data,
                 n.chains=3,burnin = 5000, sample =
                 10000, thin=5, method="parallel")
```

JAGS (and BUGS and Stan) requires that the data be given as a list. Via the run.jags() function, JAGS was called with three independent chains in parallel (using three CPUs), where each chain ran with a burn-in of 5,000 samples and collecting 50,000 = (10,000 × 5) posterior samples. After thinning by 5, 10,000 posterior draws were saved for each chain, for a total of 30,000 MCMC posterior draws. Printing the JAGS *fitb* object reveals summary statistics for the marginal posterior distributions and plotting the *fitb* object shows a traceplot and density (Figure 2.1).

```
print(fitb)
> JAGS model summary statistics from 30000 samples (thin = 5; chains = 3; adapt+burnin = 5000):

>        Lower95 Median Upper95 Mean    SD     Mode    MCerr MC%ofSD SSeff   AC.50    psrf
> mu     91.528 95.583 99.435 95.59 1.9926 95.614 0.011505  0.6    30000 -0.00534 1.0001
> sigma  3.5949 5.7205 9.0102 5.9876 1.5032 5.3586 0.008693  0.6    29901 0.000293 1.0004
>lambda  2.6513 3.4881 4.4659 3.5226 0.46841 3.4848 0.002704  0.6    30000 0.000215 1.0004
> Total time taken: 4.8 seconds
```

As described in the run.jags() manual (Denwood 2016), the JAGS output shows the posterior median and 95% credible interval (Lower95, Upper95), mean, standard deviation (SD), and mode. For diagnostics, it shows the Monte Carlo standard error of the mean estimate (MCerr), effective sample size (SSeff), autocorrelation with a lag of 50 (AC.50), the Monte Carlo standard error as a percent of the standard deviation (MC%ofSD), and the potential scale-reduction factor of the Gelman–Rubin statistic, sometimes called R-hat (psrf). For diagnostics, we typically like for SSeff to be at least 10,000 for each variable, an AC.50 close to 0 and a psrf value close to 1. To see the MCMC summary statistics using the *coda* library in R, use the syntax *summary(fitb[[1]])*. Note that the 95% credible interval is a highest posterior

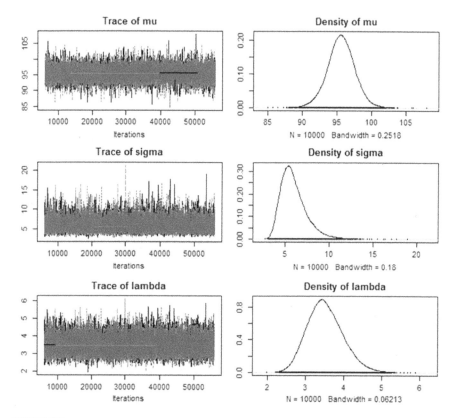

FIGURE 2.1

Traceplot and density for posterior distribution from three MCMC chains of μ (mu), σ (sigma), and λ = ln(σ²) (lambda).

density (HPD) interval and may not be equal to the (2.5%, 97.5%) marginal posterior quantiles.

For graphical diagnostics, we prefer the plots from the coda library. The function call is *plot(fitb[[1]])* instead of *plot(fitb)*, which creates a similar set of graphs. We also prefer to run two or more independent MCMC chains so that we can visualize the consistency and convergence of the chains.

To calculate the Monte Carlo probability from Section 2.3, the *fit* object must be converted to a matrix. Computer code is shown below. The JAGS-based posterior probability = 0.175, which is within Monte Carlo error of the true value. The Monte Carlo 2.5%, 50%, and 97.5% marginal posterior quantiles of μ are also close to their respective true values.

```
th.post = as.matrix(as.mcmc.list(fitb))
mean(th.post[,"mu"] > 95 & th.post[,"mu"] < 105 &
                    th.post[,"lambda"] < log(25))
```

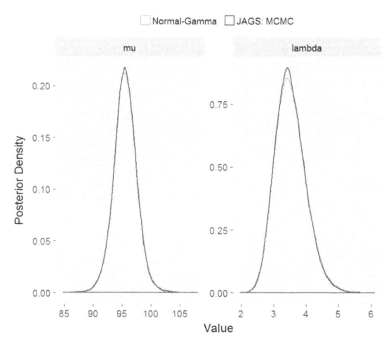

FIGURE 2.2
Posterior marginal densities of μ (mu) and $\lambda = \ln(\sigma^2)$ (lambda).

```
>  0.1752333

## Marginal quantiles of mu
quantile( th.post[,"mu"], p=c(0.025, 0.5, 0.975))

>     2.5%       50%        97.5%
>  91.59526  95.58335   99.51119
```

The marginal posterior distributions for μ and λ via JAGS (MCMC) and via the true density generated in Section 2.2 are shown to be equivalent in Figure 2.2. The sampled true density is given by R objects *mu.ng* and *lambda. ng = −log(tau.ng)*.

2.5 Concluding Remarks

An overview of Bayesian analysis is provided in this chapter. Special focus is on the concepts of Bayes' Theorem; prior, posterior, and predictive distributions; selection of priors; inferences based on posterior and predictive probabilities; and Bayesian computational tools. Some key differences between frequentist and Bayesian thinking are highlighted. The topics discussed in this chapter lay the ground for understanding Bayesian methods that are discussed in other chapters of the book. Since drug research and development are carried out through series of experimentation, Bayesian study design and analysis are likely to play more important roles in decision-making by leveraging historical data, personal beliefs, and observational data from the current studies.

3

Bayesian Estimation of Sample Size and Power

3.1 Introduction

Sample size determination is an important aspect in study design, especially in the planning of clinical trials due to regulatory requirements. An accurately and sufficiently sized study enables the investigator to detect practically meaningful differences in comparative studies or provide precise estimates of the issue at hand. The frequentist sample size calculation relies on the assumption that the true values of parameters under the alternative hypothesis are known. In practice, this assumption is rarely true. In fact, depending on available data, there are varying degrees of uncertainties around these unknown parameters. By modeling the parameters through prior distributions, Bayesian methods can account for these uncertainties in the sample size calculations, thus mitigating the risk of underpowering a study. In literature, in the context of estimating population prevalence with the desired precision, three criteria were proposed to obtain the so-called minimal sample size determination. These criteria, which are based on highest posterior density (HPD) intervals, are the average coverage criterion (ACC), the average length criterion (ALC), and the worst outcome criterion (WOC) (Joseph and Belisle 1997; Joseph, du Berger, and Belisle 1997). As these methods have been extensively discussed, in this chapter we concern ourselves with sample size determination for the purpose of testing hypotheses. Sample size calculations based on Bayesian concepts are discussed through three examples, one related to product lot release and the other two regarding futility and interim analysis in sequential trials.

3.2 Sample Size Determination

3.2.1 Frequentist Methods

In drug research, the objective of a comparative study is to collect data to test a specific hypothesis. An important aspect of the study planning is sample size determination. Given the null hypothesis of no difference, to estimate the sample size a frequentist procedure requires specification of a significance level for the test, a meaningful difference of δ, which is usually stated in an alternative hypothesis, and the expected power or probability of rejecting the null hypothesis when the true difference is δ.

As an example, consider a drug manufacturing process that produces a large number of units (e.g., tablets), some of which are defective. The batch may be released to the market if the percent of defect p equals 1%. It is desired that the lot should be rejected with a high probability if the percent of defect p equals 2%. In this situation, the hypotheses of interest are:

$$H_0: p = 1\% \text{ vs. } H_a: p = 2\%,$$

which implies that $\delta = 1\%$. The 1% defect rate in the null hypothesis is the producer's quality level or average percent of defect of batches produced by the manufacturer; whereas the 1% increase in the alternative hypothesis is selected based on consumer's risk. In reality, however, δ is often unknown. Suppose a test procedure is given such that the batch may be released if no defects are detected in a random sample of N units. In addition, the testing for defects is carried out by randomly selecting a maximum of N units and testing the units sequentially until either a defective unit is detected or none of the N units are found to be defective. The significance level and power of the above test correspond to the probabilities of rejecting the null hypothesis when the true defect rate $p = 1\%$ and accepting the alternative hypothesis when the true defect rate $p = 2\%$. Obviously, these probabilities are dependent on the sample size. For a given sample size, the appropriateness of the test described above can be evaluated through an operating characteristic OC), which defines the long-term probability of the success of a binary event with respect to the proportion of defective units in a batch. For example, consider $N = 10$. In testing of up to ten units in a newly manufactured batch, let X denote the index of the first detected defective unit. Then X follows a negative binomial distribution with probability p with stopping rule at the first observed failure so that $X \sim NB(1, p)$. Because a batch is released only when zero out of 10 sampled units are defective, the long-term probability to release a batch is $p_{rel} = (1-p)^{10}$. Conditioned on a value $p = p_0$, the OC is $(1-p_0)^{10}$. For example, if $p_0 = 0.08$ (i.e., 8% of units in a batch are defective), the probability of releasing the batch $(1-0.08)^{10} = 0.43$. By considering different values of p, one may generate an OC curve, given in Figure 3.1.

From the plot, it can be easily obtained that the probabilities of accepting a batch when $p = 1\%$ and 2% are 90% and 82%, respectively. This implies a significance level of 10% (= $1-90\%$) and power of 82%. Depending on the values of the prespecified significance level and power, the test including the sample size of 10 may or may not be acceptable. For example, if the expected significance level is 10% and power 80%, the test is adequate in providing protection from both the consumer's and producer's risk.

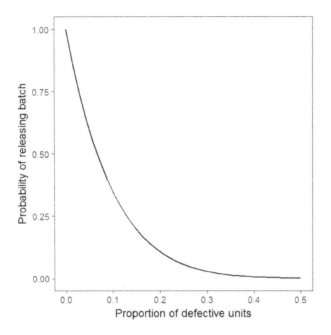

FIGURE 3.1
OC curve for probability of releasing a manufactured batch.

3.2.2 Bayesian Considerations

One of the challenges of sample size determination using the frequentist framework is that the true values of the parameters, such as the meaningful difference δ, are unknown. In practice, these parameters are often estimated from prior studies, published results in the literature, or expert opinions, and are viewed as the "true" values. Since the frequentist method does not consider the variability in those estimates in the sample size calculations, overconfidence in the "true" values may result in an underpowered study. In addition, the ad-hoc practice to determine the "true" values of those parameters makes it more challenging to carry out the frequentist test method with consistency. Bayesian procedures, which incorporate uncertainties in the parameters, provide a natural remedy for this issue.

3.2.2.1 Prior Information

In the above example, the manufacturer would like to estimate the long-term probability of releasing batches of a drug to the public; however, this requires knowledge of either p or p_{rel}. Before full-scale manufacturing, knowledge about the parameters p or p_{rel} may be obtained (Chapter 2) from expert opinion (e.g., operators of other manufacturing processes may be able to give a range for p based on experience) or possibly by estimating the parameter value from development data. This information may be encapsulated as the prior distribution for p. For example, suppose that the operators estimate that no more than 2% of the units in a batch are defective and, through a process of prior elicitation, settle on the prior distribution for $p \sim$ Beta(2, 198). This Beta prior has a mean of 1% and an upper 95th percentile of about 2%. The mean batch-release probability is calculated as $E[(1-p)^{10}] = 0.91$, which may be quickly approximated by Monte Carlo methods by generating $p_b \sim$ Beta(2, 198), $b = 1, 2, \ldots, B$, and calculating $(1/B)\sum_{b=1}^{B}(1-p_b)^{10}$. The R computer code for the Monte Carlo method using $B = 10000$ is

```
mean ( (1-rbeta(10000, shape1=2, shape2=198))^10 )
>  0.9056183
```

Thus, given only prior information, the manufacturer can expect to release its batches of a drug to the public about 91% of the time.

3.2.2.2 Use of Historical Data

After testing five full-scale manufactured drug batches, the prior information for p may be updated. Suppose zero out of ten defects were discovered in the first four batches, but a defect was discovered in the sixth unit of the fifth batch so that four of the five batches are released. The density of p (and hence p_{rel}) may be updated with the new data using the JAGS statement given by computer code [3.1]. In [3.1], X_i is the number of units tested before detecting a defect in the ith batch, so that X_i follows a negative binomial distribution with probability p, stopping at the first detected defect; i.e., $X_i \sim$ NB(1, p). Since the maximum number of tested units is ten, when no units are identified as defective, the value for X_i is right-censored and known to be bigger than 10. For $0 \le X_i \le 10$, the JAGS likelihood statement is "X[i] ~ dnegbin(1, p)". For the case $X_i > 10$, the likelihood takes the complement of the cumulative distribution function; i.e, Pr(X[i] > 10). In JAGS, special coding is required to specify right-censoring using the function call *dinterval*(X[i], 10). A new variable, *rightCens*[i], is created so that when $0 \le X_i \le 10$, *rightCens*[i] = 0, and when $X_i > 10$, *rightCens*[i] = 1. Additionally, when $X_i > 10$, the value in the data statement is set to *NA*.

[3.1]

```
require(rjags) ; require(runjags)

model.txt = "
model{

   p ~ dbeta(2, 198) ## Prior for p

   pRel <- (1-p)^10
```

```
  for ( i in 1:N )
  {
     X[i] ~ dnegbin(p, 1)
     ## rightCens: = 0 if X[i] <= 10; = 1 if X[i] > 10
     rightCens[i] ~ dinterval( X[i], 10 )
  }
}"
data = list( N=5, X=c(NA, NA, NA, NA, 6),
             rightCens=c(1, 1, 1, 1, 0) )
fitb = run.jags( model.txt, data=data, monitor=
             c("p", "pRel"),n.chains=3,burnin=10000,
             sample=10000, thin=5, method="parallel" )
```

Alternatively, one may update p_{rel} with a simpler approach by noting that four out of five batches were released. Let Y be the number of released batches out five. Then Y follows a binomial distribution with probability $(1-p)^{10}$; i.e., $Y \sim$ binomial$(5, (1-p)^{10})$. The JAGS code is shown in computer code [3.2].

[3.2]

```
model.txt = "
model{

  p ~ dbeta(2, 198) ## Prior for p

  pRel <- (1-p)^10
  Y ~ dbin(pRel, 5) ## Likelihood
}"

data = list( Y=4 ) ## Four batches out of five are
             released
fitb = run.jags( model.txt, data=data, monitor
             =c("p", "pRel"), n.chains=3, burnin=10000,
             sample=10000, thin=5,  method="parallel" )
```

Running the code statements from [3.1] and [3.2], one obtains the posterior distribution for p_{rel}, shown with the prior distribution for p_{rel} in Figure 3.2. Comparing the two approaches, the differences in the posterior distribution for p_{rel} are very slight, both yielding a slight drop to 89% in the expected batch-release probability.

3.2.3 Bayesian Approaches

As discussed by Spiegelhalter et al. (2004), there are three types of Bayesian approaches to sample size determination, namely, "hybrid classical–Bayesian", "proper Bayesian", and "decision-theoretic Bayesian". The "hybrid

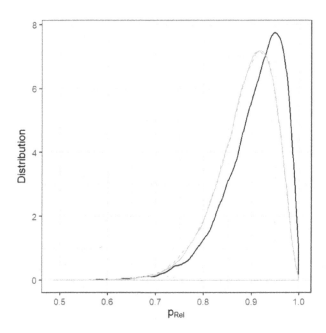

FIGURE 3.2
Black density is prior distribution of p_{rel}. Grey solid and grey dashed densities show the p_{rel} posterior, respectively, from [3.1] and [3.2].

classical–Bayesian" method utilizes a prior of unknown parameters for study design but performs the analysis entirely based on a frequentist test. In this context, the power of the test is the average of the frequentist power obtained through integration with respect to the prior distribution. This unconditional power is also referred to as predictive power (Whitehead et al. 2008) and assurance (O'Hagan et al. 2005). A sample size is chosen to achieve the desired unconditional power. By contrast, the "proper Bayesian" method determines the sample size by making use of the Bayesian framework to incorporate uncertainties of unknown parameters in the design stage. After the data are collected, a Bayesian test is carried out to test the hypotheses. Lastly, the "decision-theoretic Bayesian" approach determines a sample size that maximizes a utility function for the cost of the study and potential benefit of the new intervention or improved process (Spiegelhalter et al. 2004). Care should be taken in specifying the utilities as misspecifications can lead to suboptimal designs (Whitehead et al. 2008).

3.3 Power and Sample Size

As previously discussed, statistical power curves are operating characteristics used to compare two competing hypotheses H_0 and H_a via a test statistic.

The statistical power of a test is the long-term probability to declare H_a using a statistical decision rule, conditioned on the value of population parameters. In the following, through an example, we illustrate the use of both the "hybrid classical–Bayesian" and "proper Bayesian" approaches to the estimation of sample size and power.

3.3.1 Phase II Study

Consider a Phase II clinical trial for chronic obstructive pulmonary disease. Patients are enrolled into the trial, randomly assigned to either a placebo or a treatment arm. The gauge of the success of such a trial depends on the mean increase in lung capacity (often measured by *forced expiratory volume in the first second*, or FEV1) of the treated group over the placebo group. Let μ_{Trt} and μ_{Pla} denote the true FEV1 mean values for the treated and placebo groups and Δ be a prespecified testing limit. The binary outcome of the trial rests on the efficacy of the drug, with failure defined by $H_0: \mu_{Trt} - \mu_{Pla} \le \Delta$ and success defined by $H_a: \mu_{Trt} - \mu_{Pla} > \Delta$.

3.3.1.1 Test Procedure

Given treatment-arm data and placebo-arm data, each consisting of N patients, one may test the two possible outcomes via a two-sample Z test (a T test with known variance parameter). If, say, the p-value from the Z test is less than 0.05, one may declare H_a.

3.3.1.2 Sample Size Calculations

Conditioned on parameter values $\mu_{Trt} - \mu_{Pla} = \delta$ and sample sizes (N), one may calculate the long-term probability of success for the binary event $\mu_{Trt} - \mu_{Pla} > \Delta$. Conditioned on δ and N, the probability of success is the operating characteristic, also called statistical power. Before enrolling patients, the sponsor of the clinical trial usually calculates the smallest sample size (N) needed so that, if the drug is efficacious, statistical power will be high (ideally, equal to 1.0).

To illustrate this problem, let $\bar{Y}_{Trt}$ and $\bar{Y}_{Pla}$ denote the sample mean FEV1 values from the treated and untreated (placebo-controlled) groups, each of sample size N. Assume that, conditioned on the true mean difference $\mu_{Trt} - \mu_{Pla} = \delta$, the sample difference $\bar{Y}_{Trt} - \bar{Y}_{Pla}$ follows a normal distribution with mean δ and variance $2/N$. The test statistic is

$$Z = \sqrt{\frac{N}{2}} \left(\bar{Y}_{Trt} - \bar{Y}_{Pla} - \Delta \right)$$

with associated p-value given by $1 - \Phi(Z)$, where $\Phi(.)$ is the standard normal cumulative distribution function. Using a p-value cutoff of 0.05, trial success is declared whenever $Z > \Phi^{-1}(0.95) = 1.645$, where $\Phi^{-1}(.)$ is the inverse function of $\Phi(.)$. Conditioned on the true mean difference δ_0, the long-term probability of trial success is

$$\Phi\left(-1.645 - \sqrt{\frac{N}{2}}(\Delta - \delta)\right).$$

Letting $\Delta = 1.5$, statistical power (i.e., OC) may be calculated for different values of N and δ_0, as shown in Figure 3.3.

The clinical trial sponsor can use Figure 3.3 to determine the minimum sample size that would permit a high probability of trial success. Just as in the manufacturing problem of Section 3.1, the sponsor would like to know the value of the mean FEV1 difference δ needed to ensure a successful trial. For example, if the true value of $\delta = 3.0$, the sponsor may opt for the smallest sample size, $N = 10$. On the other hand, if $\delta = 2.25$, the sponsor may require the largest sample size under consideration, $N = 30$.

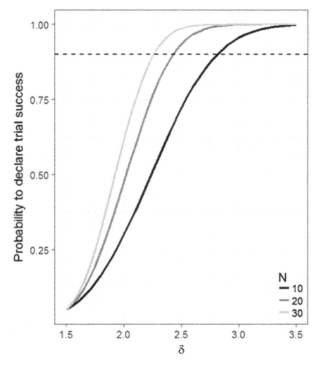

FIGURE 3.3
Statistical power curves for three sample sizes (N) and true mean difference δ. Dashed horizontal line drawn at 0.95 probability.

3.3.1.3 Incorporation of Prior

It may be a difficult task to determine a single value for δ, let alone a range of reasonable values for δ. The sponsor might elicit knowledge of δ, for example, by examining pre-clinical experimental results or by considering the range of results from clinical trials that use a similar class of drug. Suppose that the sponsor found literature for three similar, independent Phase II drug trials with results shown in Table 3.1. Assuming that the FEV1 measurements follow a normal distribution and that the variance of mean differences is still $2/N$, one can derive a distribution for δ via Bayesian methods with vague prior information. Assume that

$$\overline{W}_i = \delta + e_i,$$

where $\overline{W}_i$ is the sample mean of the ith trial and $e_i \sim N\left(0, \dfrac{2}{N}\right)$. Using the data from Table 3.1, it follows that the weighted sample mean

$$\overline{W} \mid \delta \sim N\left(\delta, \dfrac{2}{72}\right).$$

Placing the vague prior on

$$\delta \sim N(2.5, 1000),$$

it can be shown that the posterior distribution for $\delta \mid \overline{W} = 2.4$ is normal with mean and variance, respectively, given by

$$\left(\dfrac{1000}{\left(\dfrac{2}{72}\right) + 1000}\right) 2.4 + \left(\dfrac{\left(\dfrac{2}{72}\right)}{\left(\dfrac{2}{72}\right) + 1000}\right)(2.5) = 2.4$$

$$\left(\dfrac{1}{1000} + \dfrac{72}{2}\right)^{-1} = 0.028.$$

TABLE 3.1

Mean FEV1 Differences and Sample Sizes from Three Independent Phase II Clinical Trials

Mean Difference Treated vs. Placebo	Sample Size per Arm (N)
2.7	25
2.6	14
2.1	33

Figure 3.4 shows the power curves from Figure 3.3 along with the prior distribution $\delta \sim N(2.4, 0.028)$. With the prior density overlaid, it is easy to see that a sample size between $N=20$ and $N=30$ is necessary for a successful clinical trial.

Given the posterior distribution of δ, the expected probability for a successful clinical trial is

$$E_\delta\left[\Phi\left(-1.645 - \sqrt{\frac{N}{2}}(\Delta - \delta)\right)\right] \approx \left(\frac{1}{B}\right)\sum_{b=1}^{B}\Phi\left(-1.645 - \sqrt{\frac{N}{2}}(\Delta - \delta_b)\right),$$

where $\delta_b \sim N(2.4, 0.028)$.

Using $\Delta = 1.5$ and $N=30$, the R computer code for the Monte Carlo integration using $B=10,000$ is

```
mean( pnorm( -1.645 - sqrt(30/2)*
             (1.5 - rnorm(10000, 2.4, sqrt(0.028))) ) )
> 0.9385701
```

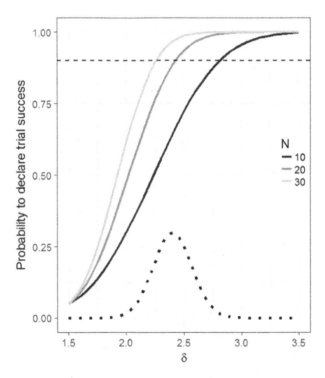

FIGURE 3.4
Statistical power curves for three sample sizes (N) and true mean difference δ with testing limit $\Delta = 1.5$. Dotted density shows the prior $\delta \sim N(2.4, 0.028)$. Dashed horizontal line drawn at 0.95 probability.

and yields the value of about 0.94. Thus, the sponsor can expect to declare H_a with 94% probability with a sample size of 30 in each arm. To achieve a different desired success rate, one may solve for N using the following code:

```
> f.opt = function(N, pr){
  ( mean( pnorm( -1.645 - sqrt(N/2)*
        (1.5 - rnorm(10000, 2.4, sqrt(0.028))) ) )
        - pr )^2
}
```

To solve for N with a target of 80% power, use

```
optimize( f.opt, interval=c(20, 50), pr=0.8)
```

resulting in (rounded up) $N = 21$ per arm.

3.3.1.4 Proper Bayesian Procedure

So far in this section, a frequentist testing approach was laid out to choose between H_0 and H_a for the Phase II clinical trial. By applying a prior distribution to the true mean difference in FEV1 (δ), a sample size could be calculated for a given expected statistical power value. The same thought process can be applied to a Bayesian testing approach for choosing between H_0 and H_a. For example, let $p = Pr(\mu_{Trt} - \mu_{Pla} > \Delta \mid data)$ denote the posterior probability of H_a with declaration of H_a if, say, $p > 0.95$. The expected statistical power of the Bayesian test is the probability that $p > 0.95$, evaluated over the prior $\delta \sim N(2.4, 0.028)$. The steps for this evaluation will be shown next.

3.3.1.5 Two Prior Distributions

Given clinical trial data, the prior distribution that we established for δ may not be conservative enough to allow for better-than-expected or worse-than-expected possibilities when evaluating the posterior probability p. A distinction must now be made between the *design prior*, which may be used to simulate the future clinical trial data, and the *analysis prior*, which will be used to evaluate the posterior probability p. The use of different priors for study design and data analysis has been broadly discussed in the literature (Tsutakawa 1972; Etzioni and Kadance 1993; Spiegelhalter and Freedman 1986). It was argued that having a separate prior for design and analysis makes sense as the individuals who design the experiment and collect data may not be those who evaluate the data. The issue was further discussed in more recent publications (Wang and Gelfand 2002; Sahu and Smith 2006; De Santis 2006, 2007; Brutti and De Santis 2008, Sambucini 2008; Brutti et al. 2008). It is recommended that an informative prior be used for the design prior to generate data more in line with what was previously observed and a non-informative prior for the analysis prior so as to let data drive the final analysis (Wang and Gelfand 2002).

In this spirit, for the above example, the design prior was constructed as $\delta \sim N(2.4, 0.028)$ so that, conditioned on a sample from the design prior, one may generate virtual clinical trial as

$$\bar{Y}_{new} \mid \delta \sim N\left(\delta, \frac{2}{N}\right).$$

A conservative, yet informative analysis prior may be given as a T distribution with location 2.0, scale $= 0.6$, and three degrees of freedom; i.e., $\delta \sim T(2.0, 0.6, 3)$. This analysis prior was chosen with a median of 2.0 and middle 95% ranging from roughly 0 to 4, so that its midpoint is slightly worse than any of the three trial results given in Table 3.1 and its tails are wide enough to essentially cover the full range of possibilities in which the drug effect is no worse than that of a placebo. The analysis prior is robust to the possibility of $\delta \leq 0$ (i.e., the placebo arm performs better than the drug-treated arm) with zero expected probability of success for the cases $N \geq 10$. On the other hand, assuming the design prior is reasonable, the chosen analysis prior should provide a significantly higher success rate relative to using the frequentist Z test. Steps for calculating the expected statistical power of $p = \Pr(\mu_{Trt} - \mu_{Pla} > 1.5 \mid data)$ with the analysis prior are given in Table 3.2.

Following the steps in Table 3.2 can be a time-consuming proposition because the non-conjugate prior in step 3 requires a sampling method such as MCMC. Table 3.2 was followed using $B = 500$ for values of N between 10 and 30 with MCMC performed in JAGS using the code shown below. Relative to the expected success rate from the frequentist Z test, the wide-tailed, reasonable analysis prior $\delta \sim T(2.0, 0.6, 3)$ provides a significant boost in the expected success rate of the future clinical trial. Comparisons of expected statistical power using the frequentist Z test and the Bayesian test method, each paired with the design prior $\delta \sim N(2.4, 0.028)$, are shown in Table 3.3.

TABLE 3.2

Algorithm for Calculating the Expected Statistical Power

Step 1	Sample from the design prior $\delta \sim N(2.4, 0.028)$.
Step 2	Generate a virtual clinical trial summary statistic as $\bar{Y}_{new} \mid \delta \sim N\left(\delta, \frac{2}{N}\right)$, using the design prior from Step 1.
Step 3	With the analysis prior $\delta \sim T(2.0, 0.6, 3)$, calculate the posterior probability $p = \Pr(\mu_{Trt} - \mu_{Pla} > \Delta \mid data)$.
Step 4	Repeat Steps 1–3 a large number of times (e.g., $B = 500$). Expected statistical power is the proportion of cases in Step 3 that resulted in $p > 0.95$.

TABLE 3.3

Expected Statistic Power with Z Test and with Bayesian Test, Paired with the Design Prior $\delta \sim N(2.4, 0.028)$

N	Expected Power with Z Test	Expected Power with Analysis Prior: $\delta \sim T(2.0, 0.6, 3)$
10	0.63	0.71
15	0.77	0.87
20	0.86	0.89
25	0.91	0.95
30	0.94	0.96

```
model.txt = "
model{

 ## Analysis prior for delta
 delta ~ dt(2., 2.78, 3 )    ## 2.78 = 1/0.6^2, where
    scale = 0.6

 ybar ~ dnorm( delta, 0.5*N ) ## Likelihood: Var(ybar)
    = 2/N
}"

N = 10 ## Sample size (repeat code with other
  sample sizes)
B = 500 ## Monte Carlo runs

delta.prior = rnorm(B, mean=2.4, sd=sqrt(0.028))
 ## Design prior
 ## Predictive dist for ybar
ybar.new = rnorm(B, mean=delta.prior, sd=sqrt(2/N))

res = rep(NA, B)
for ( b in 1:B )
{
  data = list(N=N, ybar=ybar.new[b])
  fitb = run.jags(model.txt, data=data, monitor="delta",
             n.chains=3, burnin=4000, sample=8000,
             thin=1, method="parallel")
 th.post = as.matrix(as.mcmc.list(fitb))
    ## Posterior probability that delta > 1.5
 res[b] = mean( th.post[,"delta"] > 1.5 )
}
pr = mean( res >= 0.95 ) ## Expected statistical power
```

3.4 Interim Analysis

3.4.1 Futility and Sample Size

The thought of a lengthy Phase III clinical trial can make any investigator uneasy. Consider the devastating cost of a multi-year clinical trial that fails, yielding no benefit to patients and no return on investment for the sponsor. In such a situation, an interim analysis may be performed to assess the probability of the success (or futility) of continuing the full trial, on one or two occasions before the end of the study. Should the ultimate probability of trial success appear to be low, the trial may be stopped for futility in the absence of treatment effect, saving the patients from an ineffective drug regimen and the sponsor from further monetary expense. In this context, the term "futility" refers to unlikeliness for the trial to achieve statistical significance for its primary endpoints.

When conducting a futility analysis, several considerations need to be given. For example, futility analysis is typically carried out at very low levels such as one-sided alpha of 0.0025. In addition, it may be advantageous to use endpoints other than the overall survival (Goldman, LeBlanc, and Crowley 2008) as this may result in a higher probability of stopping early for futility. In the literature, there are various approaches proposed to assess futility. They include stochastic curtailment, predictive power, predictive probability, and group sequential methods (Snapinn et al. 2006). Snapinn et al. (2006) provide a detailed discussion on several issues related to futility analyses, including ethical considerations, preservation of Type I error, one-sided against two-sided futility rules, and the impact of futility analyses on power. As noted by Lakatos (2016), sample size re-estimation and futility are intercorrelated. Although a trial may be declared futile due to a low probability of success, sample size re-estimation can be used to increase the probability of success for the trial. Hence, the conclusion of futility needs to consider the costs associated with an increased sample size.

Consider the clinical trial example in Section 3.3 with the Z testing procedure and higher testing limit of $\Delta = 2.6$. Power curves were generated for sample sizes $N = 10$, 30, and 100. Using the statistical power formula from Section 3.2, it is clear that the trial will not be successful unless the true mean difference $\delta > 3$. The power curves with the design prior of $\delta \sim N(2.4, 0.028)$ are plotted in Figure 3.5.

With $N = 100$, the expected probability of a successful trial is a paltry 2%; and with the impossibly high $N = 1,000$, the probability of success only rises to 5%. This no-hope situation illustrates the concept of *futility*. That is, because there is virtually no chance of success, the clinical trial should not be carried out under these conditions. Futility represents an important extension of the Bayesian viewpoint of sample size/power calculations. In the next section, through a case example, we illustrate the effect of sample size on utility analysis.

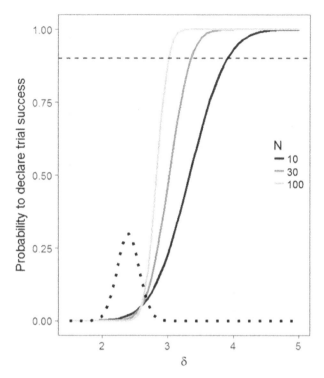

FIGURE 3.5

Statistical power curves for three sample sizes (N) and true mean difference δ with testing limit $\Delta = 2.6$. Dotted density shows the prior $\delta \sim N(2.4, 0.028)$. Dashed horizontal line drawn at 0.95 probability.

3.5 Case Example

3.5.1 Modeling of Overall Survival

Consider, for example, a two-arm oncology trial with patients randomly enrolled into standard-of-care (soc) or a novel drug treatment (trt). The trial is considered successful if median patient survival time on the treated arm is at least 15% longer than for those on the SOC arm. The intention is to enroll 200 total patients per arm. To keep the problem simple, an exponential distribution is used to model the survival distribution so that, conditioned on parameter λ, the probability to survive up until time t (months) is $S(t) = e^{-\lambda t}$. Median survival is the time point $t = t_{50}$ that results in $S(t) = 0.5$; i.e., $t_{50} = \ln(2)/\lambda$.

3.5.2 Maximum Likelihood Estimation

Letting λ_{soc} and λ_{trt} denote the exponential survival model parameters for SOC and treated arms, the competing hypotheses for the oncology trial are given by

$$H_0: \theta_{soc} - \theta_{trt} \leq \ln(1.15) \text{ and } H_a: \theta_{soc} - \theta_{trt} > \ln(1.15),$$

where $\theta_i = \ln(\lambda_i)$, $i = $ soc, trt.

Let $\{(T_{ij}, \delta_{ij})\}$ be the clinical data with T_{ij} denoting the time of death (months) of the jth patient on the ith treatment arm ($i = $ soc, trt) or, if the patient is alive at the end of the study period, the enrollment time of that patient, and δ_{ij} to indicate that the patient is dead ($\delta_{ij} = 0$) or alive ($\delta_{ij} = 1$). Suppose that for treatment i ($i = $ soc, trt), $\delta_{ij} = 0$ for m_i patients and $\delta_{ij} = 1$ for n_i patients. Each parameter θ_i is estimated via maximum likelihood estimation (MLE) (Rodriguez 2010) as

$$\hat{\theta}_i = \log(m_i) - \log\left(\sum_j T_{ij}\right)$$

with associated standard error $\sqrt{\exp(-\hat{\theta}_i)/\sum_j T_{ij}}$.

Under the supremum conditions of H_0, the test statistic

$$Z = \frac{\hat{\theta}_{soc} - \hat{\theta}_{trt} - \ln(1.15)}{\sqrt{\dfrac{\exp(-\hat{\theta}_{soc})}{\sum_j T_{soc,j}} + \dfrac{\exp(-\hat{\theta}_{trt})}{\sum_j T_{trt,j}}}}$$

asymptotically follows a standard normal distribution. The investigator will declare H_a if the observed value of $Z > \Phi^{-1}(0.95) = 1.645$.

3.5.3 Futility Analysis

The interim analysis is scheduled after the first 100 patients per arm are enrolled, with survival data collected at 18 months. The investigators wish to know if they should continue the trial, ultimately enrolling an additional 100 patients (or more) per arm. Results from the first 100 patients per arm are shown in Table 3.4.

Using Table 3.4, $\hat{\theta}_{soc} = \ln(1/12)$ and $\hat{\theta}_{trt} = \ln(1/18)$, resulting in an observed value $Z = 1.57 < 1.645$. The results are promising, but insufficient to declare H_a. Assuming that other patients will respond similarly to the SOC or treatment, the interim results can be used to predict the remaining trial results by generating additional patients via the posterior predictive distribution.

TABLE 3.4

Summary Statistics of Interim Data for First 100
Patients per Arm

	SOC	Treated
# patients dead (m_i)	75	65
# patients alive (n_i)	25	35
$\sum_{m_i} T_{ij}$ (sum of times for dead patients)	450	540
$\sum_j T_{ij}$ (sum of times for all patients)	900	1170

The posterior distribution of θ_{soc} and θ_{trt} may be sampled by running the JAGS code given below. As in Section 3.2.2, JAGS provides a special method for right-censored data in the form of the *dinterval()* function. For the right-censored observations, we must look over each surviving patient. Priors were chosen to be normally distributed with means at the MLEs and standard deviation approximately equal to four times the standard errors of the MLEs. An interesting survival statistic is the median survival, given by $\ln(2)/\exp(\theta)$. The posterior densities for median survival are shown in Figure 3.6.

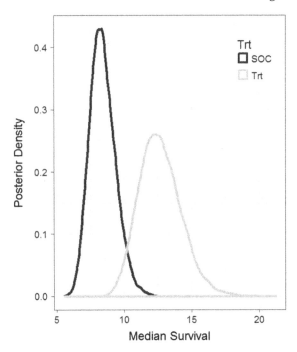

FIGURE 3.6
Posterior densities of median survival.

```
model.txt = "
model{

  for ( i in 1:2 )
  {
     ## Prior for theta ~ N( MLE, 4*SE )
    theta[i] ~ dnorm(Est[i], 4.)

      ## Likelihood for those who died: Tsum ~
         gamma( m, exp(theta) )
     Tsum[i] ~ dgamma( m[i], exp(theta[i]) )
  }
  ## Likelihood terms for those who survived
     beyond 18 months
  for ( j in 1:25 ) ## SOC group
  {
    surv1[j] ~ dexp( exp(theta[1]) )
    rightCens1[j] ~ dinterval( surv1[j], 18 )
  }
  for ( k in 1:35 ) ## Trt group
  {
    surv2[k] ~ dexp( exp(theta[2]) )
    rightCens2[k] ~ dinterval( surv2[k], 18 )
  }

}"
data = list(Tsum=c(450, 540), Est=c(log(1/12),
            log(1/18)), m=c(75, 65), surv1=rep(NA, 25),
            rightCens1=rep(1, 25),
            surv2=rep(NA, 35), rightCens2=rep(1, 35) )
fitb = run.jags( model.txt, data=data,
            monitor="theta", n.chains=3,burnin=10000,
            thin=10, sample=5000, method="parallel" )
```

Given a sample from the posterior θ_{soc} and θ_{trt}, the remaining data from the clinical trial may be generated from the exponential distribution; i.e., $\tilde{T}_{ij} \mid \theta_i \sim \exp(e_i^\theta)$, for $j = 101, 102, \ldots, 200$. Since the survival data are collected at 18 months, if $\tilde{T}_{ij} \le 18$, $\tilde{\delta}_{ij} = 0$ and if $\tilde{T}_{ij} > 18$, then $\tilde{T}_{ij}$ is right-censored at 18 months and $\tilde{\delta}_{ij} = 1$. Thus, the "full" data set consists of the original measured data on 100 patients per arm, $\{(T_{ij}, \delta_{ij})\}_{j=1}^{100}$, and a sample from the posterior predictive distribution for the virtual set of 100 patients per arm, $\{(\tilde{T}_{ij}, \tilde{\delta}_{ij})\}_{j=101}^{200}$. From the data set with 100 real and 100 virtual subjects, the Z statistic is again calculated. This process is repeated for all (or a large number of) draws of θ_{soc} and θ_{trt} from the posterior distribution in order to generate a posterior predictive distribution of the Z statistic. Code is shown below.

```
Tsum.soc.1 = 900
Tsum.trt.1 = 1170
m.soc.1 = 75
m.trt.1 = 65
th.post = as.matrix(as.mcmc.list(fitb)) # Put JAGS
    results into matrix
 ## Z.tilde= posterior predictive distribution of Z
Z.tilde = rep(NA, nrow(th.post))

N = 100   ## add 100 virtual patients

for ( b in 1:nrow(th.post) )
{
  ## SOC virtual patient times
 T.tilde.soc = rexp( N, exp(th.post[b,"theta[1]"]) )
  ## Virtual patients dead or alive?
 delta.tilde.soc = ifelse( T.tilde.soc <= 18, 0, 1)
  ## Right-censored value
 T.tilde.soc[delta.tilde.soc==1] = 18
  ## Trt virtual patient times
 T.tilde.trt = rexp( N, exp(th.post[b,"theta[2]"]) )
  ## Virtual patients dead or alive?
 delta.tilde.trt = ifelse( T.tilde.trt <= 18, 0, 1)
  ## Right-censored value
 T.tilde.trt[delta.tilde.trt==1] = 18

  ## Sum of SOC times for "full" data
 Tsum.soc = Tsum.soc.1 + sum(T.tilde.soc)
  ## Sum of Trt times for "full" data
 Tsum.trt = Tsum.trt.1 + sum(T.tilde.trt)
  ## Sum SOC dead for "full" data
 m.soc = m.soc.1 + sum(delta.tilde.soc==0)
  ## Sum Trt dead for "full" data
 m.trt = m.trt.1 + sum(delta.tilde.trt==0)

 theta.hat.soc = log(m.soc) - log(Tsum.soc) ## New SOC MLE
 theta.hat.trt = log(m.trt) - log(Tsum.trt) ## New Trt MLE
 Z.tilde[b] = (theta.hat.soc - theta.hat.trt - log(1.15)) /
            sqrt( exp(-theta.hat.soc)/Tsum.soc +
                  exp(-theta.hat.trt)/Tsum.trt )
}
## Probability of success
mean(Z.tilde > qnorm(0.95))
```

Unfortunately, after adding 100 virtual patients, the posterior predictive probability of declaring H_a is only 72%. Re-running the code, but with 250 additional virtual patients, achieves an expected 80% success rate. The investigators must make a tough decision, whether to enroll only 100 more patients or to lengthen the trial time (and cost) to boost the chance of success with an additional 250 patients.

3.6 Concluding Remarks

As illustrated by the manufacturing and the Phase II clinical trial problems, the design prior provides a means of directly evaluating the OC and statistical power curves. By calculating the expected probability of success of a binary decision process over the possible values of the design prior, investigators are given direction in choosing the sample size that will likely lead to a successful outcome. The same tool can be used to steer investigators away from no-hope situations of futility. Finally, interim analyses can also be enhanced via the same thought process, as shown in the Phase III oncology trial example.

As noted in Chapter 2, for some problems, there is little prior information. In such a case, a vague prior or a prior with dispersion wider than the uncertainty from the likelihood may be appropriate. In the pharmaceutical industry, however, prior information often abounds for manufacturing problems, non-clinical research, and clinical trials. The formation of design and analysis priors should result from thorough discussion and mutual agreement within a team.

Section II

Pre-Clinical and Clinical Research

4

Pre-Clinical Efficacy Studies

4.1 Introduction

Pre-clinical studies are an integral part of drug research and development. Since testing a new drug in humans carries a significant safety risk, regulatory guidance requires safety data from animal testing before clinical trials or marketing application begin (ICH 19941-2011b). The primary objective of animal studies is to identify potential toxicities and determine a safety dose, which can be used in clinical trials. It is also necessary, however, to characterize the efficacy profile of drug candidates in the pre-clinical stage to justify further evaluations in human subjects. On the other hand, because of ethical reasons and economic considerations, investigators are often urged to use as few animals as possible to achieve pre-clinical study objectives. *In-vivo* (cell-based) efficacy and toxicity experimentation is used to circumvent most of the animal testing by weeding out impotent or harmful drug compounds. Additionally, *in-vivo* dose ranging may provide a reasonable starting dose for the testing of promising compounds in animal models. For ethical, economic, and safety concerns, animal studies need to be well designed and methods of data analysis carefully chosen. Although there is vast published literature on statistical design and analysis in animal studies (Chow and Liu 1998), it is primarily focused on safety evaluations. In addition, the small sample sizes of these studies greatly diminish the power of the traditional frequentist methods such as t-test and ANOVA to detect biologically meaningful difference. To ameliorate these challenges, historical knowledge about the drugs under evaluation must be brought to bear. In this chapter, through two real examples, we demonstrate the use of Bayesian analysis to conduct efficacy assessments of drug combination (in-vitro and in-vivo) and monotherapies with censored data.

4.2 Evaluation of Lab-Based Drugs in Combination

4.2.1 Background

Cancers are heterogenous diseases known to have various signaling pathways. Therefore, inhibition of such pathways individually by a single targeted therapy often leads to compensation by other pathways, resulting in a loss of efficacy (Ramaswamy 2007; Flaherty et al. 2010). In the clinic, this type of compensation leads to innate and/or acquired tumor resistance and relapse. In recent years, there is an increasing trend to use combination therapies to achieve better treatment effect (Pourkavoos 2012). In addition, safety risks may be mitigated by pairing lower dose levels of two combined drugs that, together, provide a sufficient level of efficacy for the patient population. Furthermore, as pointed out by Pourkavoos (2012), development of combination drugs is an integral part of lifecycle management of marketed products and new drugs. In general, drug combinations can yield activity that is synergistic, independent, or antagonistic Zhao and Yang (2017). *In-vitro* and *in-vivo* animal studies can play a very important role for assessing the effects of a drug combination. Various experimental designs, including factorial and response surface designs, were described by Novick and Peterson (2015).

4.2.2 Statistical Methods

Commonly used statistical models to evaluate drug combination efficacy are the Bliss (Bliss 1939) independence and Loewe additivity models (Loewe 1928). Greco, Bravo, and Parsons (1995) have discussed these two reference models in detail. Conceptually, the Loewe additivity model focuses on dose reduction and the Bliss independence model focuses on treatment effect enhancement. The two methods essentially address the same question, albeit from two different perspectives.

4.2.2.1 Loewe Additivity

Consider two drugs A and B such that the potency R of drug A relative to drug B is a constant. Let $D_{y,1}$ and $D_{y,2}$ be the respective doses of Drugs A and B acting alone, resulting in an effect y. For the combination dose (d_1, d_2) to produce an equivalent effect y, it must satisfy:

$$d_1 + Rd_2 = D_{y,1}$$

$$\frac{d_1}{R} + d_2 = D_{y,2}$$

After some algebraic manipulations, the above equations can be re-expressed as

$$\frac{d_1}{D_{y,1}} + \frac{d_2}{D_{y,2}} = 1.$$

The above relationship between doses d_1 and d_2 is commonly referred to as Loewe additivity. Let $\tau = \frac{d_1}{D_{y,1}} + \frac{d_2}{D_{y,2}}$. When $\tau < 1$, it means that the same treatment effect can be achieved at a lower combination dose level (synergism); when $\tau > 1$, it implies that high-dose levels have to be given to achieve the same treatment effect (antagonism); and when $\tau = 1$, it indicates that the treatment effects are additive and there is no advantage or disadvantage in combining them (additivity). One advantage of the Loewe additivity model is that serves as the basis for the isobologram, a graphical tool for synergism or antagonism analysis.

4.2.2.2 Bliss Independence

Bliss independence, which is also referred to as the fractional product method in literature, is an alternate method for assessing drug interaction. It relies on the assumption that the two inhibitors possess independent mechanisms of action. The effect of the combination drug is represented probabilistically as the union of two independent events due to monotherapies. Consider two monotherapy inhibitors with normalized mean signals μ_1 and μ_2, $0 < \mu_1, \mu_2 < 1$, evaluated at respective concentrations x_1 and x_2. The expected mean evaluated at the combination (x_1, x_2) under the null state of the Bliss independence model is $\mu_1 \times \mu_2$. Letting μ_{12} denote the true combination mean, synergism is declared whenever $\mu_{12} < \mu_1 \times \mu_2$ and antagonism is declared whenever $\mu_{12} > \mu_1 \times \mu_2$. A similar equation can be constructed for Bliss synergism/antagonism for two agonist compounds.

Whether Bliss independence or Loewe additivity is a better reference model has been a subject of much debate. Detailed discussions can be found in Berenbaum (1989) and Graco et al. (1995). The former showed that when the dose–response curves are characterized through simple exponential functions, Bliss independence implies Loewe additivity and vice versa. Note that neither the Bliss nor Loewe model relies on a particular underlying dose–response model, used to describe the components of the combination. Greco (1995) typically paired the synergy model (Bliss or Loewe) with an Emax model for the monotherapies. In general, Bliss and Loewe systems are not equivalent. While the debate continues, some consensus was reached among a group of scientists in the Sarriselka agreement which recommends the use of both Bliss independence and Loewe additivity as reference models (Greco et al. 1992).

4.2.3 Antiviral Combination

Combination therapies have long been used to treat viral infections. For example, the introduction of highly active antiretroviral therapy (HAART) enabled effective suppression of HIV viruses, making the incurable disease manageable (Delaney 2006). In the following, we discuss an in-vitro combination study intended to evaluate the effect of antiviral combination drug consisting of two agents, namely, Cpd1 and Cpd2.

4.2.3.1 Data

Two antiviral agents were tested on human cells in each of three 96-well plates. A grid of 64 levels (x_1, x_2) of the two agents, consisting of seven positive concentrations from each monotherapy, a control, and all combinations of the monotherapies were plated. Each treated well contained human cells, the HIV virus, and a concentration or one or both drug agents. All three plates also contained eight wells each of a negative control (no drug) and a positive control (no virus). On a per-plate basis, the assay signals were normalized as a percentage of the negative and positive control means. The means of the normalized signals (each with $N = 3$) for each drug combination pairing (x_1, x_2) are shown in Figure 4.1. All concentrations were standardized to the largest concentration so that standardized concentrations for both drug agents range from $0 - 1$.

4.2.3.2 Model

For each pair of concentrations, the mean assay responses are described using the following model:

$$\bar{y}_{ij} \mid \mu(x_{1i}, x_{2j}), \sigma^2 \sim N\left(\mu(x_{1i}, x_{2j}), \sigma^2\right)$$

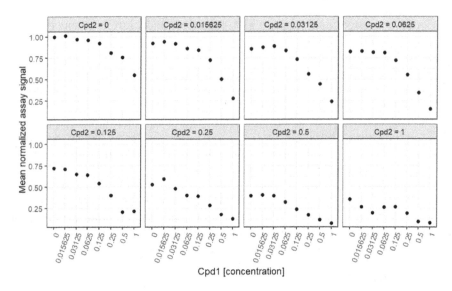

FIGURE 4.1
Drug combination data. Mean values shown ($N = 3$).

with

$$\mu(x_{1i},0) = y_{\min,1} + \frac{y_{\max} - y_{\min,1}}{1 + \exp\left(s_1 \log(x_{1i}) - s_1\theta_1\right)}$$

$$\mu(0,x_{2j}) = y_{\min,2} + \frac{y_{\max} - y_{\min,2}}{1 + \exp\left(s_2 \log(x_{2j}) - s_2\theta_2\right)}$$

for the first and second monotherapies, and $\mu(x_{1i},x_{2j}) = \mu_{ij}$ for the combinations. Sample standard deviation values are given alongside each sample mean, each associated with $N=3$ replicates. Conditioned on σ^2, a distribution for the pooled variance $\hat{\sigma}^2$ is

$$128 \frac{\hat{\sigma}^2}{\sigma^2} \sim \chi^2(128),$$

with the 128 degrees of freedom stemming from the 64 unique drug combinations, each providing two degrees of freedom. The pooled standard deviation estimate is $\hat{\sigma} = 0.10$. By placing a prior distribution on the parameters, one may test for Bliss synergy at each combination by calculating the posterior probability

$$p_{ij} = \Pr\left(\mu(x_{1i},x_{2j}) < \mu(x_{1i},0) \times \mu(0,x_{2j}) | \text{data}\right).$$

4.2.3.3 Assessment of Drug Effect

One frequentist method (Novick 2013) relies on several asymptotic assumptions and requires box constraints on the parameters ($y_{\min,1}, y_{\min,2}, y_{\max}, \mu_{ij}$) in order to ensure that mean responses stay within the range 0–1. With Bayesian methods, the statistical distributions are exact and the constraints are placed on the marginal prior distributions. We initially apply weak prior distributions to illustrate the concept of the prior constraints with normal and truncated normal priors given by

$$y_{\max} \sim TN\left(\text{Mean} = 0.9, \text{SD} = 10, L = 0.5, U = 1\right)$$

$$y_{\min,1}, y_{\min,2} \sim TN\left(\text{Mean} = 0.1, \text{SD} = 10, L = 0, U = 0.5\right)$$

$$\theta_1, \theta_2 \sim N\left(\text{Mean} = 0.5, \text{SD} = 10\right)$$

$$s_1, s_2 \sim TN\left(\text{Mean} = 1, \text{SD} = 2, L = 0, U = \infty\right)$$

$$\mu_{ij} \sim TN\left(\text{Mean} = 0.5, \text{SD} = 10, L = 0, U = 1\right)$$

These priors truncate all means to fall between 0 and 1 and, since the two monotherapies are known inhibitors, also force the shape parameters to

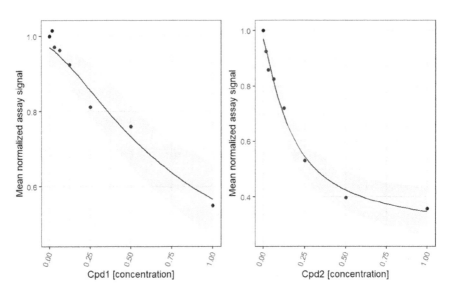

FIGURE 4.2
Posterior median and 95% credible bands for monotherapy data.

take on positive values while also preventing their values from ballooning. Though we decided against it, one may similarly constrain the responses to fall between 0 and 1 in the likelihood.

A graph of the monotherapy data with posterior median fitted values and 95% credible bands is shown in Figure 4.2.

Computer code for MCMC is provided below.

```
d = read.csv("Drug Combo Data.csv") ## Load the data

model.txt = "
model{

  ## Priors
  yMax ~ dnorm(0.9, 0.01)T(0.5, 1.)

  ## Compound 1
  yMin1 ~ dnorm(0.1, 0.01)T(0., 0.5)
  theta1 ~ dnorm(0.5, 0.01)
  s1 ~ dnorm(1., 0.25)T(0., )

  ## Compound 2
  yMin2 ~ dnorm(0.1, 0.01)T(0., 0.5)
  theta2 ~ dnorm(0.5, 0.01)
  s2 ~ dnorm(1., 0.25)T(0., )

  sigma ~ dt(0., 100., 1)T(0., ) ## Half-cauchy with
      scale=0.1
```

```
  tau <- 1/(sigma*sigma)

  ## Likelihood
  SigSqHat ~ dgamma( 0.5*degFree, 0.5*degFree/
                     (sigma*sigma) )

  ## Negative control
  y0 ~ dnorm( yMax, N0*tau )

  ## Monotherapy for Cpd 1
  for ( i in 1:m1 )
  {
   mu1[i] <- yMin1 + (yMax-yMin1)/
           ( 1 + exp( s1*log(x1[i]) - s1*theta1 ) )
   y1[i] ~ dnorm( mu1[i], N1[i]*tau )
  }

  ## Monotherapy for Cpd 2
  for ( j in 1:m2 )
  {
   mu2[j] <- yMin2 + (yMax-yMin2)/
           ( 1 + exp( s2*log(x2[j]) - s2*theta2 ) )
   y2[j] ~ dnorm( mu2[j], N2[j]*tau )
  }

  ## Combinations
  for ( k in 1:mc )
  {
   muC[k] ~ dnorm(0.5, 0.01)T(0., 1.) ## Prior for muC
   yc[k] ~ dnorm( muC[k], Nc[k]*tau ) ## Likelihood for yc
  }

  }"

  ## Split up the data into negative control (NC),
monotherapies, and combinations
  d1 = split( d, d$Type )

  ## Get pooled sample variance with pooled degrees of
freedom
  degFree = sum(d$N-1)
  sigSq.hat = sum( (d$N-1)*d$SD^2 )/degFree

  ## Set up data for JAGS
  data = list( N0=d1[["NC"]]$N, y0=d1[["NC"]]$Mean,
               m1=nrow(d1[["Mono1"]]),
               x1=d1[["Mono1"]]$Cpd1,
```

```
y1=d1[["Mono1"]]$Mean,
            N1=d1[["Mono1"]]$N,
            m2=nrow(d1[["Mono2"]]),
            x2=d1[["Mono2"]]$Cpd2,
y2=d1[["Mono2"]]$Mean,
            N2=d1[["Mono2"]]$N,
            mc=nrow(d1[["Combo"]]),
yc=d1[["Combo"]]$Mean, Nc=d1[["Combo"]]$N,
        SigSqHat=sigSq.hat, degFree=degFree
        )


        ## Call JAGS
fitb = run.jags( model.txt, data=data,
            monitor=c("yMax", "yMin1", "theta1", "s1",
            "yMin2",  "theta2", "s2", "muC", "sigma"),
            n.chains=3, burnin=10000,
            sample=20000, thin=10, method="parallel" )

## Place results into a matrix
th.post = as.matrix( as.mcmc.list(fitb) )
```

The following code was created to calculate the posterior probability of synergism.

```
stats = matrix(NA, nrow(d1[["Combo"]]), 6)
for ( i in 1:nrow(d1[["Combo"]]) )
{
 x1 = d1[["Combo"]][i,"Cpd1"]
 x2 = d1[["Combo"]][i,"Cpd2"]
 ## Posterior distribution for monotherapy means
 mu1 = th.post[,"yMin1"] + (th.post[,"yMax"]-
            th.post[,"yMin1"]) /
            (1+exp(th.post[,"s1"]*log(x1)-
            th.post[,"s1"]*th.post[,"theta1"]))
 mu2 = th.post[,"yMin2"] + (th.post[,"yMax"]-
            th.post[,"yMin2"]) /
            (1+exp(th.post[,"s2"]*log(x2) -
            th.post[,"s2"]*th.post[,"theta2"]))
 ## Posterior distribution for combination mean
 muC = th.post[,paste("muC[", i, "]", sep="")]
 stats[i,] = c( x1, x2, median(mu1), median(mu2),
                median(muC), mean(muC < mu1*mu2) )
}
 ## stats column: "Prob.syn" = probability of synergy
colnames(stats) = c("Cpd1", "Cpd2", "mu1", "mu2",
                "muC", "Prob.syn")
```

Figure 4.3 provides the posterior medians for the combinations, colored dark if $p_{ij} > 0.95$, indicating that the combination shows Bliss synergism. From the figure, one may conclude that synergism between these two compounds occurs whenever $x_1 \geq 0.5$.

4.2.3.4 Use of Historical Data as Priors

For drug combination analyses, another advantage of the Bayesian method is the natural ability to include prior information for the monotherapy parameters. It is uncommon for a drug combination analysis to proceed without historical knowledge of one or both of the monotherapy curves. For example, the second compound was previously run ten times, providing ordinary least-squares (OLS) estimates for $(y_{\min,2}, \theta_2, s_2, y_{\text{Max}})$. Ranges of the OLS estimates are shown in Table 4.1.

In the JAGS code, we replaced the priors for the parameters shown in Table 4.1 with uniform priors across each range. For example, we replaced $s_2 \sim dnorm(1., 0.25)T(0.,)$ with $s_2 \sim dunif(0.5, 2)$. As expected, the resulting 95% credible band around the monotherapy curve of the second compound is slightly narrower than shown in the right side of Figure 4.2. One additional mid-concentration combination was identified as synergistic while the synergism claim for combinations (0.03125, 1) and (1, 1) was dropped. Although we cannot be sure, presumably, the historical information provides additional statistical power to make the correct decision.

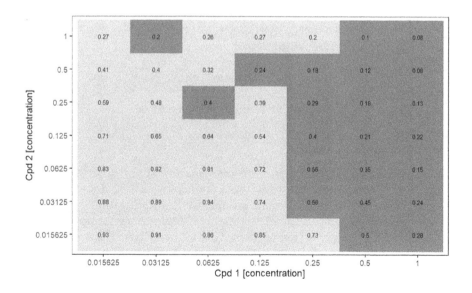

FIGURE 4.3
Posterior medians of the combinations. Dark color indicates $p_{ij} > 0.95$.

TABLE 4.1

Range of Parameter Estimates

Parameter	Range
y_{Max}	(0.9, 1.0)
y_{Min2}	(0, 0.2)
θ_2	(−2, −1)
s_2	(0.5, 2)

4.2.4 Evaluation of Fixed Dose Combination

In a fixed-dose combination study, the key question to address is whether each component contributes to the combination effect. Suppose that the drug effect is measured in terms of rate of undesired events such as death. Define

$$\theta = \mu_{11} - \min(\mu_{10}, \mu_{01}).$$

Therefore, $\theta < 0$ implies that there is a synergistic effect. The above question can be answered through testing the hypotheses

$$H_0: \theta \geq 0 \quad \text{vs.} \quad H_1: \theta < 0.$$

Various frequentist procedures were proposed, focusing on preserving Type I error (Lehmann 1952; Berger 1982; Snapinn 1987; Laska and Meisner 1989; Hung 1993). It is, however, more straightforward to apply Bayesian test methods. For example, based on the posterior probability, one may claim that the combination is synergistic if

$$\Pr(\theta < 0 | \text{data}) \geq p_0,$$

where p_0 is a predefined positive number between (0, 1).

4.2.4.1 Follow-up Experiment

Based on the success of the in-vitro combination study described in the previous section, an in-vivo study was conducted with 32 mice randomly assigned to each of four treatment groups. By translating the results from the in-vitro experiment to a mouse model, a single concentration for each of Cpd1 and Cpd2 was tested so that the study consists of a 2x2 factorial of Cpd1 = 0/1 (no/yes) and Cpd2 = 0/1. The goal of the study is to show a reduction in a mean biological measurement that could be interpreted for a potential human clinical trial. Conditioned on the parameter values, the data model for the future study will be

$$Y_{ijk} \mid \mu_{ij}, \sigma^2 \sim N\left(\mu_{ij}, \sigma^2\right),$$

where Y_{ijk} is the measured response from the kth animal with Cpd1 $= i$ and Cpd2 $= j$, μ_{ij} is the mean of a group with Cpd1 $= i$ and Cpd2 $= j$, and σ^2 is the common variance.

Prior information will be determined from historical studies. Available data stem from five studies with a control arm and one study each for Cpd1 and Cpd2. A summary of the data is given in Table 4.2.

The historical data are modeled as

$$\hat{\sigma}_e^2 \mid \sigma_e^2 \sim \text{gamma}\left(\text{shape} = \frac{\lambda}{2}, \text{rate} = \frac{\lambda}{2\sigma_e^2}\right),$$

$$\bar{Y}_{s,t} \mid \theta_s, \eta_t, \sigma_e^2 \sim N\left(\theta_s + \eta_t, \sigma_e^2 / N_{s,t}\right) \text{ and}$$

$$\theta_s \mid \sigma_s^2 \sim N\left(0, \sigma_s^2\right),$$

where $\bar{Y}_{s,t}$ is the sample mean from study s and treatment t from $N_{s,t}$ animals, $\hat{\sigma}_e^2$ is the pooled variance across studies with λ associated degrees of freedom, θ_s denotes a study effect, and η_t denotes the mean treatment effect. Weakly informative priors were assigned to the historical-data parameters as

$$\eta_t \sim N\left(\text{Mean} = 5, \text{SD} = 2\right),$$

$$\sigma_S, \sigma_e \sim \text{half-Cauchy}\left(0, \text{Scale} = 0.1\right).$$

TABLE 4.2

Historical Mouse Study Data

Study	Control Mean	Cpd Mean	Pooled SD	Pooled Degrees of Freedom (DF)
1	4.7 ($N=8$)		0.5	14
2	4.9 ($N=8$)		0.3	14
3	5.0 ($N=6$)		0.3	19
4	5.1 ($N=6$)	Cpd1: 4.5 ($N=8$)	0.4	19
5	4.8 ($N=6$)	Cpd2: 4.4 ($N=8$)	0.4	19
		Pooled SD and DF	0.38	85

Computer code for MCMC is provided below.

```
model.txt = "
model{

  ## Prior distribution
  for ( i in 1:nTrt )
  {
   eta[i] ~ dnorm(5, 0.25) ## SD=2
  }
  sigmaS ~ dt(0., 100., 1)T(0., )
  sigmaE ~ dt(0., 100., 1)T(0., )

  tauS <- 1/(sigmaS*sigmaS)
  tauE <- 1/(sigmaE*sigmaE)

  ## Likelihood
  SigSqHat ~ dgamma( 0.5*degFree, 0.5*degFree/
                     (sigmaE*sigmaE) )

  ## Hierarchical likelihood for mean
  for ( j in 1:nStudy )
  {
   thetaS[j] ~ dnorm(0., tauS)
  }

  for ( k in 1:nObs )
  {
   mu[k] <- eta[ trt[k] ] + thetaS[ study[k] ]
   tauN[k] <- N[k]*tauE
   ybar[k] ~ dnorm( mu[k], tauN[k] )
  }
}"
 ## Set up data for JAGS
data = list( nObs=7, nStudy=5, nTrt=3,
       ybar=c(4.7, 4.9, 5.0, 5.1, 4.8, 4.5, 4.4),
       N=c(8, 8, 6, 6, 6, 8, 8),
       SigSqHat=0.38^2, degFree=85,
       trt=c(1, 1, 1, 1, 1, 2, 3),
       study=c(1, 2, 3, 4, 5, 4, 5) )

       ## Call JAGS
fitb = run.jags( model.txt, data=data,
   monitor=c("eta", "sigmaS", "sigmaE"),
   n.chains=3, burnin=10000, sample=20000, thin=20,
   module="glm", method="parallel" )

th.post = as.matrix( as.mcmc.list(fitb) )
```

For the future study, the prior distribution for the mean should take into account both between-study variance and within-study variance. That is, the prior distribution for μ_{ij} should reflect knowledge of the treatment means η_s and the between-study variability σ_S via its posterior predictive distribution. For example, the posterior predictive distribution of μ_{00} is generated as

```
eta1 = rnorm(nrow(th.post), mean=th.post[,"eta[1]"],
                            sd=th.post[,"sigmaS"])
```

A reasonable prior distribution for μ_{00} that covers the distribution of *eta1* is

$$\mu_{00} \sim T(\text{center} = 4.9, \text{scale} = 0.15, \text{df} = 8).$$

This is seen by plotting

```
plot( density(eta1) )
eta.seq = seq(3, 7, length=100)
lines( eta.seq, dt( (eta.seq-4.9)/0.15, 8 )/0.15,
       col="red" )
```

Continuing similarly, priors for μ_{10} and μ_{01} are derived as

$$\mu_{10} \sim T(\text{center} = 4.45, \text{scale} = 0.2, \text{df} = 8) \text{ and}$$

$$\mu_{01} \sim T(\text{center} = 4.4, \text{scale} = 0.2, \text{df} = 8).$$

Because there is no *in-vivo* prior information for μ_{11}, we continue to use

$$\mu_{11} \sim N(\text{Mean} = 5, \text{SD} = 2).$$

Note, however, that prior information for the combination effect may be translated from the in-vitro experimental results through a prior elicitation exercise. The prior for σ for the future study comes from the posterior distribution of σ_e from the historical data analysis. A good-fitting distribution for σ_e | data is log-normal(-0.97, cv = 8%). Widening this slightly, a prior for σ is given as

$$\sigma \sim \text{log-normal}(-0.97, \text{cv} = 10\%).$$

Admittedly, while much tighter than the original weak priors, because there are only five studies to draw from, this set of distributions is only modestly informative for the future data.

The combination study sample means with $N = 8$ animals per treatment group are given in Table 4.3. The pooled standard deviation across the four treatment groups is 0.37 with 28 degrees of freedom. Armed with the data

TABLE 4.3

Sample Means ($N = 8$) from the
Combination Study. The Values 0
and 1 Correspond to Situations
Where the Agent is Not Used and
Used, Respectively

		Cpd1	
		0	1
Cpd2	0	4.9	4.6
	1	4.5	4.1

and priors, we can set out to estimate $\Pr(\mu_{11} < \min(\mu_{10}, \mu_{01}) \mid \text{data})$ using the
computer code below.

```
model.txt = "
model{

## Prior distribution
mu[1] ~ dt(4.9, 44.44, 8) ## mu[0,0]
mu[2] ~ dt(4.45, 25., 8)  ## mu[1,0]
mu[3] ~ dt( 4.4, 25., 8)  ## mu[0,1]
mu[4] ~ dnorm( 5., 0.25)  ## mu[1,1] -- vague

lsigma ~ dnorm( -0.97, 100. )
sigma <- exp(lsigma)

tau <- 1/(sigma*sigma)
tauN <- N*tau

## Likelihood
SigSqHat ~ dgamma( 0.5*degFree, 0.5*degFree/
                   (sigma*sigma) )

for ( i in 1:4 )
{
  ybar[i] ~ dnorm( mu[i], tauN )
}
}"
## Set up data for JAGS
data = list( ybar=c(4.9, 4.6, 4.5, 4.2), N=8,
            SigSqHat=0.37^2, degFree=28 )

## Call JAGS
fitb = run.jags( model.txt, data=data,monitor=c("mu",
                "sigma"),
```

```
n.chains=3, burnin=10000, sample=10000, thin=5,
module="glm", method="parallel" )

th.post = as.matrix( as.mcmc.list(fitb) )

## Posterior probability that mu[1,1] < min( mu[1,0],
    mu[0,1] )
pr = mean(th.post[,"mu[4]"] < th.post[,"mu[2]"] &
            th.post[,"mu[4]"] < th.post[,"mu[3]"])
```

Because $\Pr(\mu_{11} \le \min(\mu_{10}, \mu_{01}) \mid \text{data}) = 0.98$, the combination treatment is declared to be synergistic and may be considered for an animal safety and eventually, human trials.

4.3 Bayesian Survival Analysis

4.3.1 Limitations of Animal Data

The goal of many pre-clinical oncology studies is to discover compounds that produce a tumor-size reducing effect in animals. Various animal models have long been used to study the effects of anti-cancer therapies and fulfill regulatory requirements before the therapies are advanced to human testing. The utility of these models largely depends on how predictive of treatment effect in humans they are. To this end, various animal models have been developed. For example, in xenograft animal models, a human tumor is transplanted and grown under the skin (or tissue of tumor origin) of an immunocompromised animal. Syngeneic models, where spontaneous animal tumors have been propagated in immunocompromised animals, have also been developed for study. Merits of various types of murine oncology models were discussed by Richmond and Su (2008). A typical animal efficacy study includes testing multiple agents or the same agent at different dose levels along with a control. The drug effects are measured in terms of tumor growth. Subsequent to dosing, the tumor size or volume of each animal is measured repeatedly over the course of the experimental period.

Oftentimes, relative efficacy is assessed through comparisons of mean tumor sizes among the treatment group. Treatment groups are rank-ordered, and the 'winner' with the highest rank-order picked. When no animal is sacrificed during the course of a study, an appropriate statistical model may be fitted to the data (e.g., analysis of variance or analysis of covariance) to facilitate the comparison of mean tumor size at a time point of interest. One challenge, however, in murine oncology studies, is the small number of animals used in the study. Thus, it is important to properly design and model the data to provide sufficient statistical power to differentiate the treatment effects of two or more drug compounds. Posing an addition challenge, animals may be sacrificed during the course of the study for reasons that are treatment dependent, including large tumor size, tumor ulceration, and significant body weight loss. The non-random missingness of tumor volume data at later time points combined with small sample sizes often presents a unique challenge to rank-order the efficacy of oncology treatments.

4.3.2 Current Methods

There are several straightforward methods based on analysis of variance that allow a direct comparison of mean tumor volumes (typically performed on log-scaled data). So long as no animal is sacrificed before the study end, the mean tumor volume comparisons permit a simple rank-ordering of compounds. Handling mean comparisons in the presence of data censoring can be difficult and may require unrealistic assumptions to be applied to the data. For example, if at the half-way point in a study, the tumor of a control animal ulcerates, the animal is sacrificed. Should the last observed tumor volume of that animal be carried forward? Should it instead be assumed that its tumor volume would have grown larger? Such assumptions require a deep understanding of the cellular mechanisms that may yet be unknown to the investigators. We list a few statistical methods that attempt to work around this impasse.

Hather et al. (2014) compare the average rate of change in log tumor volume. The average rate of change is estimated from the slope coefficient from a simple linear regression model that links the log tumor volume with time, as estimated from each animal. Large slope values suggest exponential, unimpeded tumor growth and small or negative slope values indicate therapeutic efficacy and so a comparison of the estimated slopes may be performed to rank-order the treatment effects. While Hather et al. (2014) do not specify a distribution for the slopes, one could consider the hierarchical model

$$\log\left(TV_{ijk}\right) = \alpha_{ij} + \beta_{ij}t_k + e_{ijk}$$

where TV_{ijk} is the tumor volume for the jth animal in the ith treatment group measured at the kth time point t_k, $\begin{pmatrix}\alpha_{ij}\\\beta_{ij}\end{pmatrix} \sim N\left(\begin{pmatrix}\alpha_i\\\beta_i\end{pmatrix}, V\right)$ denote the intercept and slope for the jth animal in the ith group, and $e_{ijk} \sim N\left(0, \sigma^2\right)$ denote the residual errors.

If $\beta_i < \beta_{i'}$, then treatment i is more efficacious compared to treatment i'. A frequentist may test the hypotheses by fitting a mixed-effects model to the data and calculating a p-value via asymptotic assumptions. Instead of the hierarchical model, one may separately estimate the slopes for each animal by $\{\hat{\beta}_{ij}\}$, assuming that $\hat{\beta}_{ij} \sim N\left(\beta_i, \sigma_\beta^2\right)$. Then β_i versus $\beta_{i'}$ may be examined with a two-sample t-test. For a more conservative approach, the slopes may be compared via a non-parametric Wilcoxon rank-sum test. If one or more animal is sacrificed during the course of the study, however, the slope estimates may be biased. Hather et al. propose to retain all slope values for the comparisons, regardless of the time at which the animal was sacrificed. Thus, Hather et al., perhaps unrealistically, consider censored data to be missing at random.

For clinical survival data, Stein et al. (2008, 2009, 2011) propose to model the repeated tumor size time-series measurements with one of several nonlinear growth/decay models. Stein et al. show a modest correlation between the models' growth parameters and survival time, suggesting that the growth parameter may be used to rank-order efficacy of treatments. Software for the Stein et al. method is available in the tumgr package of R (R Core Team 2018), Because the Stein et al. method discards the data from subjects that cannot be fitted by any of their proposed growth/decay models, Novick et al. (2018) found that, in practice, their procedure can throw away most or all subject data from entire treatment arms in murine experimental data sets, rendering the Stein et al. method of limited use. The Stein et al. method also indirectly assumes that tumor sizes for animals sacrificed before the final study time point follow the pattern of the growth/decay model, an assumption that may be unrealistic.

For a method that is more applicable to smaller-sized animal data sets, Vardi et al. (2001) compare area under the tumor growth curve (AUC), adjusted for right-censoring. Software is available for the Vardi et al. method in the clinfun package of R (R Core Team 2018), which utilizes a non-parametric permutation test to make pair-wise comparisons of AUC for every pair of animals. A comparison of AUC is not always desirable as it may be difficult to distinguish between two sets of tumors with the same AUC, but very different tumor growth profiles. The Vardi method compares partial AUC of two animals up to the smaller of the last observed time points, which can make the distinguishing of AUC values even harder.

Survival analysis, which examines the time to death, provides a viable alternative to a tumor size comparison. A strong benefit of survival analysis is that it does not require any presumption of a post-sacrificed animal's tumor size. However, the aforesaid issues regarding small sample size issue of tumor volume data may cause the conventional survival analysis to give rise to nonsensical parameter and variability estimates.

4.3.3 Bayesian Solution

In this section, we introduce a Bayesian survival analysis technique introduced by Novick et al. (2018) to pick the best treatment arm and to illustrate the use of the method through a real-life example.

4.3.3.1 Survival Function

In survival modeling, two outcome variables (T, δ), are observed for each subject, where T denotes the time to event (animal is sacrificed or dies) and the binary variable δ indicates if the event occurs before the conclusion of the study. When $\delta = 1$, T is set to the time at which the event occurred and when $\delta = 0$, T is set to the final time point and is called *right-censored*, indicating that the animal has not yet reached the event by the end of the study. Let the survival function for the ith treatment group $S(t \mid \theta_i) = \Pr(T > t \mid \theta_i)$ denote the probability that a subject with parameter θ_i survives beyond the time point t. Given treatment groups A and B, one would clearly favor treatment group A at time t if $S(t \mid \theta_A) > S(t \mid \theta_B)$. A common model for survival data uses the non-parametric Kaplan-Meier approach. The Kaplan-Meier method, however, is limited in scope and does not, for example, permit the modeling of a covariate, such as the baseline tumor size. Several parametric survival models are available in pre-packaged software; see, for example see the *survival* library in R, PROC LIFEREG in SAS. In the following section, the Weibull parametric survival model is studied in detail.

4.3.3.2 Weibull Modeling

Parametric models can be used to describe the survival function (e.g., exponential, Weibull, log-normal, and log-logistic distributions). In this section, we focus on the Weibull distribution. It is a straightforward exercise to fit a maximum likelihood Weibull survival model to data via in the survreg() function in the R *survival* library; however, because the Weibull parameterization differs among the dweibull() function in the R *stats* library, the survreg() function in the R *survival* library, and JAGS, we think it will be easier to focus on one parameterization. In JAGS, with parameters shape=η and rate=λ, the Weibull probability density function and cumulative density functions are given by

$$f(t \mid \eta, \lambda) = \eta \lambda t^{\eta-1} \exp\left(-\lambda t^{\eta}\right),$$

$$F(t \mid \eta, \lambda) = 1 - \exp\left(-\lambda t^{\eta}\right).$$

For Weibull survival regression with a covariate x_{ij}, data triplets are $(T_{ij}, \delta_{ij}, x_{ij})$, where T_{ij} is the final recorded timepoint for the jth subject in the ith treatment arm, $\delta_{ij} = 1$ indicates that the (i, j)th animal was sacrificed at time T_{ij} and $\delta_{ij} = 0$ indicates that T_{ij} is right-censored. The data model is

$$T_{ij} \mid \eta, \lambda_i \sim \text{Weibull}(\eta, \lambda_i),$$

where η is the shape parameter that is common across treatment arms, $\lambda_i = \exp\left(\alpha_i + \beta_i x_{ij}\right)$ with $x_{ij} = \ln(\text{baseline tumor size}) - \ln(M)$, and M is the geometric mean baseline tumor size across all animals.

The survival probability

$$S(t| \eta, \lambda_i) = \Pr(\text{Time}_{ij} > t) = \exp(-\lambda_i t^\eta).$$

Comparisons of Weibull model parameters are often made through the hazard function, which is defined as the ratio of the negative rate of change in survival and the survival function and is given by

$$h(t| \eta, \lambda) = -\frac{d}{dt} S(t| \eta, \lambda_i) / S(t| \eta, \lambda_i).$$

The hazard function for the Weibull model is

$$h(t| \eta, \lambda_i) = \eta \lambda_i t^{\eta-1}.$$

The log hazard ratio of groups 1 and 2 is

$$\ln\left\{ \frac{h(t| \eta, \lambda_2)}{h(t| \eta, \lambda_1)} \right\} = \ln(\lambda_2) - \ln(\lambda_1),$$

allowing one to compare the survival curves through the hazard with the λ_i parameters. Treatments that are associated with low hazards are considered better than those treatments that are associated with high hazards. Unfortunately, even the simple Weibull model with only one unique parameter per treatment group and one shared parameter can suffer numerical issues in the presence of small data sets.

Consider the frequentist maximum likelihood Weibull survival model fit. The maximum likelihood is

$$\prod_{(i,j):\delta_{ij}=1} f(T_{ij}| \eta, \lambda_i) \prod_{(i,j):\delta_{ij}=0} S(T_{ij}| \eta, \lambda_i).$$

For the reader's reference, the survreg() function in the R *survival* library maximizes the likelihood and is called with the following computer code.

```
d = read.csv("Survival data.csv")
fit0 = survreg( Surv(Time, !Censor)~Trt + Trt:x - 1,
                        data = d, dist="weibull" )
```

Unfortunately, the survreg parameterization is quite different from JAGS. To keep the parameterization straight, the following computer code in R is provided to maximize the log-likelihood.

```
nlogL.weib = function(theta, Trt, x, Time, Censor)
{
  ## Weibull survival regression with three treatment
    arms: A, B, C
```

```
## theta = ( alpha[A], alpha[B], alpha[C],
##     beta[A], beta[B], beta[C], log(eta) )
## Trt = [factor] A, B, C
## x = covariate
## Time = last measured time point
## Censor = [logical] If FALSE, Time is observed.
##                    If TRUE, Time is right-censored.

## JAGS Weibull pdf:
## f(t | eta, lambda) = eta*lambda*t^(eta-1)
##                         *exp( -lambda*t^eta )
## JAGS Weibull survival:
## S(t | eta, lambda) = exp(-lambda*t^eta)

Intercept = theta[1:3]
Slope = theta[4:6]
leta = theta[7]
eta = exp(leta)
trt = as.vector( unclass(Trt) )
llambda = Intercept[ trt ] + Slope[ trt ]*x
lambda = exp(llambda)

## Observed
nlogL1 = -sum(!Censor)*leta - sum(llambda[!Censor]) -
         (eta-1)*sum(log(Time[!Censor])) +
         sum( lambda[!Censor]*(Time[!Censor]^eta) )
## Right-censored
nlogL2 = sum( lambda[Censor]*Time[Censor]^eta )

nlogL = nlogL1 + nlogL2
return(nlogL)
}

## Starting values
theta0 = c( alphaA=0, alphaB=0, alphaC=-5,
            betaA=0, betaB=0, betaC=0, leta=0 )
fit0 = optim( theta0, nlogL.weib, Trt=d$Trt, x=d$x,
                      Time=d$Time, Censor=d$Censor,
                      method="BFGS", hessian=TRUE )
fit0$varBeta = solve(fit0$hessian) ## Variance-
   covariance matrix
fit0$table = data.frame(Param=names(fit0$par),
                               Est=fit0$par, SE=sqrt
                               (diag(fit0$varBeta)))
```

The Bayesian method uses the same likelihood, but adds prior information for the intercept and slope terms as well as the Weibull shape parameter. Blending the study data with prior information can help to reduce sample sizes or increase the precision in the posterior distribution, especially when information is available for one or more treatment groups, such as the control/standard of care group. In addition, while frequentist analysis of survival data typically centers on median survival or log-odds of survival, the Bayesian paradigm permits the comparison of survival probabilities without the need for asymptotic approximations. Bayesian Weibull survival modeling will next be illustrated with an example.

4.3.4 Case Example

In this section, we analyze a real example murine oncology data set and use Bayesian survival discussed above to pick the best treatment arm. The experiment employed ten animals in each of three oncology arms (A, B, or C). The animals were randomized into the treatment groups on day 10 of an 84-day study. Tumor volume was measured every 2-3 days for each animal. An animal was removed from the study if either tumor volume reached or exceeded 2,000 mm³ or the tumor was ulcerated. Tumor growth/decay data are shown for individual animals in Figure 4.4. Noting that six and ten (out of ten)

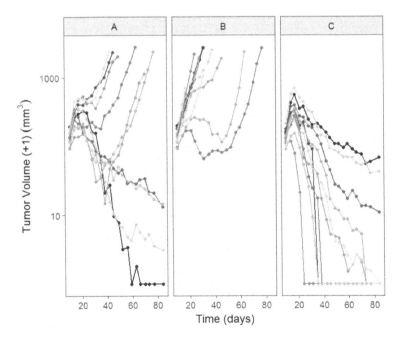

FIGURE 4.4
Tumor volumes for ten animals in each of three treatment arms. To permit log-scaling the y-axis, 1 mm³ was added to the tumor values before graphing.

animals in treatment arms A and B were sacrificed before the final time point, we decided to compare the efficacy of the three treatments via survival analysis. The survival data are shown in Table 4.4. It is clear from the data that chances of survival are best on treatment C and worst on treatment B.

Parameter estimates from the maximum likelihood with standard errors and approximate 95% confidence intervals are shown in Table 4.5.

Because all of the times in treatment C are right-censored, the likelihood is flat in the space for parameters (α_C, β_C) so that there was no guarantee that the optimization would converge. Although the *optim()* function provided a result with a positive-definite Hessian matrix, the standard error of the intercept term (α_C) for treatment C is 99.1, meaning that a comparison of hazards with, say, treatments B and C is hardly possible. For example, when the geometric mean baseline $= M$, $\lambda_i = \exp(\alpha_i)$ and so the log hazard ratio for treatments B and C is ($\alpha_B - \alpha_C$). Based on Figure 4.3, we expect that $\alpha_B > \alpha_C$; i.e., it is more hazardous to take treatment B than treatment C. A 95% confidence interval on $\alpha_B - \alpha_C$ may be approximated from the likelihood results with the following computer code.

```
X = c(0, 1, 0, 0, 0, 0, 0) - c(0, 0, 1, 0, 0, 0, 0)
Est = X%*%fit0$par
SE = sqrt( X%*%fit0$varBeta%*%X )
ci95 = c( Est - qnorm(0.975)*SE, Est + qnorm(0.975)*SE )
print(ci95)
> -180.9706 207.3827
```

Though the estimated log hazard ratio is 13.2 (treatment B is estimated to be more hazardous than treatment C), the resulting 95% confidence interval is

TABLE 4.4

Survival Data for Ten Animals in Each of Three Treatment Arms (A, B, C). Baseline Column Gives the Tumor Size on Day 10. Starting from Day 10, Time is Number of Days Until the Animal Was Sacrificed. Times Marked in Bold Are Right-Censored, Indicating that the Animal Would Have Survived Beyond the Final Time Point

	Time	Baseline		Time	Baseline		Time	Baseline
	32	109.4		14	126.19		74	115.91
	35	89.68		18	146.58		74	110.07
	39	115.65		18	98.1		74	111.26
	53	68.84		21	152.82		74	108.94
Trt	60	67.05	Trt	21	73	Trt	74	97.24
A	67	76.56	B	21	71.69	C	74	113.94
	74	134.33		28	78.62		74	94.75
	74	108.72		35	87.88		74	64.09
	74	73.19		53	65.73		74	105.1
	74	89.69		67	98.41		74	53.79

TABLE 4.5

Estimates, Standard Errors, and 95% Confidence Intervals
for Weibull Model Coefficients from Maximum Likelihood

Coefficient	Value	Standard Error	95% CI
α_A	−9.6	1.8	(−13.1, −6.1)
α_B	−7.8	1.6	(−10.9, −4.6)
α_C	−21.0	99.1	(−215.2, 173.2)
β_A	−1.0	1.8	(−4.5, 2.6)
β_B	1.8	1.4	(−0.9, 4.5)
β_C	−0.2	384.3	(−753.4, 753.0)
$\log(\eta)$	0.8	0.2	(0.4, 1.2)

a nonsensical (−181, 207). Although frequentists may be able to constrain the standard errors of the treatment C coefficients through penalized regression, Bayesians may simply constrain the parameter range through the prior distribution. We will suppose that treatments A, B, and C are novel compounds, so that we have no material prior information on the Weibull survival curve parameters other than our experiences with murine survival data. In such a case, we might assume a normal distribution for the regression parameters centered at the maximum likelihood parameter estimates, but with a reasonable standard deviation to limit the range of the posterior distribution.

If no data are right-censored, conditioned on the parameter values, JAGS models the *i*th response with a statement like *Time[i] ~ dweib(eta, lambda)*. With a mixture of observed and right-censored data, JAGS also requires an indicator variable, *is.censored[i]*, which takes the values 0 and 1, and is measured against a limit, *Lim[i]*. If *Time[i] < Lim[i]*, then *is.censored[i]* = 0. Otherwise, *is.censored[i]* = 1. Observed times *Time[i]* are paired with *is.censored[i]=0* and the *Lim[i]* = a very large value for time of sacrifice (e.g., *Lim[i]=1000*). Right-censored times *Time[i]* are paired with *is.censored[i]=1* and *Lim[i]* = *Time[i]*. Further, the right-censored *Time[i]* are treated as stochastic variables and are set to *NA* in the data list object submitted to JAGS. The JAGS code is given below with posterior medians and 95% credible intervals given in Table 4.6.

TABLE 4.6

Posterior Medians and 95% Credible
Intervals for Weibull Model Coefficients

Coefficient	Median	95% CI
α_A	−9.9	(−13.2, −6.9)
α_B	−7.9	(−11.0, −5.3)
α_C	−21.4	(−30.7, −13.7)
β_A	−1.1	(−4.8, 2.2)
β_B	1.8	(−0.9, 4.4)
β_C	−0.2	(−9.6, 9.6)
$\log(\eta)$	0.8	(0.4, 1.1)

```
model.txt = "
model
{

  ## Prior distribution
  for ( i in 1:nTrt )
  {
       Inter[i] ~ dnorm(InterEst[i], 0.04) ## SD = 5
       Slope[i] ~ dnorm(SlopeEst[i], 0.04)
  }
  eta ~ dexp(0.02)  ## Same as rgamma(1, 0.02). Mean=5,
                        Range 0 - 45
  leta <- log(eta)
  ## Likelihood
  for ( j in 1:N )
  {
   llambda[j] <- Inter[ Trt[j] ] + Slope[ Trt[j] ]*x[j]
   lambda[j] <- exp( llambda[j] )
   Time[j] ~ dweib(eta, lambda[j])

   ## If is.censored[j] = 0, then Time[j] < Lim[j]
(observed).
   ## If is.censored[j] = 1, then Time[j] >= Lim[j]
(right-censored)
   is.censored[j] ~ dinterval( Time[j], Lim[j] )
  }
 }"

 data = list( N = nrow(d), nTrt=nlevels(d$Trt),
              Trt=as.vector(unclass(d$Trt)),
              Time=ifelse(d$Censor, NA, d$Time),
              is.censored=ifelse(d$Censor, 1, 0), x=d$x,
              Lim=ifelse(d$Censor, d$Time, 1000),
              InterEst=as.vector(fit0$par[1:3]),
              SlopeEst=as.vector(fit0$par[4:6]) )
 fitb = run.jags( model=model.txt,
              monitor=c("Inter", "Slope", "eta",
              "leta"), data=data, n.chains=3,
              burnin=10000, sample=20000, thin=100,
              method="parallel" )

 th.post = as.matrix( as.mcmc.list(fitb) )
  ## Posterior median and 95% CIs
 apply(th.post, 2, quantile, p=c(0.5, 0.025, 0.975))
```

```
## log hazard ratio of B vs. C when x= 0
lhaz.BC = quantile( th.post[,"Inter[2]"]-
                    th.post[,"Inter[3]"], p=c(0.5,
              0.025, 0.975) )
```

For the case $x = 0$, the survival curves with 95% credible bands are shown in Figure 4.5.

With the exception of the variability on parameters (α_C, β_C), point estimates (posterior medians) and credible intervals are not terribly different from the maximum likelihood results given in Table 4.5. The posterior median and 95% credible interval for the log hazard ratio of B vs. C is captured in the R variable *lhaz.BC* with the values 13.4 and (5.8, 23.4), strongly suggesting that treatment B is more hazardous than treatment C.

In addition to providing more realistic uncertainty intervals around model parameters, the Bayesian process allows for testing of more complicated hypotheses. Consider the following superiority hypotheses given in Novick

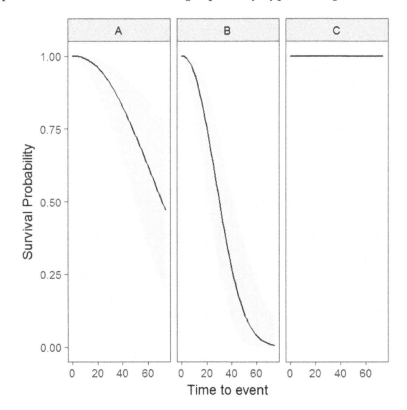

FIGURE 4.5
Weibull survival curves with 95% credible bands for the case $x=0$.

et al. (2018), which tests if the survival on treatment C is at least 10% larger than the survival on treatment B for all times points from 50 – 74 days (i.e., the latter 1/3 of the study).

$$H_0: S(t|\eta,\lambda_C) \leq 1.1\, S(t|\eta,\lambda_B) \text{ for some } 50 \leq t \leq 74 \text{ days}$$
$$H_a: S(t|\eta,\lambda_C) > 1.1\, S(t|\eta,\lambda_B) \text{ for all } 50 \leq t \leq 74 \text{ days}$$

(4.1)

Hypotheses (4.1) are tested via the posterior probability

$$p_0 = \Pr(S(t|\eta,\lambda_C) > 1.1\, S(t|\eta,\lambda_B) \text{ for all } 50 \leq t \leq 74|\text{ data}).$$

Note that $S(t|\eta,\lambda_C) > 1.1\, S(t|\eta,\lambda_B)$ for all $50 \leq t \leq 74$ if and only if

$$(\lambda_B - \lambda_C) > \frac{\log(1.1)}{50^\eta}.$$

At $x = 0$, this is easily accomplished with the following code.

```
p0 = mean( th.post[,"Inter[2]"]- th.post[,"Inter[3]"] >
                 log(1.1)/50^th.post[,"eta"] )
```

The posterior probability p_0 is 1.0, strongly suggesting that survival on treatment C is far superior to survival on treatment B.

4.4 Concluding Remarks

Pre-clinical efficacy assessment is a key component in the decision-making regarding advancing a candidate drug or drug combination into clinical development. Animal studies, however, tend to be small because of ethical and economic concerns. Despite the importance and unique challenge, there are a limited number of publications on use of novel statistical methods for pre-clinical efficacy evaluation. We describe several Bayesian methods for *in-vivo* drug combination and censored animal study data analysis.

5

Bayesian Adaptive Designs for Phase I Dose-Finding Studies

5.1 Introduction

Phase I dose-finding clinical trials are intended to find the maximum tolerated dose of a new drug for a specific mode of administration. Because of ethical concerns, it is desirable to minimize the risk of exposing patients to excessive toxicity. To this end, dose-finding studies are carried out sequentially, starting from a low dose and gradually escalating to higher doses. An implicit assumption is that the probability of experiencing toxicity increases with dose. Phase I dose-finding trials may be carried out with healthy volunteers if the drugs are relatively non-toxic. For drugs with known toxicities, it is conventional to test the drugs in the target patient population. Several considerations are given when designing a Phase I dose-finding trial. They include the selection of a starting dose, the definition of dose-limiting toxicity (DLT), the dose-escalation schedule, and inference of the maximum tolerated dose (MTD) at the end of the study. In the past decades, various dose-finding designs have been proposed, including algorithm-based, model-based, and hybrid designs. This chapter begins with a discussion of algorithm-based designs and their advantages and disadvantages. It then focuses on model-based designs, specifically the continual reassessment method and dose escalation with overdose control. It also includes a discussion of the hybrid designs such as the modified toxicity probability interval. Several examples are used to illustrate the implementation of these methods.

5.2 Algorithm-Based Designs

5.2.1 3 + 3 Design

Per the survey by Rogatko et al. (2007), the most commonly used design is the "3 + 3 design". It is aimed at determining the MTD, which is the highest dose at which a prespecified proportion of patients experience a DLT. MTD is typically in the range of 20% to 33%. A DLT is an adverse reaction to the treatment which is of safety concern and is often study specific. Figure 5.1 shows a schematic procedure of this design without dose de-escalation. In brief, at dose level i, a group of three patients are entered into the dose cohort. If zero out of three patients experience the DLT, the dose escalation takes place and three patients are entered in the next high-dose level $i+1$. If one out of three patients are observed to have DLT, three more patients are added to the current-dose group. If no DLT is observed for the additional three patients, dose escalation continues; otherwise, the dose level $i+1$ is declared as the MTD.

5.2.2 Alternate Algorithm-Based Designs

Note that in this design, the previous lower dose level is always chosen to be the MTD. The method is overly conservative and inefficient as there is no chance for the current dose to be declared as the MTD. The second deficiency of the 3 + 3 design is that it always starts from the lowest dose level, further causing inefficiency of the design. To address these issues, increase the patient's chance to receive a therapeutic dose, and provide a better estimation of MTD, several modifications of the 3 + 3 design were proposed by various authors (Lin and Shih 2001 and 2004; Storer 1989). These modified designs provide opportunities for the current dose level to be declared as the

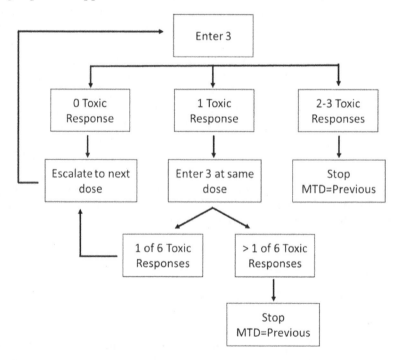

FIGURE 5.1
Dose-escalation scheme for a 3 + 3 design.

MTD, increase efficiency by starting a dose in the middle of the prespecified dose levels, and grant the investigator the ability to reach the MDT quickly through a two-stage design. The two-stage design first assigns one or two patients at each dose level until the first occurrence of toxicity is observed and then switches to the traditional dose-escalation design.

5.2.3 Advantages and Disadvantages of Algorithm-Based Designs

Although algorithm-based designs are conceptually simple and easy to imple-ment, they possess several drawbacks. Chief among these are: (1) Few patients are tested at the MTD level while too many patients are given suboptimal doses (Heyd and Carlin 1999; O'Quigley et al. 1990); (2) The probability of obtaining the MTD is low (Thall and Lee 2003); (3) Because of the small sample, there is great deal of uncertainty in the MTD estimate (Goodman et al. 1995); and (4) They have very poor operating characteristics. For example, even though a target interval for the DLT rate between 16% and 33% is widely accepted, this target range is rarely achieved in the 3 + 3 design (Lin and Shih 2001). Through a simulation study, He et al. (2006) also showed that the expected toxicity level at the MTD from the 3 + 3 design ranges between 19% and 22%; see Figure 5.2. This implies that the MTD is often an underestimate of the true MTD.

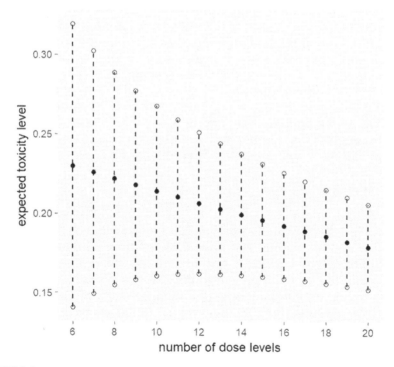

FIGURE 5.2
Expected toxicity level of 3 + 3 design [adapted from He et al. (2006)].

The issues of the traditional algorithm-based design are also noted in several regulatory documents (FDA 2011b; EMA 2007). As stated in those guidelines, alternate approaches may be used.

5.3 Model-Based Designs

5.3.1 Continual Reassessment Method

To address the difficulties encountered with the 3 + 3 designs, O'Quigley et al. (1990) introduced the continual reassessment method (CRM). Assuming that the toxic response increases as the dose level increases, the CRM uses a parametric model to describe the dose–toxicity relationship. Essentially a Bayesian approach, the CRM updates this relationship based on the posterior distribution of the model parameters after each patient response is obtained. The first patient is assigned to the dose that is closest to the MTD based on the prior probability. Subsequently, each patient is assigned to the dose that is closest to the MTD based on the updated dose–toxicity relationship. As pointed out by O'Quigley et al. (1990), when compared to the traditional algorithm-based approaches, the adaptive approach of the CRM method clearly has several advantages (O'Quigley et al. 1990; O'Quigley and Chevret 1991). It reduces the chance of allocating patients to subtherapeutic or harmful doses, has higher efficiency in finding the MTD, and eases ethical concerns. In addition, the model does not have to be accurate over the entire range of doses under study. Since each patient receives the dose that represents the best estimate of the MTD, more information is gathered for doses around the true MTD. Therefore, a reasonable estimate of the dose response is expected from any relatively flexible model, including those that perform poorly when the dose moves away from the target MTD (O'Quigley et al. 1990). For this reason, a reasonable one-parameter model can perform as well as a more complex two-parameter model.

5.3.1.1 Models

Let $D = \{d_1, d_2, \ldots, d_k\}$ and $P = \{p_1, p_2, \ldots, p_k\}$ be the range of doses to be studied in a dose-finding study and associated prior probabilities of observing DLT at those levels, respectively. P is often obtained from prior knowledge. As noted by O'Quigley et al. (1990), it is rare for such knowledge to be unavailable. Together, D and P represent a dose–toxicity relationship before the current study is conducted. It is further assumed that the MTD, $x^* \in D$. The target DLT at MTD is p_0. The study plans to enroll n patients. Let Y_j denote the random variable of whether the jth patient, who is given to dose level x_j, has a toxic response. Mathematically,

$$Y_j \sim \text{Bernoulli}\big(1, \psi(x_j, \theta)\big),$$

where $\psi(x_j, \theta)$ is a function describing the probability of observing a DLT with parameters θ.

In the literature, several single-parameter models were suggested to describe p_y as shown in Table 5.1.

5.3.1.2 Procedure for Finding MTD

Let $\pi(\theta)$ be the prior distribution of θ. The original CRM suggested by O'Quigley et al. (1990) proceeds as follows:

1. Choose a dose–response model $\psi(x, \theta)$ such as those in Table 5.1 and a set of dose levels D. Also define both the prior distribution $\pi(\theta)$ of the model parameter θ and the target probability of DLT, p_0;

2. Assign the first patient to the dose level x_1 such that the corresponding prior probability p is closest to p_0;

3. For $j \geq 2$, after the toxicity response Y_{j-1} is observed, using the Bayes theorem, update the posterior distribution of θ

$$\pi(\theta \mid Y_1, \ldots, Y_{j-1}) = \frac{f(x \mid \theta \pi(\theta)}{\int f(x \mid \theta \pi(\theta) d\theta}$$

where $f(x \mid \theta)]$ is the likelihood function:

$$f(x \mid \theta)] = \prod_{i=1}^{j-1} p_j^{Y_j} (1 - p_j)^{1-Y_j}, \text{ where } p_j = \psi(x_j, \theta);$$

4. Update the value of the dose–toxicity curve $\psi(x, \theta)$ at each dose level $d_i \in D$ $i = 1, \ldots, k$ using either of the following two estimators:

$$\hat{p}_{ij} = \int \psi(d_i, \theta) \pi(\theta \mid Y_1, \ldots, Y_{j-1}) d\theta \quad \text{or}$$

$$\hat{p}_{ij} = \psi(d_i, \hat{\theta}_j)$$

TABLE 5.1

Single-Parameter Models Used to Describe Dose–Toxicity Relationship

Model	Formula
Hyperbolic tangent (O'Quigley et al. 1990)	$\psi(x_j, \theta) = [(\tanh x_j + 1) / 2]^\theta$
Logistic (O'Quigley 1992)	$\log\left(\dfrac{\psi(x_j, \theta)}{1 - \psi(x_j, \theta)}\right) = \alpha_0 + x_j \theta$
Power (O'Quigley and Shen 1996)	$\psi(x_j, \theta) = x_j^{e^\theta}$

where $\hat{\theta} = \int \theta \pi(\theta \mid Y_1,...,Y_{j-1}) d\theta$. The jth patient is assigned to the dose level $x_j = d_l$ such that the $\hat{p}_{lj}$ is closest to the target value p_0. The closeness can be measured by several metrics such as the squared distance $\Delta(u,v) = (u-v)^2$.

5. This process is repeated until the prespecified number of patients, n, is reached.

Although the CRM has gained popularity since the publication of the original paper by O'Quigley, Pepe, and Fisher, it has also raised several controversies. Notably, it tends to expose patients to a higher dose when compared to the traditional algorithm-based design (Ratain et al. 1993). Several modifications were proposed. Several authors suggested that the lowest dose be selected as the starting dose and no more than a one-level increase be allowed for dose escalation (Korn et al. 1994; Moller 1995). In addition to the aforesaid requirements, Goodman et al. (1995) proposed to include two or three patients at each dose level. For detailed discussions and other suggestions, see O'Quigley and Chevret (1993), O'Quigley (1992), O'Quigley and Zhen (1995), Piantadosi and Liu (1996), and Heyd and Carlin (1999).

5.3.2 CRM for Phase I Cancer Trials

In this section, we provide an example to illustrate the implementation of CRM. A Phase I clinical trial in patients with metastatic colorectal cancer was conducted with the intent to determine a safe dose of a new drug for further clinical testing. The CRM design described in Section 5.5.1 was used. Patients received the drug at 400, 800, 1,200, 1,800, 2,400, or 3,000 mg once daily (QD). DLT is defined as grade 3 CTCAE (severe adverse event) or higher, with the initial probability of DLT and true probability of DLT at each dose level given in Table 5.2.

MTD was defined as the dose level at which the probability of DLT is close to 30% and the maximum number of patients to enroll in the study was 30. The single-parameter logistic model in Table 5.1 was used, with $\alpha_0 = -4.5$ and exponential prior $\pi(\theta) = 500e^{-500\theta}$. As each patient was

TABLE 5.2

Dose Levels and Corresponding Initial DLT Probability Estimates and True DLT Probabilities

	Dosing Schedule (QD)					
Dose Level (mg)	400	800	1,200	1,800	2,400	3,000
Initial Probability of DLT	0.04	0.11	0.20	0.32	0.42	0.49
True Probability of DLT	0.10	0.28	0.35	0.40	0.45	0.55

entered into the study, the posterior probability at each dose level was updated. The next dose was chosen as the one such that its associated posterior probability of DLT was closest to the targeted toxicity probability 30%, as measured by the absolute difference. The desired MDT is 800 mg (the true probability of 0.28 is closest to 0.30) and the first patient will be assigned to a dose of 1,800 mg.

The initial DLT probability is calculated as the posterior mean

$$\hat{p}_j = \int_0^\infty \frac{1}{1+\exp(4.5-\theta x_j)}\{500\exp(-500\theta)\}\,d\theta,$$

which was approximated by Monte Carlo integration with the following R code:

```
set.seed(808)
doses = c(400, 800, 1200, 1800, 2400, 3000)
a0 = -4.5
## Calculate initial posterior mean probabilities (pj)
th0 = rexp(100000, rate=500)
pj.init = sapply( doses, function(d){ mean( 1/(1+exp
                  (-(a0+th0*d))) ) })
```

The first patient is assigned to dose 1,800 mg, corresponding to an initial DLT probability of 0.32. We will computer-generate each patient response as

$$Y_j \sim \text{bernoulli}(p_{j,\text{true}}),$$

where the $p_{j,\text{true}}$ are given in the True Probability of DLT row of Table 5.2.

Computer code is given below, with the results shown in Table 5.3. For this scenario, the MDT of 800 mg could have been established after the fifth patient was enrolled. Because the true probability was not generated from the assumed exponential prior and because only zero or one patient was assigned to a dose other than 800 mg, as seen in Table 5.3, the posterior means for doses other than the MDT need not be theoretically close to their respective true values. See Table 5.4 for posterior medians and 95% credible intervals for the p_j after the last patient was enrolled.

Note that in repeated runs of the program with different random seeds, the resulting MDT was not always 800 mg. Because the R variables $p0 = 0.3$, $p.true = 0.28$ for dose = 800, and $p.true = 0.35$ for dose = 1,200, and because new patients are assigned to the dose most closely associated with $p0$, dose 1200 is a reasonable result for the MDT. If, however, a new patient is assigned to the dose with the probability closest to $p0$ from below, then the MCMC typically yields an MDT of one of 400 mg or 800 mg. To reflect the new rule,

TABLE 5.3

Estimated Probability (Posterior Mean) of DLT and Dose Assignment

			Dose					
			400	**800**	**1,200**	**1,800**	**2,400**	**3,000**
			True Probability					
			0.10	*0.28*	*0.35*	*0.40*	*0.45*	*0.55*
	Dose		Prior					
Patient	**Assigned**	**Response**	**0.04**	**0.11**	**0.20**	**0.32**	**0.42**	**0.49**
1	1,800	1	0.07	0.27	0.50	0.73	0.85	0.91
2	800	0	0.05	0.18	0.39	0.66	0.81	0.88
3	1,200	1	0.07	0.29	0.60	0.86	0.95	0.98
4	800	1	0.09	0.42	0.76	0.95	0.99	1.00
5	800	0	0.07	0.34	0.69	0.93	0.98	0.99
6	800	0	0.06	0.29	0.63	0.90	0.97	0.99
7	800	0	0.06	0.25	0.58	0.88	0.97	0.99
			.					
			.					
			.					
29	800	0	0.06	0.29	0.69	0.96	1.00	1.00
30	800	0	0.06	0.28	0.68	0.96	1.00	1.00

TABLE 5.4

Posterior Medians (Estimate) and 95% Credible
Intervals (Lower, Upper)

	Estimate	**Lower**	**Upper**
p_1	0.062	0.042	0.088
p_2	0.279	0.146	0.453
p_3	0.696	0.402	0.877
p_4	0.970	0.839	0.995
p_5	0.998	0.976	1.000
p_6	1.000	0.997	1.000
θ	0.004	0.003	0.005

the R code *index[i+1] = which.min(abs(pj[i,]-p0))* can be changed to *index[i+1]* = *max(which(pj[i,] <= p0))*.

```
set.seed(304)
p0 = 0.3
x = Y = index = rep(NA, 30)
```

```
## Set the dose for the first patient
index[1] = which.min( abs(pj.init-p0) )
x[1] = doses[ index[1] ]

p.true = c(0.10, 0.28, 0.35, 0.40, 0.45, 0.55)
pj = matrix(NA, 30, length(doses))

## JAGS model
model.txt = "
model{
 theta ~ dexp(500)      ## Prior for theta
 a0 <- -4.5
 for ( i in 1:nDose )
 {
  logit(p[i]) <- a0 + theta*dose[i]
 }
 ## Likelihood
 for ( j in 1:nObs )
 {
  Y[j] ~ dbern( p[index[j]] )
 }
}"
for ( i in 1:30 )
{
  ## Response of ith patient
 Y[i] = rbinom( 1, size=1, prob=p.true[index[i]] )
 data = list(nDose=length(doses), dose=doses, nObs=i,
                      Y=Y[1:i], index=index[1:i])

 ## Update posterior distribution of p[j]
 fitb = run.jags( model.txt, data=data, monitor="p",
        n.chains=3, thin=1, burnin=10000,
        sample=20000, method="parallel" )

 ## Get posterior mean of p[j]
 pj[i,] = fitb$summary[[1]][,"Mean"]

 if ( i < 30 )
 {
  index[i+1] = which.min( abs(pj[i,]-p0) )
  x[i+1] = doses[ index[i+1] ]
 }
}
```

5.3.3 Escalation with Overdose Control

The key feature of the CRM is that each patient is entered in the trial at the dose closest to the MTD. An alternative Bayesian method called escalation with overdose control (EWOC) was proposed by Babb et al. (1998) such that it ensures the proportion of patients who receive an overdose does not exceed a pre-chosen threshold. It was shown by Zacks et al. (1998) that EWOC is optimal from the perspective that it minimizes the predicted proportion of underdosed patients. In other words, it approaches the MTD at a rapid speed. Assume that the MTD is within the minimum and maximum dose levels $X_{\min}$ and $X_{\max}$ in the trial. Let Y be the response variable that takes a value of 1 when a DLT is observed and 0 when there is no DLT. It is further assumed that the dose–toxicity relationship can be modeled through a two-parameter function as follows:

$$\Pr(Y = 1 | \text{dose} = x) = F(\beta_0 + \beta_1 x)$$

where F is a cumulative distribution function with $\beta_1 > 0$ so that F is monotonically increasing in dose level x.

As with the CRM, EWOC allocates patients based on the updated dose–toxicity relationship derived from the posterior distribution of the parameters (β_0, β_1). Let γ and ρ_0 be the dose level at the MTD and probability of a DLT at $X_{\min}$, respectively. That is,

$$\Pr(Y = 1 | \text{dose} = \gamma) = \theta$$
$$\Pr(Y = 1 | \text{dose} = X_{\min}) = \rho_0$$

where θ is the prespecified probability of observing a DLT at MTD.

The above model is illustrated in Figure 5.3.

The model can be reparameterized in terms of γ and ρ_0. Such reparameterization has some advantages because the new parameters have practical interpretations. For example, a prior distribution for $\rho_0 = \Pr(\text{DLT} | \text{dose} = X_{\min})$ may come from studying toxicity in animal studies. In addition, a prior distribution for the MTD γ may come from historical literature on similar compounds with $\Pr(\text{DLT} | \text{dose} = \gamma) = \theta$. To illustrate, suppose that

$$\Pr(\text{DLT} | \text{dose} = x) = \frac{1}{1 + \exp(-(\beta_0 + \beta_1 x))}.$$

It can be easily derived that

$$\beta_0 = \frac{1}{\gamma - X_{\min}} \left[\gamma \log\left(\frac{\rho_0}{1 - \rho_0}\right) - X_{\min} \log\left(\frac{\theta}{1 - \theta}\right) \right]$$

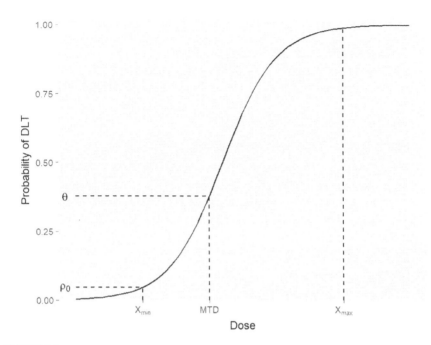

FIGURE 5.3
Probability of DLT against dose level.

$$\beta_1 = \frac{1}{\gamma}\left\{\log\left(\frac{\theta}{1-\theta}\right) - \rho_0\right\}.$$

Let $D_{j-1} = \{(x_i, y_i), \ i = 1, \ldots, j-1\}$ be the dose levels and corresponding responses of the first $j-1$ patients. After specifying a prior distribution $\pi(\gamma, \rho_0)$ of γ and ρ_0, the joint posterior distribution $\pi(\gamma, \rho_0 | D_{j-1})$ of (γ, ρ_0) can be derived. The marginal posterior distribution of MTD, γ, given D_{j-1} can be obtained by integrating over ρ_0:

$$\pi(\gamma | D_{j-1}) = \int_{\rho_0} \pi(\gamma, \rho_0 | D_{j-1}) d\rho_0.$$

Let $\pi_{j-1}(x)$ be the marginal posterior cumulative distribution function of γ given D_{j-1}. Supposing that all doses in $[X_{min}, X_{max}]$ can be used, EWOC proceeds as follows:

1. Assign the first patient to dose level $x_1 = X_{min}$.
2. The jth patient ($j = 2, \ldots, J$) receives dose level at x_j such that $\pi_{j-1}(x_j) = \alpha$, known as the feasibility bound. That is, the dose given to the patient is the $\alpha \times 100$th percentile of the posterior distribution of the MTD.

This ensures that the chance for each patient to be administered a dose higher than the MTD is bounded by α. In the case that a set of dose levels, $d_1, \ldots, d_k$, are prespecified for a particular trial, the dose level for the jth patient can be determined such that it is a value in $\{d_1, \ldots, d_k\}$ closest to the dose chosen in the continuous case. Specifically,

$$d_j = \max\left\{d_i \colon d_i - x_j \le T_1 \text{ and } \pi_{j-1}(x_j) - \alpha \le T_2\right\}$$

where T_1 and T_2 are two non-negative constants.

3. Repeat Step 2 until the prespecified sample size is reached.
4. At the end of the trial, all dose information from the study is used to estimate the MTD. For example, the MTD can be obtained by minimizing expected loss with respect to its posterior distribution.

The loss function originally suggested by Babb et al. (1998) is given by:

$$l_\alpha(x, \gamma) = \begin{cases} \alpha(\gamma - x) & \text{if } x \le \gamma \\ (1 - \alpha)(x - \gamma) & \text{if } x > \gamma. \end{cases}$$

It is an asymmetric loss function that implies that the loss caused by treating a patient at a dose higher than the MTD by δ units is $(1 - \alpha)/\alpha$ times greater than that caused by treating the patient at a dose δ units below the MTD. Therefore, the escalation scheme is more conservative for smaller values of α.

Example

An illustration of the escalation method with overdose control is provided for a drug compound with $X_{min} = 100$ and $X_{max} = 2,000$ mg. Let $\rho_0 = 0.05$, $\theta = 0.3$, and the MDT $\gamma = 680$ mg so that

$$\Pr(Y = 1 \mid \text{dose} = X_{min}) = 0.05$$

$$\Pr(Y = 1 \mid \text{dose} = \gamma) = 0.3.$$

Note that $\Pr(Y = 1 \mid \text{dose} = X_{max}) = 0.58$. Given a dose x, the true probability of DLT is given by

$$\Pr(Y = 1 \mid \text{dose} = x) = \frac{1}{1 + \exp\left(-\left\{\beta_0 + \beta_1 \ln(x)\right\}\right)},$$

with (β_0, β_1) related to (ρ_0, γ) as shown in Section 5.3.3.

Prior distributions were placed on (ρ_0, γ) so that

$$\rho_0 \sim \text{Beta}(3, 50) \text{ and}$$

$$\gamma \sim TN(6.1, 1; X_{min}, X_{max}),$$

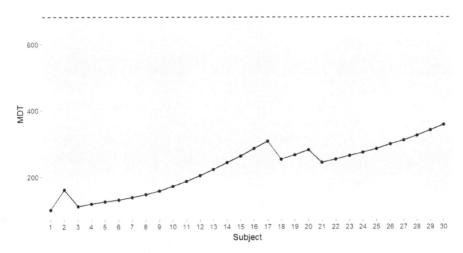

FIGURE 5.4
Assignment of subject doses for EWOC method example.

which has the truncated normal distribution. Thirty patients will be enrolled in the EWOC, one at a time, with the first patient dosed at X_{min}. After admitting a patient, the posterior distribution for (ρ_0, γ) is updated so that the next subject is assigned the lower 90% credible limit for the MDT γ. Computer code in R is shown below and results are shown in Figure 5.4.

```
## All doses are ln-scaled
## Xmin and Xmax
xmin = log(100)
xmax = log(2000)

## True probability of DLT, given a ln-dose "x"
rho0 = 0.05 ## Probability of DLT when x = xmin
theta = 0.3 ## Probability of DLT when x = MDT
lmdt = log(680)  ## = log(gamma)
beta0 = (1./(lmdt-xmin))*( lmdt*log(rho0/(1-rho0)) -
                        xmin*log(theta/(1-theta)))
beta1 = (1/lmdt)*( log(theta/(1-theta)) - beta0 )
prob.dlt = function(x){ 1/(1+exp(-(beta0+beta1*x))) }

prob.dlt(xmin)  ## This is rho0 = 0.05
prob.dlt(lmdt)  ## This is theta = 0.3

## JAGS model code
model.txt = "
model{
```

```
## Priors for rho0 and log(gamma)
lgamma ~ dnorm(6.1, 1.)T(xmin, xmax)  ## Truncated to
(xmin, xmax)
rho0 ~ dbeta(3, 50)  ## 95% of values between 0.01
and 0.13

beta0 <- (1./(lgamma-xmin))*( lgamma*log(rho0/(1.-
rho0)) - xmin*log(theta/(1.-theta)))
beta1 <- (1./lgamma)*( log(theta/(1.-theta)) - beta0 )

## Likelihood
for ( i in 1:N )
{
 logit(p[i]) <- beta0 + beta1*x[i]   ## x[i] = log(dose)
 Y[i] ~ dbern( p[i] )
}
}"

set.seed(441)
x = Y = rep(NA, 30)

x[1] = xmin ## First patient enrolled with dose = xmin

for ( i in 1:30 )
{
   ## Generate data for ith patient with true DLT
      probability
 Y[i] = rbinom( 1, size=1, prob=prob.dlt(x[i]) )

 ## Create data for JAGS
 data = list(N=i, x=x[1:i], Y=Y[1:i], xmin=log(100),
             xmax=log(2000), theta=0.3)

 ## Update posterior distribution of (rho0, lgamma)
 fitb = run.jags( model.txt, data=data,
monitor=c("rho0", "lgamma"),
        n.chains=3, thin=25, burnin=10000,
sample=20000,
        method="parallel")
 th.post = as.matrix( as.mcmc.list(fitb) )

 if ( i < 30 )
  x[i+1] = quantile(th.post[,"lgamma"], 0.10) ## Lwr
          90% CL: log(MDT)
}
```

After 30 patients, the lower 90% credible limit for γ of 356 mg underestimated the true value of 680 mg. Note that the final posterior median of γ was 682 mg and, with the trend showing a steady climb, it is likely that a larger final sample size would have led to the correct MDT. Indeed, the entire exercise was repeated, except that patients were enrolled five at a time to speed recruitment and estimation of the MDT so that the last five patients (out of the total 150 patients) were dosed with 595 mg, which is much closer to the true value. Two lines of code were changed, namely

```
## Generate data for ith recruitment with true DLT
   probability
Y[i] = rbinom( 1, size=5, prob=prob.dlt(x[i]) )
```

and in the JAGS code
```
Y[i] ~ dbin( p[i], 5 )
```

5.3.4 Escalation Based on Toxicity Probability Intervals

5.3.4.1 Toxicity Probability Intervals

There are several challenges concerning the implementation of the Bayesian dose-finding methods in the previous sections. One is that it requires in-depth statistical expertise and another is that a target toxicity probability needs to be defined by investigators. In addition, the methods may be sensitive to the selection of priors. Among the above-mentioned difficulties, it is especially challenging for the investigator to define the target toxicity. An alternate method was suggested by Ji et al. (2007) to allow investigators to specify a range of target toxicity probability, also known as toxicity probability interval. The method is a hybrid of Bayesian CRM and 3 + 3 design.

5.3.4.2 Model

Let p_0 denote the nominal target toxicity probability. Let $x_j (j = 1, ..., J)$ be the dose used to treat the current n_j patients, of whom Y_j patients have experienced toxicities. It is further assumed that

$$Y_j \sim \text{binomial}(n_j, p_j),$$

$$p_j \sim \text{beta}(a_0, b_0)$$

are used for updating p_j. As previously discussed, the posterior probability of p_j follows a beta distribution

$$p_j \mid y_J \sim \text{Beta}(a_0 + y_j, b_0 + n_j - y_j).$$

5.3.4.3 Method

The method by Ji et al. (2007) partitions the unit interval $(0, 1)$ into three intervals based on posterior toxicity probability:

$$\Delta = \left\{ \left(0, p_0 - k_1 s_j \right), \left[p_0 - k_1 s_j, 0, p_0 + k_2 s_j \right], \left(p_0 + k_2 s_j, 1 \right) \right\}$$

where s_j is the posterior standard deviation of p_j and k_1 and k_2 are small positive constants, which are defined by the investigator.

The posterior probabilities of de-escalating to the dose $x_{j-1}(D)$, staying in dose x_j (S), or escalating to the dose $x_{j+1}(E)$, are obtained as:

$$q_{D,j} = \Pr\left[p_j > p_0 + k_1 s_j \,|\, Y_j \right]$$

$$q_{S,j} = \Pr\left[p_0 - k_2 s_j \leq p_j < p_0 + k_1 s_j \,|\, Y_j \right]$$

$$q_{E,j} = \Pr\left[p_j < p_0 - k_2 s_j \,|\, Y_j \right]$$

It is natural to assign the next dose based on the maximum of the above three probabilities; however, the above rule would result in a dose escalation without considering that the next dose level might be highly toxic (Ji et al. 2007). To address this potentially ethical issue, a utility function may be introduced as follows (Ji et al. 2007; Berry et al. 2011):

$$U(d,a) = \begin{cases} 0 & \text{if } d = 1 \text{ and } a = D \\ 0 & \text{if } (d = J \text{ and } a = E) \text{ or } \left(\Pr\left[p_{d+1} > p_0 \,|\, Y_j \right] > \xi \right) \\ q_{a,j} & \text{otherwise} \end{cases}$$

where $a \in \{E, D, S\}$ and ξ is a cutoff value between 0 and 1 which is used to define an unacceptable level of toxicity. The utility function is constructed such that there is no de-escalation after the first dose being evaluated, no escalation after the last dose, and no escalation in the event that the probability of observing toxicity is higher than the acceptable threshold.

Based on the above utility function, the next dose can be selected such as

$$d \equiv \begin{cases} d-1 & \text{if } U(d,D) = \max_a U(d,a) \\ d+1 & \text{if } U(d,E) = \max_a U(d,a) \\ d & \text{otherwise} \end{cases}$$

At the conclusion of the trial, the MTD is chosen based on an isotonic regression (Robertson et al. 1988) on the posterior means $\hat{p}_j = E(p_j \,|\, \text{all data})$, which gives rise to a set of transformed values of $\hat{p}_j^*$, and which are monotonically increasing with respect to j. The MTD is estimated as $\hat{p}_0^*$ such that

$$\left|\hat{p}_0^* - p_0\right| = \min_j \left|\hat{p}_j^* - p_0\right|.$$

5.3.4.4 Method Implementation

As shown by Ji et al. (2007), the decision to either de-escalate, stay, or escalate can be constructed based on the number of patients n_j in the current cohort j, and the number of toxicities observed in the cohort. Because of this, a table of dose-assignment actions can be provided before the trial is actually carried out. Computer code for the Ji, Li, and Bekele method is available in R and Excel and may be downloaded from the following website:
https://biostatistics.mdanderson.org/softwaredownload/SingleSoftware.aspx?Software_Id=72.

Figure 5.5 shows the results from the downloaded R code.

In Figure 5.5, the row represents the number of patients treated at the current dose level, whereas the column corresponds to the number of patients experiencing toxicity. For each combination of number of patients treated and number of patients having toxicity, the corresponding decision regarding the dose escalation, stay, and de-escalation decision is listed. If the current dose level is unacceptable due to high toxicity, it is excluded from the

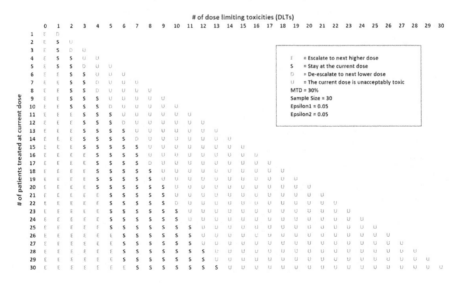

FIGURE 5.5
Dose assignment as a function of the number of patients in a cohort and the number of patients experiencing toxicity.

study. The corresponding action is labeled as "U". To illustrate, suppose five patients were entered in the current dose, and three of them experienced toxicity. From the table, an action of de-escalation should be taken and the next patient should be given the previous dose.

5.4 Concluding Remarks

Phase I dose-finding studies, aimed at an estimation of MTD, are an important part of clinical development. As reported by various authors, however, most dose-finding trials are carried out using the traditional algorithm-based designs, in which dose escalation is primarily based on toxicity response in the previous dose. Since only a small number of subjects are used for these trials, it is imperative to use dose information across all dose levels. As such, model-based approaches are advantageous when compared to algorithm-based methods. The sequential nature of dose-escalations trials makes it suitable to adopt Bayesian methods. Over the past decades, significant advances have been made in method development, particularly for model-based approaches. The methodological exploration continues to remain active. Coupled with related software development, the model-based designs will hopefully be more broadly adopted to meet the increasing demand for more efficient Phase I dose-finding trials.

6

Design and Analysis of Phase II Dose-Ranging Studies

6.1 Introduction

A dose-ranging study is a clinical trial in which two or more doses of a drug are tested to determine the most effective and safe dose to be used in the Phase III confirmatory trials. Since the doses used in the study are chosen based on MTD, the study is usually conducted after the information of MTD becomes available. Additionally, a dose-ranging study typically includes the SOC or placebo group. Through such studies, clinical researchers gain the understanding of the dose–response relationship, in terms of efficacy, which is used to guide the selection of the optimal dose. Traditionally, the dose–response relationship is obtained from two or three doses, typically permitting only pair-wise comparisons of the dose groups. A major limitation of this method is its lack of ability to interpolate the response at doses that are not evaluated in the study. More recently, dose-ranging studies have evolved to be more focused on the model-based approaches. They include general linear contrast tests among doses, modeling the dose–response curve, a hybrid between the two methods such as MCPMod (Bretz et al. 2005), isotonic regression modeling (Oron and Flournoy 2017), and Bayesian modeling (e.g., Smith and Marshall 2006). When compared to other methods, Bayesian modeling is preferential as it takes advantage of dose–response modeling that links multiple doses, shares information among doses, increases information and decreases uncertainty, and incorporates prior information from previous studies or experts' opinions. Combined, these advantages yield more powerful comparisons and more precise estimations. It is worth noting that as with other Bayesian applications, the challenge when leveraging historical data to form a prior for a new study is to determine whether the existing data are sufficiently similar to the setting of the new trial (Novick et al. 2018). The next study is rarely an exact replica of the previous one, and so it is important to account for potential heterogeneity between historical and current trial settings when building the prior distribution. In this chapter, we discuss statistical considerations in the design and analysis of phase II dose-ranging studies. Key issues discussed include the selection of dose–response curve, use of prior information for study planning, and analysis, sample-size and power calculations.

6.2 Phase II Dose-Ranging Studies

Phase III studies, often called confirmatory trials, are used to provide a definitive assessment of the effectiveness of a candidate drug. The success or failure of a Phase III clinical trial rests on many factors. Key among those is a set of doses used in the trial, which is selected through previous dose-ranging studies. As mentioned, a Phase II dose-ranging study includes the SOC or placebo and a few dose groups of the test drug, which presumably provide a range covering the most efficacious and safe dose. The study is carried out in the targeted population typically using a randomized parallel design. With a sufficient sample size, an optimal dose can be obtained through data collected from the study.

6.2.1 Criticisms of Traditional Methods

In mathematical terms, this range consists of all safe doses d such that the mean response as a function of the dose $f(d)$ achieves an acceptable efficacy target; e.g., $f(d) > f(0) + \delta$, for some clinically meaningful difference δ. The goal of the Phase II dose-range study is to estimate the function $f(d)$ and calculate the doses of clinical interest.

A traditional dose-ranging method relies on pair-wise comparison. Usually, data are statistically modeled via one-way ANOVA so that $f(d_i) = \mu_i$ for the ith study arm. Consider a design with a SOC and two different doses. Let arms $i = 1$, 2, and 3 respectively denote the SOC (i.e., $d_1 = 0$), a mid-level dose, and the highest tolerated dose groups. The Phase III trial dose would consequently be set to one of the doses (d_2 or d_3) such that $f(d_i) > f(0) + \delta$. The downsides of the design result from its inability to gain a complete understanding of the dose–response relationship. Consider the case when $f(0) + \delta < f(d_2) < f(d_3)$. Although the clinician may select either doses d_2 or d_3, one cannot discern if there may be a dose lower than d_2 that provides clinical efficacy. Even worse is the case $f(d_2) < f(0) + \delta < f(d_3)$, so that the clinician has little choice but to select the highest tolerated dose for the Phase III trial. As before, one cannot determine a dose between d_2 and d_3 that provides clinical efficacy.

6.2.2 Model-Based Approaches

6.2.2.1 Modeling Dose–Response Curve

More recently, Phase II dose-ranging clinical trial designs have evolved to include more dose groups and focus on the modeling of a dose–response curve. While the use of a dose–response curve conforms to the needs of the clinician, one difficulty is that the shape of the curve is usually unknown a priori to the Phase II study. Several approaches to this problem have been developed in the literature. Bretz et al. (2005) evaluate several credible dose–response models fitted to trial data and use a weighted-model averaging approach. Oron and Flournoy (2017) eschew the parametric model and instead propose isotonic (spline) regression. The four-parameter logistic model is a popular choice for dose–response model fitting. Several authors (Thomas et al. 2014, Thomas and Roy 2017; Wu et al. 2018) show that a three-parameter Emax curve (a three-parameter version of the aforementioned logistic curve) typically provides an adequate description of the data across a broad range of compounds and therapeutic areas. For ease of discussion, we focus on the three-parameter Emax model (hereafter, simply the Emax model). With a parametric model, a parameter θ is added to the argument in the dose–response function. The Emax curve (Seber and Wild 2003) is given by

$$f(\theta,d) = A + \frac{(B-A)}{\{1 + \exp(\log C - \log(d))\}} \tag{6.1}$$

where $\theta = (A, B, \log C)$, A = minimum mean response (when $d = 0$), B = maximum mean response (when $d = \infty$), and $\log C$ = natural log of the dose that yields a mean response of $(A+B)/2$. Define the $ED50 = e^{\log C}$. In this chapter, the Emax curve will be used to develop a Phase II study design.

6.2.2.2 Determination of Minimum Efficacy Dose

With the Emax model, theoretically, the minimum dose that provides $f(\theta, d) > f(\theta, 0) + \delta$ is given by

$$d_\delta(\theta) = ED50\left(\frac{\delta}{B-(A+\delta)}\right). \tag{6.2}$$

Because back-calculated doses are typically log-normally distributed, we let $ld_\delta(\theta) = \ln(d_\delta(\theta))$. In practice, the parameters in Equation (6.2) are estimated. When planning a study design, several considerations need to be given. One is the determination of the number of doses and the number of subjects assigned to each dose that will result in a sufficiently precise estimate of $d_\delta(\theta)$. The other is the use of historical data for the above calculations.

As described in Chapter 3, prior information for θ can enhance the trial design either by reducing the number of required subjects or by improving the precision of $d_\delta(\theta)$. In addition, with prior information, statistical power or assurance may be provided for testing the hypotheses:

$$H_0: f(\theta,d_i) \leq f(\theta,0) + \delta \text{ versus } H_a: f(\theta,d_i) > f(\theta,0) + \delta. \tag{6.3}$$

Certainly, given any dose d, the operating characteristic for testing $f(\theta, d) > f(\theta, 0) + \delta$ can be determined.

6.3 Estimating Predictive Precision and Assurance for New Trial

In this section, we describe a Bayesian procedure for evaluating predictive precision in the estimate of the minimum effective dose (Equation [6.2]) and predictive assurance in testing the Hypotheses (6.3).

6.3.1 COPD Study

To provide context, we use an example described by Novick et al. (2018) regarding the planning of a randomized, placebo-controlled parallel Phase IIb dose-ranging study for chronic obstructive pulmonary disease (COPD). The study objective is to evaluate the dose response, efficacy, and safety of five dosage regiments along with placebo and determine or two doses for Phase III clinical trials. The six treatment arms include a placebo arm (dose = 0) plus five dosing arms of 37.5, 75, 150, 300, and 600 micrograms (mcg). Three sample sizes of $N = 30$, 40, or 50 per dosing group were considered. The measured response from each subject is called FEV1, the maximal amount of air one can forcefully exhale into a specialized device in the span of one second. The clinical outcome variable is the change in FEV1 from baseline after six weeks on treatment.

6.3.2 Estimation Method

It is assumed that Equation (6.1) will provide an adequate fit to the future dose–response FEV1 data, modeled as

$$\text{FEV1}_{ij} = f(\theta, d_i) + e_{ij},$$

where FEV1_{ij} is the six-week change in FEV1 from baseline measurement of the jth patient on the ith dose ($i = 1, 2, ..., 6; j = 1, 2, ..., N$), d_i is the ith dose (i.e., $d_1 = 0, d_2 = 37.5, ..., d_6 = 600$), and the e_{ij} are independent, identically distributed Gaussian errors with zero mean and common variance σ^2.

A frequentist might employ nonlinear OLS or maximum likelihood (ML) to determine the estimate for θ. Let $\hat{\theta}$ denote the ML estimate for θ.

To examine predictive precision, let the estimated ln-dose of interest be given by $ld_\delta(\hat{\theta})$. An approximate 95% confidence interval for $ld_\delta(\theta)$ is given by

$$ld_\delta(\hat{\theta}) \pm 1.96 \times SE_{ld},$$

where SE_{ld} is the standard error of $ld_\delta(\hat{\theta})$ calculated via the delta method.

Define the precision of $ld_\delta(\theta)$ as the half-width of the confidence interval, $1.96 \times SE_{ld}$. For the comparison of Hypotheses (6.3), a p-value approach is taken. For a given study, dose d_i, the test statistic, is

$$Z = \frac{f(\hat{\theta}, d_i) - f(\hat{\theta}, 0) - \delta}{SE_f},$$

where SE_f is the standard error of $f(\hat{\theta}, d_i) - f(\hat{\theta}, 0)$ calculated via the delta method and the p-value is $1 - f(Z)$, with $\Phi(.)$ being the standard normal cumulative density function. A p-value <0.05 suggests that dose d_i provides a strong benefit over placebo; i.e., H_a is true.

For a given study design, frequentist predictive precision and power depend on direct knowledge of θ and σ^2, which are typically unknown and need to be estimated. Bayesian predictive precision and assurance (expected power) depend on the prior distribution of θ and σ^2. Because the value of θ varies from one trial to the next, assume the hierarchical model

$$\theta \sim N(\theta_0, V_0),$$

where θ_0 is the 3 x 1 population parameter average and V_0 is the 3 x 3 population variance–covariance matrix. Any predictive calculation will therefore require $(\theta_0, V_0, \sigma^2)$, which respectively represent the Emax model population parameter average, study-to-study variability, and within-study variability.

The Bayesian paradigm permits prior knowledge of $\Theta = (\theta_0, V_0, \sigma^2)$ to enter into predictive precision and power calculations. For the moment, assume that the prior distribution for Θ is known. As outlined in Chapter 3, for a given study design (i.e., sample size N per dose), the predictive precision and statistical assurance may be estimated as follows.

    i. Draw a random sample Θ_b from Θ.

    ii. Generate the Emax model parameters for study b as $\theta_b \sim N(\theta_{0,b}, V_{0,b})$.

    iii. Generate pseudo FEV1 dose–response data as $FEV1_{ij}^{(b)} = f(\theta_b, d_i) + e_{ij}^{(b)}$, where $e_{ij}^{(b)} \sim N(0, \sigma_b^2)$.

    iv. From the pseudo-trial data in Step iii, estimate the Emax model parameters by ML as $\hat{\theta}_b$.

    v. Repeat steps i–v, yielding the set $\{\hat{\theta}_b\}$, $b = 1, 2, \ldots, B$.

For each $\hat{\theta}_b$, one may calculate $SE_{ld,b}$ and $SE_{f,b}$, respectively, the standard error of $ld_\delta(\hat{\theta}_b)$ and the standard error of $f(\hat{\theta}_b,d_i) - f(\hat{\theta}_b,0)$. For the sake of argument, define the predictive precision of $ld_\delta(\theta)$ as the median value (with respect to the prior distribution of Θ) of $1.96 \times SE_{ld,b}$. Let

$$Z_b = \frac{f(\hat{\theta}_b,d_i) - f(\hat{\theta}_b,0) - \delta}{SE_{f,b}}.$$

Statistical assurance is the predictive probability that $\Phi(Z_b) > 0.95$. Given the set $\{\hat{\theta}_b\}$, predictive precision may be estimated as the posterior predictive median of $1.96 \times \{SE_{ld,b}\}$. The Phase III clinical ln-dose might then be selected as a dose in the range of

$$ld_\delta(\hat{\theta}) \pm 1.96 \, \text{Median}\{SE_{ld,b}\}.$$

Statistical assurance is estimated by

$$\frac{1}{B}\sum 1\{f(Z_b) > 0.95\},$$

where $1(.)$ is the indicator function.

6.3.2.1 Selection of Priors

The big question, then, is how does one obtain a prior distribution for Θ? Clearly, a background in current COPD trial literature is valuable and a working knowledge of FEV1 results for the placebo arm and within-study FEV1 variability across various studies provides at least part of the big picture. It may be difficult to find historical data that permit the estimation of the distributions for both θ_0 and V_0. Imagine, for example, the historical placebo data that recorded FEV1 at week six in five different COPD studies shown in Table 6.1.

TABLE 6.1

Historical Placebo Data from COPD Trials

Study	Mean ($\bar{Y}$)	N	Pooled Standard Deviation ($\hat{\sigma}$)
1	−0.02	165	0.21 (328 df)
2	−0.01	155	0.23 (308 df)
3	0.00	200	0.24 (995 df)
4	0.01	195	0.22 (582 df)
5	0.03	130	0.24 (516 df)

Columns are placebo mean for change in fev1 from baseline at week six, placebo-arm sample sizes, and pooled standard deviation across all trial arms with associated degrees of freedom (df).

From Table 6.1, with vague priors for $(\mu_0, \sigma_S, \sigma)$, we can fit the model

$$\mu_i \mid \mu_0, \sigma_S^2 \sim N\left(\mu_0, \sigma_S^2\right),$$

$$\bar{Y}_i \mid \mu_i, \sigma^2 \sim N\left(\mu_i, \frac{\sigma^2}{N_i}\right), \text{ and}$$

$$\hat{\sigma}_i^2 \mid \sigma^2 \sim \text{Gamma}\left(\frac{df_i}{2}, \frac{df_i}{2\sigma^2}\right).$$

Computer code with priors $\mu_0 \sim N(0,1)$ and σ_S, $\sigma \sim$ half-Cauchy(0, scale = 0.1) is given below.

```
model.txt = "
model
{
## Priors
mu0 ~ dnorm( 0, 1 )          ## Placebo mean
sigmaS ~ dt(0., 100., 1)T(0., )  ## Study-to-study
variability
sigmaE ~ dt(0., 100., 1)T(0., )  ## Within-study
variability

tauS <- 1/(sigmaS*sigmaS)
tauE <- 1/(sigmaE*sigmaE)

## Likelihood
for ( i in 1:nStudy )
{
 mu[i] ~ dnorm( mu0, tauS )
 ybar[i] ~ dnorm( mu[i], tauE*N[i] )
 sigSqHat[i] ~ dgamma( 0.5*degFree[i],
                       0.5*degFree[i]*tauE )
}

}"

## Prepare data for JAGS
data = list( nStudy=5, ybar=c(-0.02, -0.01, 0, 0, 0.03),
             N=c(165, 155, 200, 195, 130),
             sigSqHat=c(0.21, 0.23, 0.24, 0.22, 0.24)^2,
             degFree=c(328, 308, 995, 582, 516) )

## Call JAGS
fitb = run.jags( model.txt, data=data,
```

```
    monitor=c("mu0", "sigmaS", "sigmaE"),
    n.chains=3, burnin=10000, sample=20000, thin=10,
    module="glm", method="parallel" )

  th.post = as.matrix( as.mcmc.list(fitb) )
```

6.3.2.2 Estimation of Dose–Response Curve

The posterior distribution of $(\mu_0, \sigma_S, \sigma)$ can partially serve as the prior information for the Emax model. The Emax model parameter A may be modeled as $A \sim N(\mu_0, \sigma_S^2)$. Given the historical data of Table 6.1, the Emax model parameters B and $logC$ are completely unknown and so their distributions must be derived through prior elicitation (i.e., expert opinion, literature review). One might assign, for example, a distribution for B with values that tend to be greater than $\mu_0 + \delta$ (or else the study is immediately futile) along with variability σ_S^2. Additionally, the distribution of ED50 ($= e^{logC}$) is presumably contained within the study design. For now, assume the priors $B \sim N(\mu_0 + 2.5\delta, \sigma_S^2)$ and $logC \sim N(4.5, SD = 0.3)$ so that, roughly speaking, 3.6 $< logC < 5.4$, meaning that the ED50 falls between 35 and 220 mcg. A graph of the prior predictive distribution of the Emax model (i.e., $f(\theta, d)$) is shown in Figure 6.1.

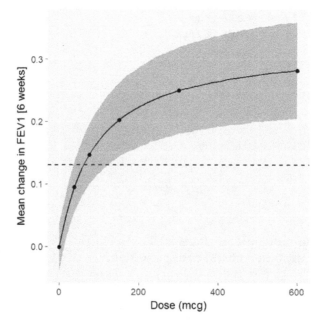

FIGURE 6.1
Prior predictive distribution of the Emax model.

6.3.2.3 **Estimation of Precision and Assurance**

Following steps i–v, computer code is given to calculate the predictive precision of $ld_\delta(\theta)$ and the assurance associated with testing (Hypotheses [6.3])
with $d_3 = 75$ mcg and $d_5 = 300$ mcg against placebo when $\delta = 0.13$ and $N = 40$
subjects/dosing arm. First, some functions are given to make the necessary
calculations.

```
## Functions for estimating Emax parameters and std
   errors of interest
emax.model = function(theta, dose)
{
 mu = theta[1] + (theta[2] - theta[1])/(1 + exp(theta
 [3]-log(dose)))
 return(mu)
}
emax.grad = function(theta, dose)
{
 ## Partial derivative of emax.model with respect to
    theta

 grad = rep(NA, 3)
 exp.term = exp(theta[3]- log(dose))
 temp = 1/(1 + exp.term)
 grad[1] = 1 - temp
 grad[2] = temp
 grad[3] = -temp*temp*(theta[2]-theta[1])*exp.term

 return(grad)
}

nlogLik = function (theta, dose, ybar, N, sSq, degFree)
{
  ## Negative log-likelihood for Emax model with summary
     statistics
  ## theta = (A, B, logC, ln(sigmaE))
  ## dose = vector of unique doses
  ## ybar = Mean FEV1 value at each dose
  ## sSq = pooled variance estimate
  ## degFree = degrees of freedom associated with sSq

  emax = emax.model(theta, dose)
  sigmaE = exp(theta[4])
  out = -sum( dnorm( ybar, mean=emax, sd=sigmaE/sqrt(N)
) ) - dgamma( sSq, shape=0.5*degFree, rate=0.5*degFree/
    sigmaE^2 )
```

```
  return(out)
}
SE.ld = function(theta, V, delta)
{
 ## delta method: standard error of ld( theta_hat )
 ## theta = parameter estimates for Emax model
 ## V = estimated variance-covariance matrix

 ## Linear contrast for delta method
 C = c( 1/(theta[2]-theta[1]-delta), -1/(theta[2]-
     theta[1]-delta), 1 )

 SE = as.vector( sqrt( C%*%V[1:3,1:3]%*%C ) )
 return(SE)
}
SE.f = function(theta, V, dose)
{
 ## delta method: std error of f(theta_hat, dose)
    - f(theta_hat, 0)

 ## theta = parameter estimates for Emax model
 ## V = estimated variance-covariance matrix

 ## Linear contrast for delta method
 C = emax.grad(theta, dose) - c(1, 0, 0)

 SE = as.vector( sqrt( C%*%V[1:3,1:3]%*%C ) )
 return(SE)
}
```

Next, computer code is given to calculate the posterior predictive precision of $ld_\delta(\theta)$ as well as the assurance for Equation (6.2) when the dose $= 75$ and 300 mcg.

```
N = 40
delta = 0.13
dose = c(0, 37.5, 75, 150, 300, 600)
degFree = length(dose)*(N-1)

set.seed(804)
B = nrow(th.jags)
res = matrix(NA, B, 5)
for ( b in 1:B )
{
```

```
## Prior distribution of (A, B, logC, sigS)
theta0 = c( A=th.jags[b, "mu0"], B=th.jags[b, "mu0"]
            +2.5*delta, logC=4.5 )
sigS = th.jags[b, "sigmaS"]
sigE = th.jags[b, "sigmaE"]
theta = rnorm(3, mean=theta0, sd=c(sigS, sigS, 0.3))

## Prior predictive distribution of (ybar, sSq)
emax = theta[1] + (theta[2] - theta[1])/
             (1 + exp(theta[3]-log(dose)))
ybar = rnorm( 6, mean=emax, sd=sigE/sqrt(N) )
sSq = sigE^2*rchisq(1, degFree)/degFree

  ## Maximum likelihood fitter
theta00 = c( theta0, lsig=log(sigE) ) ## Starting
            values
fitb = optim( theta00, nlogLik, dose=dose, ybar=ybar,
              N=N, sSq=sSq, degFree=degFree,
              hessian=TRUE, method="BFGS" )

res[b,1] = fitb$converge==0 ## Did the MLE algorithm
            converge?
  ## Estimate var(theta_hat) = inverse Hessian matrix
varTheta = try( solve(fitb$hessian), silent=TRUE )
if ( fitb$converge==0 & class(varTheta)[1] != "try-
     error" )
{
  ## Calculate log( d.delta )
 res[b,2] = fitb$par[3] + log(delta) -
                  log( fitb$par[2]-fitb$par[1]-delta )
  ## SE{ log( d.delta ) )
 res[b,3] = SE.ld( fitb$par, varTheta, delta )

  ## Calculate p-value at dose = 75
 Zb = ( emax.model(fitb$par, 75) - fitb$par[1] )/
                  SE.f( fitb$par, varTheta, dose=300 )
 res[b,4] = 1 - pnorm(Zb)  ## p-value

  ## Calculate p-value at dose = 300
 Zb = ( emax.model(fitb$par, 300) - fitb$par[1] )/
                  SE.f( fitb$par, varTheta, dose=300 )
 res[b,5] = 1 - pnorm(Zb)  ## p-value
 }
}
```

```
## Roughly 98% usable results
good.index = !is.na(res[,2]) & !is.na(res[,3]) &
                        !is.na(res[,4]) & !is.na(res[,5])

mean( good.index )
> 0.9813667

predictive.precision = 1.95 * median( res[good.index, 3] )

assurance.75 = mean( res[good.index,4] < 0.05 ) # dose=75
assurance.300 = mean( res[good.index,5] < 0.05 ) #
dose=300
```

After running the computer code, roughly 2% of the simulated results needed to be thrown away due to lack of ML convergence or the inability to calculate $ld_8(\hat{\theta}_b)$, SE_{ld}, or SE_f. The median value of $ld_8(\hat{\theta}_b)$ is 4.09 and the predictive precision (*predictive.precision*) is about 0.36, meaning that the Phase III ln-dose should be in the range of 3.73–4.45; thus, the dose is roughly in the range of 40–85 mcg. Statistical assurance for comparing mean FEV1 at dose=75 mcg vs. dose=0 is 0.992 and statistical assurance for the comparison of dose=300 mcg vs. dose=0 is 0.997. If prior assumptions are not far from the truth, a Phase II design with $N=40$ per dose seems like a sure bet in determining a useful Phase III dose. The entire exercise should be repeated to evaluate different sample sizes (N), different doses, and possibly unbalanced study designs.

As a final note, in the above analysis, it is assumed that the future Phase II study data will be analyzed by ML. Since prior information is available, the Emax model may be fitted via Bayesian methods. When calculating the predictive precision/assurance, should the same prior distribution be used to both generate the future trial data and analyze the data? Several authors (O'Hagan et al. 2005; Hobbs and Carlin 2008) propose the creation of two priors, namely the *design* prior, which is used to generate the prior predictive distribution and a more robust (i.e., less certain) *analysis* prior, used to fit the model to the future data. The calculations shown in this chapter needed only a few minutes of computer processing time. By adding Bayesian Emax model fitting, on today's typical computers, processing time can blow up quickly. Some compromises in the number of Monte Carlo runs may be necessary for the sake of reasonable computing time.

6.4 Concluding Remarks

According to a published report (Kola and Landis 2004), lack of clinical efficacy and safety amounts to about 40% of the attrition rate of drugs in the late-stage clinical development. It is important to determine the range of efficacious and safe doses through dose-ranging studies. The traditional methods based on pair-wise comparison lack the ability to extrapolate their findings from the study of doses that are not tested. The use of model-based approaches overcomes this shortcoming. Precise estimation of the dose–response curve is the foundation for a precise estimate of the minimum effective dose and the range of efficacious doses. In recent years, there has been an increasing interest from both industry and regulatory agencies in making use of external evidence in drug development, including late-stage clinical trial design and analysis. In this chapter, through a case example, we demonstrate the utility of Bayesian methods in dose-ranging studies and ease of its implementation in support of study design and analysis.

7

Bayesian Multi-Stage Designs for Phase II Clinical Trials

7.1 Introduction

Phase II clinical trials are conducted to assess the efficacy of a new drug after a safe dose is identified from Phase I studies. The optimal dose(s) determined from the Phase II studies will be tested in the Phase III trials. Because of competition from other sponsors who develop drugs targeting the same patient population, timely completion of Phase II trials is a key factor of a successful clinical program. For these reasons, interim analyses are often planned to give the sponsor the option to terminate the study early for either efficacy, futility, or safety. Many frequentist methods for interim analysis have been proposed to control Type I error. However, due to logistic issues, it can be challenging to apply these methods. For example, among many other restrictions, they typically require a fixed number of patients at the time when an interim analysis is carried out. This may be impractical for multi-site and multi-region trials. Bayesian multi-stage designs provide greater flexibility as their inference is not affected by sample sizes or early termination of the study. In the Bayesian framework, either the posterior probability or predictive probability is continuously updated as new observations become available. Interim analysis can be performed on an on-going basis without incurring practical difficulties. In this chapter, we concern ourselves with a discussion of Bayesian multi-stage designs for early Phase II studies including both single-arm and comparative studies. The designs have the advantage that the trials may be stopped early for futility or efficacy or to continue. Two examples are provided to demonstrate how to implement Bayesian designs for both single-arm and comparative trials.

7.2 Phase II Clinical Trials

After the MTD of an experimental drug is determined through the Phase I dose-finding studies discussed in Chapter 5, the primary focus of clinical development shifts from safety to efficacy. Phase II studies are carried out to investigate the activity of the drug in the target patient population while gaining additional understanding of the drug safety (Green et al. 2002). These studies can be further divided into Phase IIa and Phase IIb. The former is used to screen out ineffective drugs whereas the latter to determine the most efficacious dose. Phase IIa studies are usually single-arm open-label trials. Typically, a multi-stage design is to enhance trial efficiency. The efficacy of the drug is compared to that of SOC, based on historical data (Simon 1989; Thall and Simon 1994a). If successful, the drug is tested in Phase IIb studies. The multi-stage feature is desirable as it allows for early stopping for either futility or efficacy; in addition to that, the design requires a smaller sample size than a single-stage study. Phase IIb studies are multi-arm trials comparing the efficacy of the drug in various dose levels and regimen with the standard care. Taken together, data generated from Phase II studies are used to aid the go/no-go decision regarding whether the drug is sufficiently efficacious to further investigation in large-scale Phase III trials.

7.3 Multi-stage Designs

7.3.1 Frequentist Approaches

Multi-stage designs have long been used for Phase II efficacy studies to increase trial efficiency. Early two-stage designs include the work by Gehan (1961) and Simon (1989). Both designs render the sponsor an early termination of the study due to futility. Simon's optimal design was constructed to minimize the expected sample size under the null hypothesis. An alternate design called minimax design is also considered by Simon (1989). It is aimed at minimizing the maximum sample size. In either case, Type I and Type II errors are controlled. Using different optimization criteria, many other multi-stage designs have been proposed. For example, Fleming (1982) proposed a one-sample multiple testing procedure which allows for early termination for futility or efficacy while preserving the size, power, and simplicity of the single-stage procedure; Bryant and Day (1995) suggested a two-stage design that simultaneously assesses both clinical response and toxicity; Jung et al. (2004) developed a family of two-stage designs that are admissible according to a Bayesian decision-theoretic criterion based on an ethically justifiable loss function. Several group sequential designs were suggested by Pocock (1977, 1982), and O'Brian and Fleming (1979) to allow for repeated testing.

Wang and Tsiatis (1987) and DeMets and Lan (1994) extended the early work by introducing the concept of alpha spending, which rendered greater flexibility in conducting interim analyses.

Although frequentist multi-stage designs in general increase the trial efficiency, they have several limitations. For example, they have the rigid requirement of fixed sample size at each stage of analysis, which is difficult to adhere to particularly in multi-center trials (Green and Dahlberg 1992; Lee and Liu 2008). In addition, Type I and Type II protection is not warranted if the actual interim analysis is not performed strictly in accordance with the original design. As pointed out by Lee and Liu (2008), these designs also lack a formal mechanism to terminate the trial early before the prespecified sample size is reached. The above-mentioned challenges make it difficult to implement the frequentist multi-stage designs and argue for more flexible alternatives.

7.3.2 Bayesian Methods

Several Bayesian multi-stage designs have been proposed in the literature (Thall and Simon 1994a, 1994b, 1995; Thall et al. 1995; Heitjan 1997; Jung et al. 2004; Lee and Liu 2008). Statistical inferences under these designs are based on either posterior probability (Thall and Simon 1994a) or predictive probability (Thall and Simon 1994b; Lee and Liu 2008), which incorporate both prior knowledge of parameters of interest, and interim data. Since the inferences are not constricted by the designs, they provide greater flexibility for interim analyses. In fact, the more interim analyses are performed, the required sample sizes diminishes in size. Since Bayesian methods depend on prior information from historical data or expert opinion, it is important to use robust methods to elicit priors. Further, interim analysis requires patient response data be available at the time of analysis, which might not be realistic for some situations in which it takes a long time to assess patient responses. Cai et al. (2014) suggested an approach that treats the delayed response as missing data and copes with them using an imputation method. In the following, we focus our discussion on the Bayesian design based on predictive probability by Lee and Liu (2008) and on the Bayesian continuous monitoring design based on posterior probability by Thall and Simon (1994).

7.3.3 Bayesian Single-Arm Trials

Consider an oncology study where the patient response is binary. The study is designed to test the hypotheses concerning a new therapy:

$$H_0: p \leq p_0 \text{ vs. } H_1: p > p_1$$

where p is the overall response rate of the new therapy, p_0 is the response rate of the standard of care, p_1 is the rate that represents a meaningful improvement of the new therapy over the SOC.

Assume that throughout the study, the treatment responses out of n patients enrolled follows a binomial distribution, binomial(n, p) with a prior distribution $p \sim \text{Beta}(a, b)$. The quantity $a / (a + b)$ is the mean of the prior distribution; whereas $a + b$ measures how informative the prior is. The above beta distribution can be parameterized in terms of these two quantities. Let $N_{\max}$ be the maximum number of patients to be entered in the study and let X_n be the number of responses observed in n patients currently in the study. Consequently, the posterior distribution of the response rate p follows a beta distribution,

$$p \mid X_n = x_n \sim \text{Beta}(a + x_n, b + n - x_n).$$

7.3.3.1 Go or No-Go Criteria

One set of "go or no-go criteria" is based on posterior probabilities of efficacy and futility. They are defined as follows:

1. Go criterion is met if $\Pr[p > p_1 \mid x_n] > P_E$;
2. No-Go criterion is met if $\Pr[p > p_1 \mid x_n] < P_F$;
3. Continue enrollment until one of the above decisions or the maximum sample size N_{Max} is reached,

where P_E and P_F are thresholds of efficacy and futility, respectively.

7.3.3.2 Predictive Probability

Let $m = N_{\text{Max}} - n$ be the number of potential patients to be enrolled in the second stage of the trial and Y the number of patients who respond to the therapy. Hence

$$Y \mid X_n = x_n \sim \text{Beta} - \text{binomial}(n, a + x_n, b + n + 1 - x_n - y).$$

Lee and Liu (2008) suggested that the decision of futility and efficacy be made based on the predictive probability of efficacy. The predictive probability measures the strength of a decision, given by

$$PP_E = E\{I(\Pr[p > p_1 \mid x_n, Y] > P_E)\}$$

$$= \int I\left(\Pr[p > p_1 \mid x_n, Y] > P_E\right) dP[Y \mid x_n]$$

$$= \sum_{i=0}^{m} \Pr[y = i \mid x_n] \times I\left(\Pr[p > p_1 \mid x_n, Y = i] > P_E\right)$$

where $I(.)$ is an indicator function, which assumes 1 or 0 depending on whether the event in the parentheses is true or not, and $\Pr[p > p_1 | x_n, Y = i]$ is the posterior probability.

Likewise, the predictive probability of futility can be estimated by

$$PP_F = \sum_{i=0}^{m} \Pr[y = i \mid x_n] \times I\left(\Pr[p > p_0 \mid x_n, Y = i] > P_F\right).$$

Efficacy and futility criteria are given below:

1. Declare efficacy if $PP_E > P_{1E}$;
2. Declare futility if $PP_F < P_{1F}$;
3. Continue enrollment till one of the above decisions or the maximum sample size $N_{\max}$ is reached,

where the cut points P_{1E} and P_{1F} are values between 0 and 1, e.g., 95% specified by the investigator.

In practice, the above continuous assessment is carried out after the data of an initial number of patients become available to render reliable estimates of probabilities (Cai et al. 2014). There are other methods suggested by various authors based on predictive probability. For example, Spiegelhalter et al. (2004) suggested a method using a prior and current data to calculate predictive probabilities of eventual classical conclusions.

7.3.4 Continuous Monitoring of Single-Arm Trials

Thall and Simon (1994) considered the setting of a single-arm study where the aim is to determine if a new therapy is promising relative to the SOC. The study can be terminated at any time for futility or efficacy. The decision is made based on the posterior probability $\Pr(x, n, \delta_0) = \Pr[p_1 > p_0 + \delta_0 | x_n = x]$ where δ_0 is a clinically meaningful difference. It was suggested that an informative prior and a flat or weakly informative prior be used for response rates p_0 and p_1 of the standard care and experimental drug, respectively. Assume that $p_i \sim \text{Beta}(a_i, b_i)$, $i = 0, 1$. Note that

$$p_1 \mid X_n = x_n \sim \text{Beta}(a_1 + x_n, b_1 + n - x_n).$$

the posterior probability Pr can be obtained by

$$\Pr(x_n, n, \delta_0) = \int_{0}^{1-\delta_0} \left[1 - F\left(p + \delta_0; a_1 + x_n, b_1 + n - x_n\right)\right] f\left(p; a_0, b_0\right) dp$$

where the functions $F(\cdot)$ and $f(\cdot)$ are the cumulative probability and density functions of Beta distributions.

Define

$$U_n = \text{the smallest integer } x \text{ such that } \Pr(x,n,0) \geq P_{2E}$$

$$L_n = \text{the largest integer } x \text{ such that } \Pr(x,n,\delta_0) \leq P_{2F}$$

where P_{2E} and P_{2F} are prespecified probabilities between 0 and 1 with P_{2E} being close to 1 and P_{2F} close to zero. It is worth noting that although these two probabilities resemble Type I error and power in the classical hypothesis testing setting, they bear very different meanings (Thall and Simon 1994).

Efficacy and futility decisions are made based on the following decision rules:

1. If $X_n \geq U_n$, declare efficacy.
2. If $X_n \leq L_n$, declare futility.
3. Otherwise, continue treating another patient.

The trial is deemed to be inconclusive if neither of the above first two conditions is met by the time when the maximum sample size $N_{\max}$ is reached.

7.3.5 Comparative Phase II Studies

Single-arm Phase II studies rely on historical data of the SOC. The robustness of the data has an impact on the quality of the study design. In the absence of such data, it is necessary to conduct a randomized trial to demonstrate the efficacy of a new drug relative to the SOC. If the comparator is newly approved for the same indication, it also entails the needs of comparative trials. In these situations, the above Bayesian design with continuous efficacy and futility assessment can be extended to include "go and no-go criteria" based on either posterior or predictive probabilities of efficacy or futility. Suppose that the primary endpoint is binary. Let X_{n_1} and Y_{m_1} be the observed responses from the experiment drug arm and SOC arm, respectively, which have response rates of p_1 and p_0. The corresponding decisions of efficacy and futility rules based on posterior and predictive probabilities are detailed below.

7.3.5.1 Efficacy and Futility Based on Posterior Probability

1. Go: $\Pr\left[p_1 - p_0 > \delta_0 \mid X_{n_1} = x_{n_1}, Y_{m_1} = y_{m_1}\right] > P_{E_1}$;
2. No-go: $\Pr\left[p_1 - p_0 > \delta_0 \mid X_{n_1} = x_{n_1}, Y_{m_1} = y_{m_1}\right] < P_{F_1}$;
3. Continue enrollment till one of the above decisions or the maximum sample size $N_{\max}$ is reached,

where P_{E1} and P_{E2} are response rates of the new drug and its comparator, respectively.

7.3.5.2 Efficacy and Futility Criteria Based on Predictive Probability

1. Declare efficacy if predictive probability $PP\{\Pr[p_1 - p_0 > \delta_0 | X_{n_1} = x_{n_1}, Y_{m_1} = y_{m_1}] > P_{E_1}\} > P_1$.
2. Declare futility if predictive probability $PP\{\Pr[p_1 - p_0 > \delta_0 | X_{n_1} = x_{n_1}, Y_{m_1} = y_{m_1}] > P_{E_1}\} > P_2$.
3. Continue enrollment till one of the above decisions or the maximum sample size $N_{\max}$ is reached.

Like for the method discussed in the previous section, it is assumed that $X_{n_1} \sim \text{binomial}(n_1, p_1)$ and $Y_{m_1} \sim \text{binomial}(m_1, p_0)$ and that beta priors, $\text{Beta}(a_i, b_i), i = 0,1$, are chosen for p_0 and p_1, respectively. Under these distributional assumptions, we can obtain the posterior distributions:

$$p_0 \,|\, Y_{m_1} = y_{m_1} \sim \text{Beta}\left(a_0 + y_{m_1}, b_0 + m - y_{m_1}\right)$$

$$p_1 \,|\, X_{n_1} = x_{n_1} \sim \text{Beta}\left(a_1 + x_{n_1}, b_1 + n_1 - x_{n_1}\right).$$

Thus, the posterior probability $\Pr\left[p_1 - p_0 > \delta_0 |\, X_{n_1} = x_{n_1}, Y_{m_1} = y_{m_1}\right]$ can be calculated as follows:

$$\Pr\left(x_{n_1}, n_1, y_{m_1}, m_1, \delta_0\right)$$

$$= \int_0^{1-\delta_0} \left[1 - F\left(p + \delta_0; a_1 + x_n, b_1 + n - x_n\right)\right] f\left(p; a_0 + y_{m_1}, b_0 + m - y_{m_1}\right) dp$$

where the functions $F(\cdot)$ and $f(\cdot)$ are the cumulative probability and density functions of Beta distributions.

Likewise, the predictive probabilities of efficacy and futility can be derived:

$$PP_E = \sum_{i=0}^{n_1} \sum_{j=0}^{m_1} \Pr\left[x = i \,|\, x_{n_1}\right] \Pr\left[y = j \,|\, y_{m_1}\right]$$

$$\times I\left(\Pr\left[p_1 - p_0 > \delta_0 |\, X_{n_1} = x_{n_1}, Y_{m_1} = y_{m_1}\right] > P_{E_1}\right)$$

$$PP_F = \sum_{i=0}^{n_1} \sum_{j=0}^{m_1} \Pr\left[x = i \,|\, x_{n_1}\right] \Pr\left[y = j \,|\, y_{m_1}\right]$$

$$\times I\left(\Pr\left[p_1 - p_0 > \delta_0 |\, X_{n_1} = x_{n_1}, Y_{m_1} = y_{m_1}\right] < P_{F_1}\right).$$

7.4 Examples

In this section, we use an example to illustrate the Bayesian continuous monitoring for a single-arm study. The early stopping rules are based on the predictive probability method described in Section 7.3.5. The second example concerns a multi-stage Bayesian Phase II trial, which is used to demonstrate the efficacy of an anti-inflammatory drug and determine an optimal dose for Phase III trials. The Bayesian design was used to shorten the time of the Phase II study.

7.4.1 Oncology Trial

Consider a Phase II oncology trial with treated and control arms with 2:1 allocation, in which a maximum of 60 patients is planned and the first interim look takes place when the responses of the first 24 treated-arm subjects and 12 control-arm subjects are observed. Let p_C and p_T respectively denote the probability of a response in the control and treated arms. Efficacy, futility, or continuation rules are given by:

1. Declare efficacy if predictive probability $PP\{\Pr[p_T - p_C > 0.2|\,\text{data}] > 0.7\} > 0.9$.
2. Declare futility if predictive probability $PP\{\Pr[p_T - p_C > 0.2|\,\text{data}] < 0.1\} > 0.9$.
3. Otherwise, continue to full enrollment of 40 total treated-arm and 20 total control-arm patients.

Let x_C and x_T denote the number of responders (out of n_C and n_T) at interim. Assume uninformative priors $p_C, p_T \sim \text{Beta}(\tfrac{1}{2}, \tfrac{1}{2})$. Assume that historical literature/data point to $p_C = 0.2$ and $p_T = 0.45$. This information is used to identify the most likely final set of trial observations.

Note that for $i = C, T$,

$$p_i \,|\, \text{data} \sim \text{Beta}\left(\frac{1}{2} + x_i, \frac{1}{2} + n_i - x_i\right).$$

Thus,

$$\Pr[p_T - p_C > 0.2 \,|\, \text{data}]$$

$$= \int_0^1 \left\{ 1 - F\left(0.2 + p; \frac{1}{2} + x_T, \frac{1}{2} + n_T - x_T\right) \right\} f\left(p; \frac{1}{2} + x_C, \frac{1}{2} + n_C - x_C\right) dp,$$

where $f(.)$ and $F(.)$ denote the beta distribution pdf and cdf.

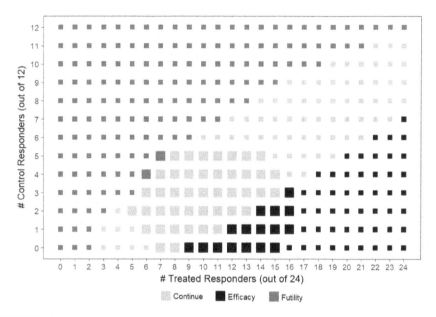

FIGURE 7.1
Conditioned on the interim data (x and y axes), the graph shows areas of high probability to stop for efficacy and futility or to otherwise continue the trial. Conditioned on $p_C = 0.2$ and $p_T = 0.45$, the larger box size shows a zone that is 95% likely to be observed.

Conditioned on the interim data, the predictive probability calculations are given in the computer code that follows. Figure 7.1 shows the zones of (x_C, x_T) that are 95% likely under $p_C = 0.2$ and $p_T = 0.45$ and the conditions under which the trial should be stopped early for efficacy/futility or continued.

```
## Clinicians best guess at probability of responder
for control and treated arms
pC = 0.2
pT = 0.45

  ## nC, nT = number of control and treated subjects
  at interim
  ## xC, xT = number of control and treated responders
  at interim
d.grid = expand.grid( nC=12, nT=24, xC=0:12, xT=0:24 )

  ## Determine a zone for which 95% of subjects will
  fall
  ## Probability that xC out of nC and xT out of nT
  are observed
d.grid$Prob.obs = dbinom(d.grid$xC, size=d.grid$nC,
                   prob=pC) *
```

```
                              dbinom(d.grid$xT, size=d.grid$nT,
                              prob=pT)
  p.seq = seq(0, 0.05, length=1000)
  pr = sapply( p.seq, function(p0){
              sum( d.grid$Prob.obs[d.grid$Prob.obs >=
              p0] ) })
  p.lim =p.seq[ which.min( abs(pr-0.95) ) ]
  d.grid$Zone95 = d.grid$Prob.obs >= p.lim

  ## Function for Pr( pT - pC > 0.2 )
  prob.diff = function(a0, b0, a1, b1)
  {
    ## Pr( Y - X > 0.2 ), where X ~ beta(a0, b0), y ~
       beta(a1, b1)
    int.func = function(z){ exp(
                pbeta(0.2+z, a1, b1, lower.tail=FALSE,
                log.p=TRUE) +
                                      dbeta(z, a0, b0,
                                      log=TRUE) ) }

    integrate(int.func, lower=0, upper=1)$value
  }

  d.grid$Prob.pp.go = d.grid$Prob.pp.no.go = NA
  d.grid$pp.go = d.grid$pp.no.go = NA
  set.seed(554)
  for ( i in 1:nrow(d.grid) )
  {

    ## Posterior distribution of pC and pT
    pC.post = rbeta(10000, 0.5+d.grid$xC[i], 0.5+d.
                grid$nC[i] -
                      d.grid$xC[i])
    pT.post = rbeta(10000, 0.5+d.grid$xT[i], 0.5+d.
                grid$nT[i] -
                      d.grid$xT[i])


    ## Original data + posterior predictive distribution
       for
    ##   remainder of study subjects
    ## These follow a beta-binomial distribution
    yC = d.grid$xC[i] + rbinom(10000, size=20-d.
    grid$nC[i], prob=pC.post)
```

```
yT = d.grid$xT[i] + rbinom(10000, size=40-d.
grid$nT[i], prob=pT.post)

## Posterior predictive distribution of Pr( p1-p0 >
    0.2 | data )
pdiff.pp = sapply(1:10000, function(b){
                    prob.diff(a0=0.5+yC[b],
                    b0=0.5+20-yC[b],
                            a1=0.5+yT[b], b1=0.5+40-
                            yT[b]) } )
## Posterior predictive efficacy probability
d.grid$Prob.pp.go[i] = mean(pdiff.pp > 0.7)
d.grid$pp.go[i] = d.grid$Prob.pp.go[i] > 0.9

## Posterior predictive futility probability
d.grid$Prob.pp.no.go[i] = mean(pdiff.pp < 0.1)
d.grid$pp.no.go[i] = d.grid$Prob.pp.no.go[i] > 0.9

}

d.grid$GoZone = factor( ifelse( d.grid$pp.go,
                "Efficacy",
                        ifelse(d.grid$pp.no.go,
                        "Futility", "Continue") ) )
```

Figure 7.1 provides the investigator with a convenient way to make a decision regarding terminating the trial for futility or efficacy or continuing the enrollment at the interim look where the responses of the first 24 treated-arm subjects and 12 control-arm subjects are observed. For example, suppose that 14 out of 24 patients from the treatment arm and 2 out of 12 patients from the control have positive responses. From the graph, the study should be stopped to declare efficacy.

7.4.2 Multi-Stage Bayesian Design

The drug under evaluation is an anti-inflammatory agent. One drug in the same class has been shown to have a desirable safety and efficacy profile. The objectives of this Phase II trial were to demonstrate the efficacy of the agent with an improved dose regimen. Specifically, a dosing schedule of every four weeks was to be explored as the dose regimen of the other drug was every two weeks. A Bayesian design with multiple interim looks is desirable as it would shorten the duration of Phase II trial. In addition, information from the competitor's clinical program can be used to define effect size and go/no-go criteria. A brief description of the study design is given in Table 7.1.

TABLE 7.1

Study Design of a Bayesian Phase II Trial

Objective	To demonstrate efficacy and determine an optimal dose regimen
Patient population	Patients with a severe inflammatory disease
Design	Randomized and placebo-controlled Bayesian Phase II with multiple interim looks
Treatment	Every four weeks, infusion of either drug at 100mg, 200mg, 400 mg, 800 mg, or placebo for 16 weeks
Primary endpoint	Flaring of the disease at week 16
Maximum study duration	52 weeks
Maximum sample size	200

From the results of the competitor's trial, it was determined that a difference δ of 15% between the treatment arm and placebo is deemed to be a clinically meaningful improvement. Therefore, the go/no-go decision was defined based on posterior probability of δ:

1. Go if $\Pr[\delta \geq 15\%] > 80\%$ for any dose;
2. No-go if $\Pr[\delta \geq 15\%] < 20\%$ for all doses,

where $\Pr[\delta \geq 15\%]$ is the posterior probability for the difference in response rate between a dose of the drug and the placebo.

Patients are assumed to enroll in the trial at a constant rate of 20 subjects per week and are randomized into the five treatment arms with 1:1:1:1:1 allocation. Measurements are taken on each patient every four weeks over the course of 16 weeks, yielding four observations per patient. To ensure the reliability of the interim analysis, the first interim look takes place after 16 weeks, after the first 80 subjects have been enrolled so that 20 patients provide a full four weeks of data, 20 patients provide three weeks of data, and so on. Further interim looks occur every eight weeks until a total of 200 patients provide the full four weeks of data.

Patients are evaluated at each time point and are given binary ratings by investigators with observations $Y_{ij}=1$ if the disease state showed improvement or $Y_{ij}=0$ otherwise, with $i=1$ (placebo), 2, ..., 5 (dose = 800 mg) indexing the doses and $j=1, 2, ..., n_i$ indexing the patients on dose i and with $(n_1 + ... + n_5) = 200$.

The dose–response relationship among the treatment groups was described through a random-effect logistic model with $\Pr(Y_{ij}=1)=p_{ij}$ and

$$\log\left[\frac{p_{ij}}{1-p_{ij}}\right] = \theta_{ij}$$

TABLE 7.2

Specifications of Prior Distributions

Prior	Parameter Specification
$E_0 \sim N(\mu_0, \sigma_0^2)$	$(\mu_0, \sigma_0^2) = (-2, 0.5^2)$, with $\mu_0 = -2$ corresponding to 12% response rate of the placebo observed in the competitor's study
$E_{max} \sim N(\mu_m, \sigma_m^2)$	$(\mu_m, \sigma_m^2) = (2, 0.5^2)$.
$E_{50} \sim N^+(\mu_{50}, \sigma_{50}^2)$	E_{50} follows a truncated normal distribution with $(\mu_{50}, \sigma_{50}^2) = (200, 50^2)$
$\sigma_e^2 \sim IG(sh_0, sc_0)$	$(sh_0, sc_0) = (2, 0.3)$. Median value of σ_e is 1.4 with middle 95% of distribution from 0.8 to 3.8

where θ_{ij} is a random variable following a normal distribution with Emax-model mean given by

$$\theta_{ij} = E_0 + \frac{dose_i E_{max}}{dose_i + E_{50}} + \epsilon_{ij}$$

with $\epsilon_{ij} \sim N(0, \sigma_e^2)$ denoting the subject-to-subject errors.

The posterior probability at each interim look can be estimated using the MCMC method and the priors in Table 7.2. At each interim, the random-effect logistic model was fitted to the data using the JAGS model code given below.

```
model.txt = "
  model{
    ## Priors
    E0   ~ dnorm(-2, 4.)   ## SD = 0.5
    Emax ~ dnorm(2, 4.)    ## SD = 0.5
    E50  ~ dnorm(200., 0.0004)T(0., )   ## SD = 50
    tau  ~ dgamma(2, 0.3)

    sigma <- 1/sqrt(tau)   ## sigma has median 1.4, 95%
    range: 0.8 - 3.8.

    ## Likelihood
    for ( i in 1:nDose )   ## Population mean for each
                                dose
    {
       mu[i] <- E0 + Emax*x[i]/(E50+x[i])
    }
    for ( j in 1:nSubject )   ## Subject errors
    {
       thetaSubj[j] ~ dnorm( 0., tau )
```

```
    }

    for ( k in 1:N )   ## Logistic model
    {
        ## p[k] = 1/(1+exp(-(mu+error)))
        logit(p[k]) <- mu[ dose[k] ]
        + thetaSubj[ subject[k] ]
        Y[k] ~ dbern( p[k] )
    }

}"
```

To evaluate the go/no-Go probabilities for a particular scenario, a small Monte Carlo study was run with 100 computer-generated data sets. Data were generated so that the respective true probabilities to show improvement are 12%, 20%, 28%, 35%, and 48% for placebo, 100mg, 200mg, 400mg, and 800 mg, respectively. The subject error standard deviation was set to $\sigma_e = 1.25$, with errors assigned around the logit link function to the true probabilities. Finally, the four patient responses were assumed to be independent. Data were generated according to the following R function:

```
create.data = function()
{
  nSubj = 200
  dose = c(0, 100, 200, 400, 800)          ## Doses
  p = c(0.12, 0.2, 0.28, 0.35, 0.48)     ## Probability
                                          of improvement
  theta = log(p/(1-p))   ## Logit of p.

  ## Create full data set
  d = data.frame(Subject=rep(1:nSubj, each=4),
                  Time=rep(1:4, nSubj), Y=NA)
  d$Period = ceiling(d$Subject/20)-1 + d$Time
                  ## Set period = 4 weeks
  dose.index = sample(1:4, nSubj, replace=TRUE)
                  ## Randomly assign dose
  d$Dose.index = dose.index[d$Subject]
  d$Dose = dose[d$Dose.index]

  ## Assign hierarchical probability model with
     subject errors
  theta.subj = rnorm(nSubj, mean=0, sd=sigma)
  d$p.subj = 1/(1+exp(-(theta[d$Dose.index] + theta.
             subj[d$Subject])))
```

```
## Get four indepedent binary responses per patient
d = do.call("rbind", by(d, d$Subject, function(d0){
            d0 = d0[order(d0$Time),]
            d0$Y = rbinom(4, size=1, prob=
            d0$p.subj[1])
            return(d0) }))

return(d)
}
```

Finally, the Monte Carlo simulation code in R is given below. Note that, given the long-run time for the simulation, we opted to run the code on a computer that would permit the use of eight independent MCMC.

```
B = 100    ## number of Monte Carlo runs
res = matrix(NA, B*4, 8)   ## Hold the results
k = 1
for ( b in 1:B )
{
  d = create.data()   ## Create full data set
  for ( period in seq(4, 13, by=3) )
                    ## Each period = 4 weeks
  {
    d0 = subset(d, Period <= period)
                    ## Interim data set

    ## The data for JAGS
    data = list( N=nrow(d0), nSubject=max(d0$Subject),
                nDose=length(dose), x=dose,
                subject=d0$Subject,
                dose=d0$Dose.index, Y=d0$Y )
    ## Run JAGS
    fitb = run.jags( model.txt, data=data,
            monitor=c("mu", "E0", "Emax", "E50",
            "sigma"),
            n.chains=8, burnin=5000, sample=7000,
            thin=15,
            modules="glm", method="parallel" )
    ## Get posterior of population probabilities for
      each dose
    th.post = as.matrix( as.mcmc.list(fitb) )
    p.post = 1/(1+exp(-th.post[,c("mu[1]", "mu[2]",
                                "mu[3]", "mu[4]",
                                "mu[5]")])))
```

```
## Calculate P( delta > 0.15 ) for each dose.  P >
   80% = Go
prob.go.15 = sapply(2:5, function(i){
                    mean( p.post[,i] - p.post[,1] >=
                    0.15 ) })

res[k,] = c(b, period, max(d0$Subject),
sum(d0$Time==4),
                                          prob.go.15)

k = k + 1
  }
}
```

The "go probabilities" (i.e., Pr[δ ≥ 15%]) are shown via box plot in Figure 7.2 and summarized in Table 7.3. Given the simulated scenario, the results are quite promising, showing a borderline chance for a "go" to occur for the

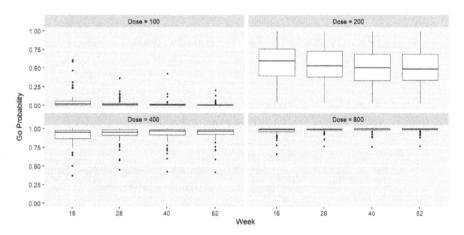

FIGURE 7.2
Box plot of Pr[δ ≥ 15%] for each dose at selected interim looks.

TABLE 7.3

Average Value of Pr[δ ≥ 15%] and, Parenthetically, Percentage of Runs (Out of 100) that Pr[δ ≥ 15%] > 80%

	Dose (mg)			
	100	200	400	800
Week 16	3% (0%)	38% (15%)	79% (70%)	93% (93%)
Week 28	1% (0%)	34% (10%)	80% (66%)	94% (96%)
Week 40	1% (0%)	31% (12%)	80% (66%)	95% (97%)
Week 52	1% (0%)	30% (9%)	81% (67%)	95% (98%)

400 mg dose and high likelihood for a "go" to occur at the highest (800 mg) dose. In fact, the "go" probability is high throughout the interim looks, which can prompt investigators to halt the trial for efficacy at an early time point.

In a final note to this example, given the Emax dose–response model in the JAGS code, it is also possible to calculate "go" posterior probabilities for interpolated doses. For example, for a dose of 600 mg, the following code might be inserted.

```
dose.600 = 600
mu.600 = th.post[,"E0"] + th.post[,"Emax"]*dose.600 /
                          (th.post[,"E50"]+dose.600)
p.600 = 1/(1+exp(-mu.600))
go.600 = mean( p.600- p.post[,1] > 0.15 )
```

In fact, taking one more step, the smallest dose that produces $\Pr(\delta \geq 15\%)$ > 80% may be reported for each Monte Carlo run so that the strategy may change to a dose-finding exercise.

7.5 Concluding Remarks

The primary focus of Phase II trials is to screen out inefficacious drugs and determine an optimal dose regimen of an efficacious drug for larger-scale Phase III confirmatory studies. Phase II studies are typically conducted with 100–300 patients. To increase the efficiency of Phase II programs, Phase II trials are sometimes carried out in two parts: Phase IIa and Phase IIb. The former is used to demonstrate the activity of the drug; whereas the latter is to find the optimum dose regimen. Phase IIa studies are typically conducted using a single-arm design, in which the efficacy of the drug is compared with that of the standard care based on historical controls. The conclusions drawn from Phase IIa studies depend on the reliability of the efficacy data of the comparator therapy. By comparison, Phase IIb are multi-arm studies which compare the efficacy of different doses (regimens) of the drug against the standard care. Phase II studies often use multi-stage designs to shorten the duration of studies. The efficiency is gained by utilizing information from the interim data to make an early go or no-go decision based on efficacy, futility, or safety. Although both frequentist and Bayesian multi-stage designs are readily available, Bayesian designs afford greater flexibility in trial conduct and are more advantageous in decision-making through utilizing relevant information both internal and external to the current trial. Therefore, they are much more suitable for Phase II clinical trials.

Section III

Chemistry, Manufacturing, and Control

8

Analytical Methods

8.1 Introduction

Analytical methods are broadly used across all aspects of drug research and development to quantify risk and aid decision-making. In early drug discovery, analytical results provide critical information for lead drug selection. During clinical development of the lead drug, analytical tests are performed to qualify clinical trial materials, evaluate clinical performance, and determine optimal dosing regimens. For a marketed product, analytical testing is an integral component of lot release to ensure the quality, safety, and efficacy of the product. In recent years, analytical methods have risen to prominence in biosimilar development as the analytical similarity between the proposed biosimilar and reference product became the foundation for marketing approval (EMA 2014, 2017; FDA 2015, 2016, 2017). For these reasons, analytical methods are a critical component of pharmaceutical quality systems. Because of its potential impact, an analytical method must be validated for its intended purposes. In addition, an analytical method should demonstrate sufficient robustness to be transferred from R&D labs to manufacturing sites. For these reasons, various statistical methods have been developed, albeit the majority of them based on frequentist methodologies. The validity of these methods often depends on normality assumptions of the random components of the analytical response. When a closed-form solution is unattainable, statistical inference based on these methods can be intractable. Bayesian methods, aided by the simulation-based computation tool, provide flexibility in model assumptions. This chapter focuses on Bayesian approaches for both analytical method validation and transfer. Several examples are also included to illustrate the Bayesian methods.

8.2 Method Validation

8.2.1 Background

Analytical methods play an important role in assessing the quality, safety, and efficacy of a drug product throughout its lifecycle. As such, analytical methods need to be validated for their intended purposes. Validation of analytical methods is also a regulatory requirement (EMA 1995; FDA 2015. ICH 1995, 2005). For example, it is clearly stated in the FDA guidance (2015) that "[e]ach NDA and ANDA must include the analytical procedures necessary to ensure the identity, strength, quality, purity, and potency of the drug substance and drug product. Each BLA must include a full description of the manufacturing process, including analytical procedures that demonstrate the manufactured product meets prescribed standards of identity, quality, safety, purity, and potency. Data must be available to establish that the analytical procedures used in testing meet proper standards of accuracy, sensitivity, specificity, and reproducibility and are suitable for their intended purpose." The regulatory guidelines also provide general concepts for method validation and stipulate on specific requirements for performance characteristics. For example, ICH Q2 (R1) (2005) recommends lists of validation characteristics for four types of analytical methods, namely, identification tests for active product ingredients (APIs), quantitative test for APIs, quantitative tests for impurity, and qualitative or limit tests for impurity content. Typical performance characteristics include accuracy, precision, specificity, linearity, range, detection limit, and quantitation limit.

Traditionally, method validation was viewed as a one-time exercise. As such, it lacked the ability to provide a high degree of assurance that the method would perform well after being transferred from the development lab to the quality control department (Borman et al. 2007). Ermer and Nethercote (2015) further noted that validation studies conducted under a strictly controlled environment do not capture all sources of variations which may be encountered in the real-life setting. Consequently, it is challenging to develop control strategies to mitigate the potential risk of performance drift of the analytical method. In recent years, in keeping with the regulatory initiatives of applying quality by design (QbD) principles for developing robust manufacturing processes, various researchers suggested the use of the QbD concepts to gain enhanced understanding of sources of variability and better control of analytical method performance (Borman et al. 2007; Nethercote et al. 2010; Nethercote and Ermer 2012; Martin et al. 2013).

Method validation and transfer consist of a series of experiments, aimed at assessing various aspects of the method performance. A systematic approach for using DOE for analytical method development and validation is discussed by Little (2014). Key considerations include experimental objectives, sample size, experimental conditions, and ranges, all of which need to be defined in a study protocol. Statistical methods of data analysis and acceptance criteria need to be well described before the experiments are carried out (Yu and Yang 2017). It is equally important to verify the assumptions of the models used to describe the data. Various statistical methods have been suggested for method validation and transfer. Burdick et al. (2013a, 2013b) discussed methods for the setting of acceptance criteria and the use of confidence interval approaches for method accuracy and precision. Based on Fieller's Theorem (Fieller 1944), LeBlond et al. (2013) proposed a test for testing linearity over a range. The test, however, does not control the overall Type I error. To address this issue, alternate tests based on generalized confidence intervals were suggested by Novick and Yang (2013) and Yang, Novick, and LeBlond (2015). For method transfer, equivalence testing is usually recommended to demonstrate comparable performance of the analytical method between sites (Kringle et al. 2001). More recently, spurred on by the QbD concepts in ICH Q8(R2) (ICH 2008), several authors proposed a total error approach to determine the range of concentrations for which the analytical method jointly provides acceptable accuracy, intermediate precision, and repeatability (Kringle and Khan-Malek 1994; Findlay et al. 2000; Miller et al. 2001; Boulanger et al. 2003; DeSilva et al. 2003; Lee et al. 2006; Hubert et al. 2004, 2007a, 2007b; Yang and Zhang 2015). These researchers explored a range of interval methods including β-expectation tolerance intervals, β-content tolerance intervals, and generalized pivotal quantities (GPQ) for validation based on total error. Rozet et al. (2011) and more recently Sondag et al. (2016) discussed the utility of Bayesian inference in method validation. Zeng et al. (2018) proposed a general framework for equivalence testing and applied the method for assay transfer. In the following sections, we primarily concern ourselves with method validation with respect to accuracy and precision and method transfer using Bayesian approaches.

8.2.2 Study Design for Validation of Accuracy and Precision

8.2.2.1 Design Considerations

As discussed above, in method validation, it is important to consider the DOE so that statistical inferences can be made regarding validation parameters. Factors that impact method accuracy and precision need to be identified through a risk assessment process, based on prior knowledge and data collected during the method development (Little 2014). The concentration levels or range to be validated also need to be defined beforehand. The range typically includes three levels with the third given as the expected results for the sample. If the range is not firmly determined before validation, it is advisable to include more than three levels for the validation (Burdick et al. 2013a, 2013b).

To estimate intermediate precision, levels of typically uncontrolled experimental factors (e.g., operator, day, device) must be varied.

In the following, for the sake of simplicity, we assume that the analyst and day are deemed to be important factors impacting the method accuracy and precision. A typical validation experiment involves multiple analysts testing replicate samples for multiple days (runs). The response can be described by the model:

$$Y_{ijk} = \mu_i + A_j + R_k + e_{ijk}, \tag{8.1}$$

where Y_{ijk} is the measured assay response (e.g., relative potency) for the ith dilution/concentration, jth analyst, and kth run, μ_i is the mean assay response for the ith dilution/concentration, $A_j \sim N(0, \sigma_A^2)$, is the analyst effect, $R_k \sim N(0, \sigma_R^2)$ is the run effect, and $e_{ijk} \sim N(0, \sigma_e^2)$ is the residual error.

Balancing between statistical rigor and costs, a planned validation experiment often contains measurements from 1 to 3 analysts who, through a nested design, measure samples across 3–4 days. Such an undertaking, however, provides little independent information on the analyst-to-analyst variance component and only a modest amount of information on day-to-day variability. Thus, prior knowledge of the variance components can play an important role in the analysis and interpretation of method validation data. For these reasons, Bayesian methods are well suited for analytical method validation.

8.2.3 Current Statistical Methods

8.2.3.1 Definitions

In regulatory guidance (ICH 1995; FDA 1995), it is defined that "the accuracy of an analytical procedure expresses the closeness of agreement between the value which is accepted either as a conventional true value or an accepted reference value and the value found." Additionally, precision is defined as "the closeness of agreement (degree of scatter) of a series of measurements obtained from multiple sampling from the same homogenous sample under the same conditions." It is the degree of agreement among individual response values of the analytical method. There are various sources of variations such as analyst and day that may contribute to the overall variability of the measurements. Precision can be evaluated at three levels: repeatability, intermediate precision, and reproducibility. Repeatability corresponds to variability due to replicate testing of the same sample by a single analyst, who uses the same instrument on the same day. In other words, repeatability is intra-instrument variation. Variations due to factors within a single laboratory are called intermediate precision. Reproducibility is related to the difference among different testing laboratories running the same method.

8.2.3.2 Methods

Let μ_T denote the true value of the analytical method response. From Model (8.1) we obtain:

$$Y_{ijk} - \mu_T = \mu_i - \mu_T + A_j + R_k + e_{ijk}.$$

It is evident that the closeness between the measurement and true value can be quantified by the difference $\mu_i - \mu_T$ and the precision related to the three random components A_j, R_k, and e_{ijk}. As a result, validation of accuracy can be achieved through the validation of method bias and precision. Current statistical methods used for validation of accuracy and precision fall in two categories: point and interval estimates (Yang 2015). The point estimate approach considers accuracy and precision acceptable if their respective estimates fall within prespecified ranges. For example, in the FDA guidance (FDA 2001), it is recommended that the precision determined at each concentration level should not exceed 15% of the coefficient of variation (CV). This method, however, obviously lacks in statistical rigor as it does not consider the sample size and associated uncertainties in the point estimates. Various confidence interval-based approaches have been proposed (Burdick et al. 2013a, 2013b). These methods are appealing as they not only provide an informative summary of the accuracy and precision but can also be used to perform a statistical hypothesis testing against predefined acceptance criteria. For detailed discussion, see Burdick et al. (2013a, 2013b) and Yang (2015).

8.2.4 Total Error Approach

The validation of accuracy and precision of the analytical method is often carried out with separate specifications for each validation parameter. This approach lacks the direct link between the assay performance and its intended purpose, which is a guarantee that a high percentage of the test results of future samples will be close to their true values. The "total error" approach (Boulanger et al. 2003; DeSilva et al. 2003) provides an alternative to the examination of each validation model parameter. Consider the hypotheses

$$H_0: \Pr\left[-\lambda < Y - \mu_T < \lambda\right] \leq \beta \text{ vs. } H_a: \Pr\left[-\lambda < Y - \mu_T < \lambda\right] > \beta \qquad (8.2)$$

where Y is the assay response on the original scale, μ_T is the true value, which is assumed to be known, $\lambda > 0$ is an acceptable limit consistently defined based on the intent of the method, and β is the desired probability for a future measurement to have the total error $Y - \mu_T$ within the limits of $\pm\lambda$.

Hubert et al. discussed a testing strategy for Hypotheses (8.2) based on a β-expectation tolerance interval (2004, 2007a, 2007b). Since a β-expectation tolerance interval is the same as the commonly known $100\beta\%$ prediction interval for a single future observation (Hahn and Meeker 1991; Yang 2015), the above strategy intuitively makes sense. Various β-expectation tolerance interval approaches were also suggested by other authors (Govaerts et al. 2008; Hoffman and Kringle 2007). Alternatively, based on similar probabilistic considerations, several β-content tolerance intervals were also proposed for method validation based on total error (Boulanger, Devanaryan et al. 2007; Boulanger, Dewe et al. 2007; Govaerts et al. 2008; Hoffman and Kringle 2007). Yang and Zhang (2015) developed a method based on generalized pivotal quantity analysis (2015), demonstrating that, when the acceptance criterion in Hypotheses (8.2) is one-sided, the β-content tolerance interval is an exact method that retains a test size of 0.05, thus protecting Type I error or consumer's risk. Through simulation, among other findings, Yang and Zhang (2015) also show that the GPQ method and the method based on a β-content tolerance interval with a confidence level of 90% both control Type I error, while a survey of five existing methods showed that the historical methods do not. The paper by Yang and Zhang (2015) provides a useful guide for selecting test methods for testing the hypotheses in Hypotheses (8.2).

8.2.5 Bayesian Solutions

Bayesian credible intervals based on posterior distributions, $\pi(\mu_i \,|\, \text{data})$, $\pi(\sigma_A^2 \,|\, \text{data})$, $\pi(\sigma_R^2 \,|\, \text{data})$, $\pi(\sigma_e^2 \,|\, \text{data})$ can be used to validate accuracy and precision. For example, the method is validated if the 95% credible intervals for μ_i and the total %CV (i.e., the %CV based on the sum of σ_A^2, σ_R^2, and σ_e^2) are within the ranges of $\mu_T - 10\%$, $\mu_T + 10\%$ and [0, 20%], respectively. If the validation were to be based on the total error, a Bayesian β-expectation tolerance interval can be constructed and used for the validation. For balanced designs, Wolfinger (1998) suggests a simulation-based method to obtain the Bayesian intervals. The method is also discussed by Krishnamoorthy and Mathew (2009). Other Bayesian methods for method validation were proposed (Rozet et al. 2011; Saffaj and Ihssane 2012; Burdick et al. 2013b). Following Krishnamoorthy and Mathew (2009), Saffaj and Ihssane (2011) describe an algorithm for constructing β-expectation tolerance intervals, based on simulation. A β-expectation tolerance interval is a 100β% credible interval for the posterior predictive distribution for the assay response. In other words, it is a Bayesian 100β% prediction interval.

For the purpose of illustration, we briefly describe the method by Saffaj and Ihssane (2011). Assume that prior knowledge suggests that the run to run variability is negligible. Therefore, Model (8.1) can be reduced to a one-factor random model:

$$Y_{ij} = \mu_i + A_j + e_{ij}. \tag{8.3}$$

Let $\bar{\bar{X}}$, SSA, and SSE be the sample mean, between-run, and within-run sum of squares:

$$\bar{\bar{X}} = \sum_{i=1}^{n_a} \sum_{j=1}^{n_w} X_{ij}$$

$$SSA = n_w \sum_{i=1}^{n_a} \left(\bar{X}_i - \bar{\bar{X}} \right)^2$$

$$SSE = \sum_{i=1}^{n_a} \sum_{j=1}^{n_w} (X_{ij} - \bar{X})^2$$

where $\bar{X}_i = \dfrac{1}{n_a} \sum_{j=1}^{n_w} X_{ij}$.

Hence, conditioned on the parameters,

$$\bar{\bar{X}} \sim N\left(\mu, \frac{n_w \sigma_a^2 + \sigma_e^2}{n_a n_w} \right)$$

$$\frac{SSA}{n_w \sigma_a^2 + \sigma_e^2} \sim \chi_{n_a}^2$$

$$\frac{SSE}{\sigma_e^2} \sim \chi_{n_a(n_w-1)}^2.$$

Therefore, the likelihood of the observed data is the product of the joint distributions of the three sufficient statistics of Equation (8.3). Paired with a Jeffrey's non-informative prior of $(\mu, \sigma_a^2, \sigma_e^2)$,

$$p(\mu, \sigma_a^2, \sigma_e^2) \propto \frac{1}{\sigma_e^2 (n_w \sigma_a^2 + \sigma_e^2)} \tag{8.4}$$

it can be shown that the posterior distributions of $\sigma_A^2 (\equiv n_w \sigma_a^2 + \sigma_e^2)$ σ_e^2 and the conditional posterior distribution of μ are given by Krishnamoorthy and Mathew (2009),

$$\sigma_A^2 \mid \bar{\bar{X}}, SSA, SSE \propto IG\left(\frac{n_a - 1}{2}, \frac{SSA}{2} \right), \tag{8.5}$$

$$\sigma_e^2 \mid \bar{\bar{X}}, SSA, SSE \propto IG\left(\frac{n_a(n_w - 1)}{2}, \frac{SSE}{2} \right), \tag{8.6}$$

$$\mu \mid \bar{\bar{X}}, SSA, SSE, \sigma_A^2, \sigma_e^2 \propto N\left(\bar{\bar{X}}, \frac{\sigma_A^2}{n_a n_w} \right), \tag{8.7}$$

where $IG(u, v)$ is an inverse-gamma distribution with parameters (u, v).

To simulate samples from the predictive density $p(X_f \mid \bar{\bar{X}}, \text{SSA}, \text{SSE})$, where X_f is a future observation, one may generate an observation from $p(X_f \mid (\mu, \sigma_a^2, \sigma_e^2)^*, \bar{\bar{X}}, \text{SSA}, \text{SSE})$ for each observation $(\mu, \sigma_a^2, \sigma_e^2)^*$ from $p(\mu, \sigma_a^2, \sigma_e^2 \mid \bar{\bar{X}}, \text{SSA}, \text{SSE})$. This is a valid approach because under the one-way random effect Model (8.3) (see Wolfinger 1998),

$$X_f \mid (\mu, \sigma_a^2, \sigma_e^2, \bar{\bar{X}}, \text{SSA}, \text{SSE}) \sim N(\mu, \sigma_a^2 + \sigma_e^2). \tag{8.8}$$

Using the distributions in Models (8.5)–(8.6), the following procedure can be employed to construct Bayesian β-expectation tolerance interval:

1. Simulate $\left(\sigma_A^2\right)^*$ and $\left(\sigma_e^2\right)^*$ from Models (8.5) and (8.6), for m_0 times. Retain the sample only if $\left(\sigma_A^2\right)^* \geq \left(\sigma_e^2\right)^*$ Let m denote the number of times for the above condition to hold;

2. Generate μ^* from the distribution in Model (8.7);

3. Simulate X_f from Model (8.8) for each observation of $\left(\mu^*, \left(\sigma_A^2\right)^*, \left(\sigma_e^2\right)^*\right)$ out of a total of m.

The posterior medians and upper limits of the credible intervals of $(\mu, \sigma_a^2, \sigma_e^2)$ can be generated based on the simulated samples. Let η_1 and η_2 denote the lower β_1^{th} upper β_2^{th} percentiles $(\beta_2 - \beta_1 = \beta)$ of the above simulated sample X_f so that the Bayesian β-expectation tolerance interval for a future observation is given by (η_1, η_2). The β-expectation tolerance interval can be used to assess if the analytical method can be deemed to be validated. For example, the null hypothesis in Hypotheses (8.2) is rejected if the (η_1, η_2) is contained within $(-\lambda, \lambda)$. Similarly, a β-content, γ-confidence tolerance interval of the future observations can be constructed (see Krishnamoorthy and Mathew 2009 for detail) to compose an analogous test. Note that there are many situations for which non-conjugate priors may be required. Even when there is no closed-form expression of the posterior or predictive distribution, the above analysis can still be carried out using the MCMC methods discussed in Chapter 3.

8.2.6 Example

8.2.6.1 Data

Consider the following real-data method validation experiment in which two analysts measured the relative potency of samples of a biological drug substance (Tables 8.1 and 8.2). For each of four independent runs, each analyst created five separate dilutions and concentrations of an independent sample and then measured the relative potency of each dilution/concentration.

TABLE 8.1

Method Validation Relative Potency Data for Biological Drug Substance

Analyst	Run	67%	82%	100%	122%	150%
A	1	61	82	96	112	141
A	2	68	77	101	125	143
A	3	68	80	105	129	159
A	4	66	76	97	115	140
B	1	68	84	104	124	147
B	2	64	81	107	113	141
B	3	64	83	99	110	139
B	4	62	80	101	112	148

Numerical column headers are the experimental diluted/concentrated relative potency of samples. Values are the measured relative potencies.

TABLE 8.2

Method Validation Relative Potency Data for Biological Drug Substance Shown on Natural Log Scale

Analyst	Run	67%	82%	100%	122%	150%
A	1	4.11	4.41	4.56	4.72	4.95
A	2	4.22	4.34	4.62	4.83	4.96
A	3	4.22	4.38	4.65	4.86	5.07
A	4	4.19	4.33	4.57	4.74	4.94
B	1	4.22	4.43	4.64	4.82	4.99
B	2	4.16	4.39	4.67	4.73	4.95
B	3	4.16	4.42	4.60	4.70	4.93
B	4	4.13	4.38	4.62	4.72	5.00

Assuming Model (8.1) after ln-transforming the measured relative potency, relative accuracy for the ith concentration/dilution is defined as the percent difference between $\exp(\mu_i)$ and its known concentration/dilution. Acceptance limits for the method validation require that the mean relative accuracy fall between 90 and 110%, the %CV for variance components due to each of analyst, run, and assay/sample fall below 15%, and the total %CV fall below 30%.

8.2.6.2 Analysis

Realistic but minimally informative priors were assigned to the parameters by

$$\mu_i \sim N(\tilde{\mu}_i, 1),$$

$$\sigma_A, \sigma_R, \sigma_e \sim \text{half-Cauchy}\left(\text{Location} = 0, \text{Scale} = 0.1\right),$$

where $\tilde{\mu}_i$ is the natural log expected value of the ith dilution/concentration.

Computer code for sampling from the posterior of $(\mu_i, \sigma_A, \sigma_R, \sigma_e)$ follows.

```
require(rjags); require(runjags)

## Create the JAGS model
model.txt = "
model{
    ## Prior distributions
   sigmaA ~ dt(0., 100., 1)T(0., )   ## half-Cauchy with
                                           scale = 0.1
   sigmaR ~ dt(0., 100., 1)T(0., )
   sigmaE ~ dt(0., 100., 1)T(0., )
   tauR <- 1/(sigmaR*sigmaR)
   tauA <- 1/(sigmaA*sigmaA)
   tauE <- 1/(sigmaE*sigmaE)

   for ( i in 1:nConc )
   {
      mu[i] ~ dnorm(mu0[i], 1)      ## On ln scale, SD=1
                                       is large
   }
   sigmaTotal <- sqrt( sigmaA^2 + sigmaR^2 + sigmaE^2 )

   ## Likelihood
   for ( j in 1:nRun )
   {
      thetaR[j] ~ dnorm(0, tauR)
   }
   for ( k in 1:nAnalyst )
   {
      thetaA[k] ~ dnorm(0, tauA)
   }
   for ( m in 1:N )
   {
      Mean[m] <- thetaR[ run[m] ] + thetaA[ analyst[m] ]
                               + mu[ conc[m] ]
      y[m] ~ dnorm( Mean[m], tauE )
   }
}"

## Load the validation data
d.val = read.csv("Validation Data.csv")

## Prepare data for JAGS
```

```
data = list( N=nrow(d.val), nRun=nlevels(d.val$Run),
             nAnalyst=nlevels(d.val$Analyst),
             nConc=nlevels(d.val$Conc),
             run=as.vector(unclass(d.val$Run)),
             analyst=as.vector(unclass(d.val$Analyst)),
             conc=as.vector(unclass(d.val$Conc)),
             y=log(d.val$Observed.RP),
             mu0=log(c(67, 82, 100, 122, 150) ) )

## Call JAGS
fitb = run.jags( model.txt, data=data,
          monitor=c("mu", "sigmaR", "sigmaA",
                  "sigmaE", "sigmaTotal"),
          n.chains=3, burnin=10000, sample=20000,
          thin=100,
          module="glm", method="parallel" )
th.post = as.matrix( as.mcmc.list(fitb) )
```

8.2.6.3 Results

Precision, through %CV, is calculated and compared to the acceptance limits by looking at an upper 95% credible limit for each variance component and for the total variance by

```
sd.95ci = apply(
            th.post[,c("sigmaA", "sigmaR", "sigmaE",
                  "sigmaTotal")],
            2, quantile, p=c(0.5, 0.95) )
cv.95ci = round( 100 * sqrt( exp(sd.95ci^2) - 1 ), 1 )
```

Results in Table 8.3 show that the point estimates (posterior medians) meet with the %CV acceptance limits, but the upper 95% credible limit for analyst is well over 15%.

Relative accuracy (also called % recovery) is examined via two one-sided testing (TOST) calculated and compared to the acceptance limits 90–110%.

TABLE 8.3

Posterior Medians and Upper 95% Credible Limits of %CV for Variance Components

Component	Relative Accuracy	Pass
Analyst	2.9 (18.1)	N
Run	3.2 (6.2)	Y
Assay/Sample	3.8 (4.8)	Y
Total (IP)	6.3 (18.1)	Y

The TOST method operationally is equivalent to the use of a 90% confidence interval approach, which declares that accuracy is acceptable if the 90% confidence interval is contained within (90, 100). The calculations were carried out with a 90% credible interval using the code below.

```
mu.90ci = exp(apply(th.post[,1:5], 2, quantile,
        p=c(0.5, 0.05, 0.95)))
conc.true = c(67, 82, 100, 122, 150)
rel.acc = round( 100*mu.90ci / matrix(conc.true, 3, 5,
        byrow=TRUE),   0)
```

Though no acceptance criterion was created for the total variance approach, 95% β-expectation tolerance intervals for relative accuracy are calculated for each concentration/dilution.

```
sigma.total = th.post[,"sigmaTotal"]
y.95pi = sapply(1:5, function(i){
            quantile( rnorm( nrow(th.post),
            mean=th.post[,i],
                    sd=sigma.total ),
                    p=c(0.025, 0.975) ) })
rel.acc.pi = round( 100*exp(y.95pi) /
                matrix(conc.true, 2, 5, byrow=TRUE), 0)
```

Results in Table 8.4 show that the point estimates (posterior medians) for relative accuracy fall within 90–110%, but the TOST barely passes for the first three dilutions and fails for the last two concentrations.

Based on statistical hypothesis testing, the validation experiment fails to meet the acceptance criteria, primarily because the posterior distribution for the standard deviation for the analyst term relied on data from only two analysts. From a total variance perspective, with 95% probability, the next relative accuracy measurement will roughly fall in the range of 80–120% across all concentrations/dilutions.

TABLE 8.4

Posterior Medians with Two-sided 90% Credible Intervals for Relative Accuracy and 95% Prediction Intervals

True Concentration/ Dilution	Relative Accuracy	Pass	95% β-Expectation Interval
67	97 (90, 105)	Y	(78, 122)
82	98 (91, 106)	Y	(79, 123)
100	101 (94, 109)	Y	(81, 127)
122	96 (89, 104)	N	(77, 120)
150	96 (89, 104)	N	(77, 121)

8.2.6.4 *Analysis Based on More Informative Priors*

The above analysis was performed almost in the absence of prior knowledge of the method. It is rare, however, for a validation experiment to occur without development work. Therefore, it is sensible for the Bayesian to consider incorporating meaningful priors to inform the variance components and, if applicable, the mean values of a validation experiment.

For the above analytical method validation, it turned out that an earlier experiment was conducted in the development laboratory run by two analysts, each producing three independent runs for a set of concentrations. The development data are shown in Table 8.5 with relative potency data on the natural log scale. The development data can be leveraged to determine a prior distribution for parameters σ_R, σ_A, and σ_e.

Computer code for MCMC sampling from the posterior distribution of (μ_i, σ_R, σ_A, σ_e) from the development data follows.

```
## Load the development data
d.dev = read.csv("Development Data.csv")

## Prepare data for JAGS
data = list( N=nrow(d.dev), nRun=nlevels(d.dev$Run),
             nAnalyst=nlevels(d.dev$Analyst),
             nConc=nlevels(d.dev$Conc),
             run=as.vector(unclass(d.dev$Run)),
             analyst=as.vector(unclass(d.dev$Analyst)),
             conc=as.vector(unclass(d.dev$Conc)),
             y=log(d.dev$Observed.RP),
             muExp=log(c(67, 100, 150) ) )

## Call JAGS
fitb = run.jags( model.txt, data=data,
            monitor=c("mu", "sigmaR", "sigmaA",
                   "sigmaE", "sigmaTotal"),
```

TABLE 8.5

Development Experiment Relative Potency Data for Biological Drug Substance Shown on Natural Log Scale

Analyst	Run	67%	100%	150%
A	1	4.25	4.62	5.04
A	2	4.23	4.62	4.83
A	3	4.29	4.65	5.00
B	1	4.20	4.67	5.00
B	2	4.28	4.78	5.12
B	3	4.28	4.75	5.05

```
        n.chains=3, burnin=10000, sample=20000,
        thin=100,
        module="glm", method="parallel" )
   ## Posterior of one experiment becomes prior for
      the next experiment
th.prior = as.matrix( as.mcmc.list(fitb) )
```

The development-data posterior distributions for the μ_i were Gaussian-like densities with ln-scaled posterior means of 4.3, 4.7, and 5.0 and standard deviations of roughly 0.1. Since the expected mean values were, respectively 4.2, 4.6, and 5.0, the root mean-squared error from the expected mean values is less than $0.14 = \sqrt{0.1^2 + 0.1^2}$. In light of the development-data results, the validation-data prior precision for the μ_i was raised from 1.0 to 16.0, corresponding to a standard deviation of 0.25. For the development-data posterior distributions for σ_R, σ_A, and σ_e, a log-normal distribution provided a reasonable fit, yielding validation-data prior densities of

$$\ln(\sigma_R) \sim N(\text{Mean} = -3.3, \text{SD} = 0.9),$$

$$\ln(\sigma_A) \sim N(\text{Mean} = -3.0, \text{SD} = 1.2),$$

$$\ln(\sigma_e) \sim N(\text{Mean} = -2.9, \text{SD} = 0.2).$$

With real prior information, computer code for sampling from the validation-data posterior of $(\mu_i, \sigma_A, \sigma_R, \sigma_e)$ follows.

```
## Create the JAGS model
model.txt = "
model{

   ## Prior distributions
   lsigmaR ~ dnorm( sEst[1], sTau[1] )
   lsigmaA ~ dnorm( sEst[2], sTau[2] )
   lsigmaE ~ dnorm( sEst[3], sTau[3] )

   sigmaR <- exp(lsigmaR)
   sigmaA <- exp(lsigmaA)
   sigmaE <- exp(lsigmaE)

   tauR <- exp(-2*lsigmaR)
   tauA <- exp(-2*lsigmaA)
   tauE <- exp(-2*lsigmaE)

   sigmaTotal <- sqrt( sigmaA^2 + sigmaR^2 + sigmaE^2 )
```

```
for ( i in 1:5 )
{
  mu[i] ~ dnorm(mu0[i], 16.)      ## Based on prior
                                  data, higher prec
}
## Likelihood
for ( j in 1:nRun )
{
  thetaR[j] ~ dnorm(0, tauR)
}
for ( k in 1:nAnalyst )
{
  thetaA[k] ~ dnorm(0, tauA)
}
for ( m in 1:N )
{
  Mean[m] <- thetaR[ run[m] ] + thetaA[ analyst[m] ]
                             + mu[ conc[m] ]
  y[m] ~ dnorm( Mean[m], tauE )
}
}"

data = list( N=nrow(d.val), nRun=nlevels(d.val$Run),
             nAnalyst=nlevels(d.val$Analyst),
             run=as.vector(unclass(d.val$Run)),
             analyst=as.vector(unclass(d.val$Analyst)),
             conc=as.vector(unclass(d.val$Conc)),
             y=log(d.val$Observed.RP),
             mu0=log(c(67, 82, 100, 122, 150)),
             sEst=c(-3.3, -3.0, -2.9),
                  sTau=1/c(0.9, 1.2, 0.2)^2 )
```

Running the computer code as before, prior-informed validation results are shown in Tables 8.6 and 8.7. Now, the validation experiment meets all acceptance criteria thanks to the development-data prior information. From a total

TABLE 8.6

Prior-informed Posterior Medians and Upper 95% Credible Limits of %CV for Variance Components

Component	Relative Accuracy	Pass
Analyst	2.1 (10.0)	Y
Run	2.7 (5.2)	Y
Assay/Sample	4.3 (5.3)	Y
Total (IP)	5.9 (11.5)	Y

TABLE 8.7

Posterior Medians with Two-sided 90% Credible Intervals for
Relative Accuracy and 95% β-Expectation Tolerance Intervals

True Concentration/ Dilution	Relative Accuracy	Pass	95% β-Expectation Tolerance Interval
67	97 (93, 102)	Y	(84, 114)
82	98 (93, 103)	Y	(84, 114)
100	101 (96, 107)	Y	(87, 118)
122	96 (92, 101)	Y	(83, 112)
150	96 (92, 102)	Y	(83, 113)

variance perspective, with 95% probability, the next relative accuracy measurement will roughly fall in the range of 85–115% across all concentrations/dilutions.

8.3 Method Transfer

8.3.1 Background

Method transfer can take place between laboratories and sites. In recent years, as more and more clinical trials are conducted globally, and drug products reach markets in different regions, companies increasingly utilize contract manufacturing organizations to ensure adequate drug supply. Accordingly, analytical method transfer has become an on-going effort. To ensure that the methods maintain validation status and provide consistent results between laboratories, a formal method transfer plan needs to be developed. The plan includes a written document describing the method transfer plan, acceptance criteria, personnel training at the receiving laboratory, implementation of validation/transfer experiments, and statistical analysis. In addition to the demonstration of an acceptable method performance at the receiving laboratory, assay transfer also requires the demonstration of comparable assay performance over a range of expected responses. The comparability of method performance is often referred to as reproducibility, which is one of the validation characteristics of analytic method stipulated by regulatory guidance (FDA 1995; ICH 1995). In this section, we describe a Bayesian method for demonstrating comparable performance when the assay response can be described through a linear model (Zeng et al. 2018).

8.3.2 Model

For the sake of simplicity, we consider a balanced parallel design, modeled by

$$Y_{ijk} = \theta_{ij} + e_{ijk}, \tag{8.9}$$

where Y_{ijk} is the assay response for the ith method (i = A,B), jth level (j = 1, ..., J), and kth replicate (k = 1, 2, ..., K) and where the independent errors follow the distribution given by $e_{ijk} \sim N(0, \sigma^2)$.

A successful transfer can be demonstrated through testing the hypotheses:

$$H_{0,j} : |\theta_{Aj} - \theta_{Bj}| \geq \delta$$
$$H_{a,j} : |\theta_{Aj} - \theta_{Bj}| < \delta \tag{8.10}$$

where δ is an equivalence limit.

Either the interval-based approach comparing mean response at each concentration level (Yang and Schofield 2014) or a Bayesian method similar to that presented in Section 8.2 can be used to establish equivalence between the sending and receiving labs at each level. There are, however, situations in which the test by Yang and Schofield (2014) cannot be carried out, such as when there is no measurement in some of the levels at one of the laboratories or a single measurement at all levels. This issue can be resolved if linearity of the response can be assumed.

8.3.3 Linear Response

Many analytical methods are required by regulatory guidance to show linearity in response over a range of concentration or dilution (ICH 2005). A comprehensive review of statistical methods for linearity validation is provided by Yang (2005). Under the linearity assumption,

$$\theta_{ij} = \theta_i(x_j) = a_i + b_i x_j,$$

where (a_i, b_i) are the intercept and slope for the ith method and the $\{x_j\}$ are a set of controlled experimental factor levels. Thus, $H_{a,j}$ in Hypotheses (8.10) may be written as $|(a_A + b_A x_j) - (a_B + b_B x_j)| < \delta$. Instead of testing Hypotheses (8.10) at each level j, a more stringent hypothesis would be $|(a_A + b_A x) - (a_B + b_B x)| < \delta$ for all $L = x_1 < x < x_J = U$. Zeng et al. (2018) show these new hypotheses are equivalent to

$$H_0 : |\beta + \eta L| \geq \delta \text{ or } |\beta + \eta U| \geq \delta$$
$$H_a : |\beta + \eta L| < \delta \text{ and } |\beta + \eta U| < \delta \tag{8.11}$$

where $\beta = (a_A - a_B)$, $\eta = (b_A - b_B)$.

As in Novick et al. (2012) and Novick and Yang (2013), one may test overall equivalence with a Bayesian posterior probability

$$p(\delta, L, U) = \Pr\left(\left|\beta + \eta L\right| < \delta \text{ and } \left|\beta + \eta U\right| < \delta \mid \text{data}\right).$$

If, say, $p(\delta, L, U) \geq 0.95$, overall equivalence is declared and analytical method reproducibility claimed.

8.3.4 Case Example

A reporter gene bioassay for measuring the potency of a biological product was transferred from a development lab (Lab A) to a QC lab (Lab B). A method transfer study was carried out, in which six independent runs were conducted in each of two labs on the same diluted samples across the assay range from 60% to 167% expected relative potency. The results along with descriptive summary statistics are given in Table 8.8.

Conditioned on model parameters, a linear hierarchical model was fitted to the data with Bayesian methods as

$$Y_{ijk} = a_{ik} + b_{ik} x_j + e_{ijk} \tag{8.12}$$

where Y_{ijk} is the ln-scaled assay response for the ith lab (A, B), jth level of x (the ln expected relative potency), and kth assay run. In addition, $(a_{ik}, b_{ik}) \sim N\left((a_i, b_i), V_i\right)$ and $e_{ijk} \sim N\left(0, \sigma_i^2\right)$. The prior distributions are chosen to be

TABLE 8.8

Observed Relative Potency Values (from Zeng et al. 2018)

Method	Assay Run	60	77	100	130	167
Lab A	1	65	82	106	134	189
	2	61	73	104	132	170
	3	62	70	97	131	157
	4	53	71	99	126	160
	5	58	76	99	128	162
	6	54	72	98	122	165
	Geo Mean	59	74	100	129	167
	%CV	8%	6%	4%	3%	7%
Lab B	1	50	68	105	83	108
	2	63	78	97	99	132
	3	54	72	95	113	142
	4	57	70	82	105	135
	5	58	69	102	107	139
	6	56	75	104	102	133
	Geo Mean	56	72	97	101	131
	%CV	8%	5%	9%	11%	10%

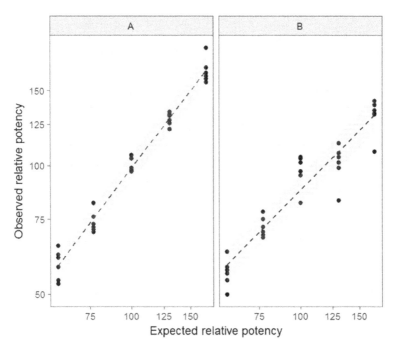

FIGURE 8.1
Scatterplot of the assay transfer data for Labs A and B. The dashed line shows the fitted line with 95% credible bands given by the grey area (adapted from Zeng et al. 2018).

$$a_i \sim N\left(\hat{a}_i, \text{SD} = 5\text{SE}\left(\hat{a}_i\right)\right),$$

$$b_i \sim N\left(\hat{b}_i, \text{SD} = 5\text{SE}\left(\hat{b}_i\right)\right),$$

$$V_i \sim \text{scaled-inverse Wishart}\left(\boldsymbol{D}, 3\right),$$

where $\hat{a}_i$ and $\hat{b}_i$ are the REML estimates, $\text{SE}(\hat{a}_i)$ and $\text{SE}(\hat{b}_i)$ are their respective standard errors, the hyperpriors for the diagonal elements of $\boldsymbol{D}$ are half-Cauchy(0, 1), and $\sigma_i \sim$ half-Cauchy(0, 1).

A Bayesian analysis was carried out to calculate the posterior $p(\delta, L, U) = \Pr(\,|\,\beta + \eta L\,|< \delta$ and $|\beta + \eta U\,|< \delta\,|\,\text{data})$ with $\delta = \ln(1.25)$. Overall equivalence is claimed if the probability $p(\delta, L, U) \geq 0.95$, with $L = 60\%$ and $U = 167\%$. Figure 8.1 shows the fitted line with 95% credible bands given by the grey area. Since $p(\delta, L, U) = 0.38$, the null hypothesis in Model (8.4) is not rejected.

```
model.txt = "
model{

    ## Priors
```

```
    for ( i in 1:2 )    ## Two sites A and B
    {
     D[i] ~ dt(0., 1., 1)T(0.,)      # Parameters in
                                       diagonal matrix D
    }
    OmegaRun ~ dscaled.wishart(D, 3)
    SigmaRun <- inverse(OmegaRun)  # SigmaRun ~ scaled
                                       inverse Wishart

    theta[1] ~ dnorm( Est[1], tauML[1] )  ## Intercept
    theta[2] ~ dnorm( Est[2], tauML[2] )  ## Slope


    sigmaErr ~ dt(0., 1., 1)T(0., )   # Residual standard
                                        deviation
    tauErr <- 1/(sigmaErr*sigmaErr)

    ## Likelihood
    for ( j in 1:nRun )
    {
       thetaRun[j,1:2] ~ dmnorm( theta, OmegaRun )
    }

    for ( k in 1:N )
    {
      mu[k] <- thetaRun[ run[k], 1]
            + thetaRun[ run[k],2 ]*x[k]
      y[k] ~ dnorm( mu[k], tauErr )
    }
}"

## Model fit for Lab A
dA = subset(d, Lab=="A")
fit0 = lmer( y~x+(1+x|Run), data=dA )   ## Get REML
                                            estimates

data = list( N=nrow(dA), nRun=nlevels(dA$Run),
             run=as.vector(unclass(dA$Run)),
             y = dA$y, x=dA$x,
             Est=as.vector(fixef(fit0)),
                       ## REML estimate
             tauML=0.04/diag(summary(fit0)$vcov)
                       ## 5x(Std Err)
               )
```

```
fitb.A = run.jags(model.txt, data=data, n.chains=3
            monitor=c("theta", "SigmaRun", "sigmaErr"),
            burnin=10000, thin=100, sample=20000,
            modules="glm", method="parallel" )

## Model fit for Lab B
dB = subset(d, Lab=="B")
fit0 = lmer( y~x+(1+x|Run), data=dB )     ## Get REML
                                                estimates

data = list( N=nrow(dB), nRun=nlevels(dB$Run),
            run=as.vector(unclass(dB$Run)),
            y = dB$y, x=dB$x,
            Est=as.vector(fixef(fit0)),
                        ## REML estimate
            tauML=0.04/diag(summary(fit0)$vcov)
                        ## 5x(Std Err)
                )
fitb.B = run.jags(model.txt, data=data, n.chains=3,
            monitor=c("theta", "SigmaRun", "sigmaErr"),
            burnin=10000, thin=100, sample=20000,
            modules="glm", method="parallel" )

th.postA = as.matrix( as.mcmc.list(fitb.A) )
th.postB = as.matrix( as.mcmc.list(fitb.B) )

L = log(60)
U = log(167)
delta = log(1.25)

## Test if means from fit1 and fit2 are equivalent
   across the entire x.range, equivalency = 25%

diff.L = abs( (th.postA[,"theta[1]"]
          +th.postA[,"theta[2]"]*L) -
              (th.postB[,"theta[1]"]
              +th.postB[,"theta[2]"]*L) )
diff.U = abs( (th.postA[,"theta[1]"]
          +th.postA[,"theta[2]"]*U) -
              (th.postB[,"theta[1]"]
              +th.postB[,"theta[2]"]*U) )

p.delta = mean( diff.L < delta & diff.U < delta )
```

8.4 Concluding Remarks

To develop a safe and effective drug and to ensure product quality, safety, and efficacy, a broad array of analytical methods is used in all stages of drug research and development and commercial use. It is critical that the methods are validated per regulatory guidance through robust study design and data analysis. When a method is transferred, a demonstration of reproducibility needs to be achieved before the method is put in routine use. It is also important to note that during the lifecycle of a product, changes in existing analytical methods may occur for the sake of improving the performance of the assay, operational ease, or reduction in cost. These changes may necessitate efforts to conduct appropriately designed studies to demonstrate the suitable or compatible performance of the new method relative to the old method which is to be replaced. The Bayesian methods discussed in this chapter can be used for revalidation or bridging purposes. Since, in the lifecycle of an analytical method, a vast amount of data is generated by the method, method validation should take full advantage of historical data to make the validation process more robust and efficient.

9

Process Development

9.1 Introduction

Process development for biopharmaceuticals consists of upstream and downstream developments. The former typically includes the creation or selection of a new cell line and a culture medium, the definition of an inoculum expansion, and the design of a production process, including a bioreactor and its operating conditions. The latter is focused on maximizing product yield and minimizing impurities. Process development is known to be labor intensive and time consuming, as a series of experiments need to be carried out to optimize the upstream and downstream developments. In the past decade, the application of QbD principles has been increasingly used to guide the process development. At the center of this new development paradigm are the identification of critical quality attributes and the development of the design space. When process parameters are controlled within the design space, product quality is warranted. Therefore, the design space not only provides grounds for effective control strategies but also lends flexibility for future improvement of the process. In certain instances, the design space may enable a manufacturer to make post-approval changes or scale up operations without prior approval from regulatory authorities. Per regulatory guidance, a manufacturing process needs to be validated for its intended purpose. The newly updated FDA guidance (2011a) recommends a risk-based approach to process validation, advocating greater use of data from process design through commercial production to establish scientific evidence that a process is capable of delivering quality. This chapter is concerned with the use of Bayesian methods to aid critical quality attribute identification, development of design space, and process validation. Wherever appropriate, we discuss frequentist statistical methods for the sake of providing the context for Bayesian alternatives.

9.2 Quality by Design

Process development relies on scientific experimentation. In the traditional development paradigm, studies are often conducted using one variable at a time. This often results in little understanding of the interdependence of variables that may impact the process performance. Likewise, the traditional process validation is often a documentation exercise, primarily focused on the initial full-scale batches from a process. The overall product quality is characterized through extensive testing, including the inspection of raw materials, in-process material testing, and final drug substance and product release testing. The lack of product and process understanding and limited knowledge of the sources of manufacture process variability can result in stringent specifications that prohibit the release of products that otherwise may have acceptable clinical performance (Yu et al. 2015). Because changes to the process and/or test methods require post-approval submissions, there are few incentives for manufacturers to improve their manufacturing processes. The QbD approach, rooted in the principle that quality should be designed into a product rather than demonstrated by testing, distinguishes itself from the traditional product and process development paradigm in many aspects. In recent years, QbD has been at the forefront of biopharmaceutical development (Kozlowski and Swann 2009). Two case studies were created to exemplify QbD approaches to product development (CMC Biotech Working Group 2009; CMC Vaccines Working Group 2012). Various applications of QbD principles to development have been discussed, regarding raw material qualification, formulation development, and purification (Rathore and Mhatre 2009). The first step in QbD-based development is to begin with predefined quality objectives which include defining the quality target product profile (QTPP). This is followed by the identification of critical quality attributes (CQAs) that have a significant impact on the drug product. Often studies are carried out to link raw material attributes (MAs) and process parameters (PPs) to CQAs. Such knowledge provides a foundation for developing robust process controls focused on the areas of high risk. It also lends the manufacturer the ability to develop a manufacturing process that is flexible and consistent in delivering a high-quality product.

After the CQAs are defined, the focus is shifted to the development of a manufacturing process that yields a QTPP-meeting product. At this stage of development, studies are carried out, using multivariate DOE strategies to evaluate the effects of process variables and their interactions on process performance. Knowledge gleaned from the results of these studies, perhaps combined with platform knowledge and data from other molecules in the same class, is used to define critical process parameters (CPPs) through a risk assessment. Based on the CPPs identified in the risk assessment, the process is optimized. This experimentation gives rise to a "design space", which is essentially an operating zone for manufacturing parameters that produces a satisfactory product with high likelihood. The above sequence of activities is repeated for each unit operation, establishing a design space for the CPPs at each operational step.

The implementation of control strategies enables a manufacturing process to consistently deliver a quality product. QbD principles call for using a risk-based approach to develop control strategies aimed at keeping the manufacturing risks at or below acceptable levels. Knowledge of CQAs and the impact of CPPs and other input materials on these CQAs enables manufacturers to avoid unnecessary testing as a means to demonstrate product quality. In essence, the level of control of each quality attribute should reflect the criticality of the attribute. Effective control strategies integrate a number of elements including input material controls, procedural controls, process parameter controls, in-process testing, specification testing, characterization/comparability testing, and process monitoring, as appropriate.

9.3 Critical Quality Attributes

A CQA is defined as "a physical, chemical, biological, or microbiological property or characteristic that should be within an appropriate limit, range, or distribution to ensure the desired product quality" (ICH 2006). CQAs collectively indicate whether the manufacturing process delivers a product that meets its QTPP. The identification of CQAs is usually accomplished through a criticality assessment that evaluates the risk associated with each attribute, including the severity (consequences to the patient) as well as the probability (likelihood of occurrence) and detectability of non-conformance of the CQAs. Both prior product knowledge and process capability are useful sources of information for such an evaluation. The former includes cumulative laboratory, non-clinical, and clinical experience related to the quality attribute under evaluation, as well as data from molecules in the same class and published literature. The latter consists of data from process development studies and relevant manufacturing experience from the same or related products. Both product knowledge and process capability serve as the basis for establishing the acceptable range for a CQA.

Since changes in CQAs might have a significant impact on product safety and efficacy, it is critical to establish the relationships between CQAs and clinical performance, and to use this knowledge to define acceptable ranges for CQAs. This knowledge provides a foundation for developing robust control strategies for the manufacturing process.

In the literature, various models have been proposed to understand the relationships between CQAs and product safety and efficacy (Schenerman et al. 2009; Yang et al. 2015). A statistical model was developed to link the composition of the active components of a drug product with bioavailability

(Yang 2013a). Yang (2013b) also used a mechanistic model to guide the control strategy of host cell DNA. In general, however, it can be difficult to link a particular quality attribute to clinical performance (safety and efficacy). In the next section, through a case example, we demonstrate how to link oncogenicity of residual host cell DNA, which is often a CQA, to clinical safety.

9.3.1 Risk of Oncogenicity

Biological medicinal products inevitably contain residual DNA from host cells. As residual DNA is a process-related impurity, it is not expected to affect product bioactivity (Schenerman et al. 2009). There is, however, a theoretical concern that cellular DNA in a medicinal product may cause oncogenic and infective events and possibly immunogenic responses (Dortant et al. 1997; Petricciani and Loewer 2001; Rothenfusser et al. 2003; Ishii et al. 2004; Peden et al. 2006; Sheng et al. 2008; Sheng-Fowler et al. 2009a, 2009b; Sheng-Fowler et al. 2010). As a result, it is critical to assess the risk of residual DNA so that an effective control strategy can be devised (Yang et al. 2015). Efforts have been made to quantify the risk associated with the residual DNA and to implement risk mitigation strategies. The culmination of these is the publication of a WHO meeting report (WHO 2007) and FDA guidance (2010). The former recommends a reduction of residual DNA in the final dose below 10 ng; whereas the latter suggests reducing DNA size below the size of a functional gene, which is approximately 200 base pair (bp). Interestingly, neither of the two guidelines issues a mandate for the above recommendation. Instead, a risk-based approach is suggested. For example, in the WHO guideline (2007), it is stated "risk assessment should be done in order to define the DNA upper limit for a particular vaccine or biological product, based on the following parameters: nature of the cell substrate, inactivation process, the method used to assess DNA content, and the size distribution of DNA fragments." Furthermore, the FDA was receptive to alternative limits of residual DNA based on the risk assessment (2010).

In The Center for Biologics Evaluation and Research (CBER)'s studies (Peden et al. 2006; Sheng et al. 2008; Sheng-Fowler et al. 2009a, 2009b, 2010), the risk factor is defined as the number of doses needed to induce an oncogenic or infective event in product recipients. A formula for the calculation of this risk factor was developed, taking into account the average DNA size and residual DNA in the final dose, as well as the oncogenic (or infective) amount of residual DNA that induces an adverse reaction. As Yang et al. (2010) pointed out, this formula fails to take into account the disruption of oncogenic sequences due to enzyme digestion and sizes of individual oncogenes. As a result, the oncogenic and infective risks are likely overstated. To counter these shortcomings, a new method was suggested by Yang et al. (2010), based on probabilistic modeling of the enzymatic degradation process. The issues with the CBER method were also noted by Krause and Lewis (1998), who proposed a remedy. The performances of the three methods were compared by Yang (2013b).

9.3.2 Bayesian Risk Assessment

In the following, we assume that a process employs an enzyme to fragment residual DNA in the product. Let p denote the probability that the enzyme cuts the phosphate ester bond between two adjacent nucleotides. Assume that each host cell genome contains I different oncogenes of size m_i and I_i copies of the oncogene, $i = 1, ..., I$. The safety factor (SF) of oncogenicity was derived as (Yang et al. 2010)

$$SF = \frac{O_m}{\sum_{i=1}^{I} I_i(1-p)^{m_i-1}(m_i / M)U}. \tag{9.1}$$

where O_m is the number of oncogene sequences required for inducing an oncogenic event, M is the genome size or total number of DNA base pairs in one copy of the host cell, and U is the average amount of residual DNA per dose of the product. A similar formula was derived for the safety factor of infectivity, but this chapter is focused on the oncogenicity risk.

Yang and Zhang (2016) formulated the safety risk as the posterior probability for the safety factor to be above an acceptable limit SF_0,

$$\Pr[SF \geq SF_0] \geq p_0 \tag{9.2}$$

where p_0 is a large, predefined probability near 1.

Selection of SF_0 and p_0 depends on both regulatory expectations as well as the intended use of the drug product. For example, for vaccines used for a large population of healthy individuals, an extremely large number should be chosen for SF_0 and a large probability value should be chosen for p_0. For a cancer population that has a higher tolerance for risk, a relatively smaller number can be set for SF_0 and a relatively larger number for p_0. In literature, $SF_0 = 10^{-6}$ were considered acceptable for an oncology drug. However, there is no guidance on the selection of p_0.

9.3.3 Modeling Enzyme Cutting Efficiency

To estimate the posterior probability in Equation (9.1), it is necessary to model the enzymatic degradation process, through which the host cell genome DNA sequence Φ is disrupted. Yang et al. (2010) and Yang and Zhang (2016) expressed the sequence Φ as

$$\Phi = B_1 c_1 B_2 c_2 ... c_{M-1} B_M$$

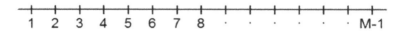

FIGURE 9.1
Genome with phosphate ester bonds being labeled as 1 to (M-1). (Adopted from Yang and Zhang 2016).

where B_is and c_is are nucleotides and phosphate ester bonds between two nucleotides. An alternate illustration of the genome DNA sequence is given in Figure 9.1.

Denote $Z_1, Z_2, \ldots, Z_{N^*}$ as the sizes of all DNA segments after enzyme digestion of Φ. It is sensible to assume that $Z_1, Z_2, \ldots, Z_{N^*}$ are independently and identically distributed according to a geometric distribution $\Pr(Z = z) = (1-p)^z p$. Assume that each bond has probability p of being broken and imagine that the phosphate ester bonds are coded from bond 1 to bond (M–1) as shown in Figure 9.1. Since each bond has equal probability p of being cut, the number of bonds being successfully cut follows a binomial distribution such that

$$N^* - 1 \sim \text{binomial}(M-1, p).$$

Furthermore, suppose that there are k genomes that go through the DNA inactivation process. The total number N of segments is the sum of segments from these k genomes, each following a binomial$(M-1, p)$. Therefore,

$$N - k \sim \text{binomial}(k(M-1), p).$$

An empirical estimate of N is obtained as

$$\hat{N} = kM / \bar{Z}$$

with $\bar{Z}$ being the average size of DNA segments, which can be measured through analytical methods. Either the estimate N or $\bar{Z}$, coupled with a prior distribution, can be used to calculate the posterior probability. In contrast, Yang et al. (2010) derived an expression for p such that $p = 1 - 2^{-1/\text{med}_0}$ where med_0 is the median size of DNA after enzymatic degradation. Therefore, both the empirical distributions of the DNA segments and p can be obtained.

9.3.4 Bayesian Solution

Let X, Y, N respectively denote the measurements of the number of oncogenes needed to induce an oncogenic event, the number of oncogenes in the final dose, and the number of DNA segments in the final dose. It is reasonable to assume that X, Y, N are independently distributed according to the following distributions (Yang and Zhang 2016):

$$X_i \mid O_m \sim N\left(O_m, \text{prec} = \tau\right),$$

$$Y_j \mid U \sim N\left(U, \text{prec} = \delta\right),$$

$$\Pr(N = t \mid p) = \binom{k(M-1)}{t-k} p^{t-k}(1-p)^{kM-t}, \quad t = k, k+1, \ldots, kM. \quad (9.3)$$

Here, $N(O_m, \text{prec} = \tau)$ denotes a normal distribution with mean O_m and variance $1/\tau$. The parameter τ is called precision, the reciprocal of variance. Assume that the parameters in Distributions (9.3) have the following conjugate prior distributions

$$O_m \mid \tau \sim N\left(O_0, n_0 \tau\right),$$

$$\tau \sim \text{Ga}(\alpha, \beta),$$

$$U \mid \tau_1 \sim N\left(U_0, n_1 \tau_1\right),$$

$$\tau_1 \sim \text{Ga}(\alpha_1, \beta_1),$$

$$p \sim \text{Beta}(a, b) \quad (9.4)$$

It can be easily verified that the posterior distribution of the parameters may be characterized by

$$O_m \mid X, \tau \sim N\left(\frac{n}{n+n_0}\bar{X} + \frac{n_0}{n+n_0}O_0, n\tau + n_0\tau\right),$$

$$\tau \mid X \sim \text{Ga}\left(\alpha + \frac{n}{2}, \beta + \frac{1}{2}\sum_{i=1}^{n}(X_i - \bar{X})^2 + \frac{nn_0}{2(n+n_0)}(\bar{X} - O_0)^2\right),$$

$$U \mid Y, \tau_1 \sim N\left(\frac{n}{n+n_1}\bar{Y} + \frac{n_1}{n+n_1}U_0, n\tau_1 + n_1\tau_1\right),$$

$$\tau_1 \mid Y \sim \text{Ga}\left(\alpha_1 + \frac{n}{2}, \beta_1 + \frac{1}{2}\sum_{i=1}^{n}(Y_i - \bar{Y})^2 + \frac{nn_1}{2(n+n_1)}(\bar{Y} - U_0)^2\right),$$

$$p \mid N \sim \text{Beta}(a + N - k, b + kM - N) \quad (9.5)$$

Note that the parameters O_m and U are positive real numbers. When stipulating priors, a positive restriction can be put on the normal prior distributions in Distributions (9.4), resulting in, for example, truncated normal distributions. The corresponding posterior distributions still have the forms in Distributions (9.5), but with positive restrictions in place.

Denote the parameter set $\theta = (O_m, \tau, U, \tau_1, p)$ and all the observables as $\tilde{X} = (X, Y, N)$. It can be easily verified that the density of the posterior distribution of $\theta | \tilde{X}$ is the product of the density functions of the above five distributions in Distributions (9.5). Let SF_0 be the acceptable lower limit of the safety factor SF. That is, the oncogenic (infective) risk of a drug product is deemed acceptable if with a high posterior probability p_0 the safety factor estimate SF satisfies $SF \geq SF_0$. In other words,

$$\Pr[SF \geq SF_0 | \tilde{X}] \geq p_0 \tag{9.6}$$

which is the posterior probability of Equation (9.2).

Let $I_{\{SF \geq SF_0\}}(\theta)$ be the indicator function of the set $\{\theta : SF \geq SF_0\}$. Thus

$$\Pr[SF \geq SF_0 | \tilde{X}] = E\left[I_{\{SF \geq SF_0\}}(\theta) | \tilde{X}\right]. \tag{9.7}$$

The above probability can be estimated using the following procedure:

1) Generate L random samples θ_l^* from the distributions in Distributions (9.5).

2) By the large number theorem,

$$\frac{\sum_{l=1}^{L} I_{\{SF \geq SF_0\}}(\theta_l^*)}{L} \rightarrow E[I_{\{SF \geq SF_0\}}(\theta) | \tilde{X}] \text{ as } L \rightarrow \infty.$$

Therefore, the probability in Inequality (9.6) can be estimated by

$$\frac{\sum_{l=1}^{L} I_{\{SF \geq SF_0\}}(\theta_l^*)}{L}.$$

9.3.5 Example

Consider the following scenario: 20 experimental measurements of the number of oncogenes (μg/dose) (X) needed to induce an oncogenic event were taken according to the normal distribution $N(9.4, precision = 2)$ and the number of oncogenes (ng/dose) in the final dose (Y) was measured 20 times following $N(1, precison = 100)$. The mean size of residual DNA ($\bar{Z}$) was 650 bp. The haploid genome size of the MDCK genome is $M = 2.41 \times 10^9$ bp and there is only one oncogene (m_1) of size 1,925 bp contained in the canine genome. The prior distributions parameters from Distributions (9.4) are set with

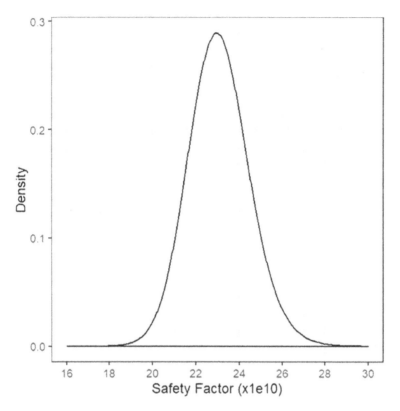

FIGURE 9.2
Posterior distribution of SF based on 5×10^7 random draws.

$\alpha = \beta = \alpha_1 = \beta_1 = 0.001$, $O_0 = U_0 = 0$, $n_0 = n_1 = 0.5$, and $a = b = 0.5$. Note that, because X and Y are given in different units (µg and ng), the posterior distribution of O_m will be multiplied by 1,000 so that its units will match with that of U.

Given the priors, the posteriors in Distributions (9.5) have known distributions and random sampling of $\theta = (O_m, \tau, U, \tau_1, p)$ is straightforward using software packages such as R (R Core Team 2018). Plugging in the random draws of parameters into the formula of SF gives 10,000 realizations from posterior distribution of SF. The mean SF is 23.1×10^{10}; see Figure 9.2 for the posterior distribution of SF based on 5×10^7 random draws. Given the lower acceptance limit $SF_0 = 10 \times 10^{10}$, the probability in Equation (9.7) was estimated to be 1. As a result, the oncogenic risk was considered acceptable when compared with prespecified acceptance limit p_0, say, 0.999. Although the Gibbs sampler shown in Distributions (9.5) could easily be carried out in R, to permit the future possibility of non-conjugate priors, the computer code is shown below using JAGS.

```
require(rjags); require(runjags)
```

```
model.txt = "
model{
  ## Prior distribution
  tau ~ dgamma(0.001, 0.001)
  Om ~ dnorm(0., 0.5*tau)

  tau1 ~ dgamma(0.001, 0.001)
  U ~ dnorm(0., 0.5*tau1)

  sigma <- 1/sqrt(tau)
  sigma1 <- 1/sqrt(tau1)

  p ~ dbeta(0.5, 0.5)

  ## Likelihood for (N-k)
  Nmk ~ dbin( p, k*(M-1) )

  for ( i in 1:20 )
  {
    x[i] ~ dnorm( Om, tau )
    y[i] ~ dnorm( U, tau1 )
  }
}"

## Testing limit
SF0 = 1e10

## Data
M = 2.41e9 ## haploid genome size
k = 20
m1 = 1925
N = k*M/650

set.seed(410) ## Generate a data set
n = 20
x = rnorm(20, mean=9.4, sd=1/sqrt(2))   ## units are ug
y = rnorm(20, mean=1, sd=1/sqrt(100)) ## units are ng

data = list(x=x, y=y, Nmk=N-k, k=k, M=M)

fitb = run.jags( model.txt, data=data, n.chains=3,
          monitor=c("Om", "sigma", "U", "sigma1", "p"),
          burnin=5000, sample=10000, thin=1,
                                    method="parallel")
```

```
th.post = as.matrix(as.mcmc.list(fitb))
th.post[,"Om"] = 1000* th.post[,"Om"] ## Convert to ng

SF = th.post[,"Om"]/( (1-th.post[,"p"])*(m1/M)
     *th.post[,"U"] )

   ## Posterior mean and posterior probability
mean(SF)
mean(SF >= SF0)
```

A sensitivity analysis was conducted to ascertain whether the posterior distribution of SF is sensitive to prior specification. Ten scenarios were considered in Table 9.1 with various hyperparameter specifications. The hyperparameters a and b have the least effect on the results. The safety factor was also insensitive to the hyperparameters (α, β, α_1, and β_1) for precision. The greatest impact was found when the pair (O_0, n_0) or (U_0, n_1) was set such that the prior was informative, as in scenarios 8–10. The posterior distribution of the safety factor changed quite a bit although the probability $\Pr[SF \geq SF_0 | \tilde{X}]$ was still above the acceptance limit of 0.999.

9.4 Design Space

9.4.1 Definition

Design space is a key concept in the implementation of QbD. According to ICH Q8 (R2) (ICH 2006), a design space is "[t]he multidimensional combination and interaction of input variables (e.g., material attributes) and process parameters that have been demonstrated to provide assurance of quality." For example, a design space for a cell culture system may have ranges for temperature, pH, feed volume, and culture duration that ensure a quality product. Design space is intimately related to quality risk management (QRM) principles. Linking manufacturing variations with the variability of CQAs sets the stage for developing effective manufacturing controls. A design space also has regulatory implications for post-approval changes as "[w]orking within the design space is not considered as a change. Movement out of the design space is considered to be a change and would normally initiate a regulatory post-approval change process" (ICH 2006). Thus, a well-developed design space may enable a manufacturer to continuously improve the manufacturing process by adapting to novel technologies without incurring additional risk and creating more regulatory hurdles. Most recently, the concept of design space has also been used in analytical method development, which will be discussed in a later section.

TABLE 9.1

Sensitivity Analysis for Safety Factor under Various Priors

Scenario/Prior Distributions	1	2	3	4	5	6	7	8	9	10
O_0	0	0	0	0	0	0	10	0	0	0
n_0	0.5	0.5	0.5	0.5	0.5	0.01	0.5	0.5	0.5	5
U_0	0	0	0	0	0	0	0	5	3	0
n_1	0.5	0.5	0.5	0.5	0.5	0.5	0.5	0.5	5	0.5
α	0.001	0	1	0.001	0.001	0.001	0.001	0.001	0.001	0.001
β	0.001	0	0.1	0.001	0.001	0.001	0.001	0.001	0.001	0.001
α_1	0.001	0	0.001	1	0.1	0.001	0.001	0.001	0.001	0.001
β_1	0.001	0	0.001	0.1	1	0.001	0.001	0.001	0.001	0.001
a	0.5	5	0.5	0.5	0.5	0.5	0.5	0.5	0.5	0.5
b	0.5	1	0.5	0.5	0.5	0.5	0.5	0.5	0.5	0.5
SF (Mean) ($\times 10^{10}$)	23.09	23.08	23.07	23.11	23.17	23.65	23.69	20.85	16.26	18.96
SF (SD) ($\times 10^{10}$)	1.44	1.41	1.40	1.50	2.31	1.17	1.16	3.15	2.60	2.43
$\Pr(SF \geq SF_0)$	1.00	1.00	1.00	1.00	1.00	1.00	1.00	1.00	1.00	1.00

9.4.2 Statistical Methods for Design Space

Several statistical methods have been proposed to determine design space through multivariate regression analysis. Of note are two traditional approaches: overlapping mean response surfaces and the composite desirability function. Both methods rely on the use of a multiple regression model to describe the relationship between the measured CQAs, *Y*, and process CQAs of the product and process parameters and other controllable inputs, such as material attributes *x*. Suppose that the relationship between *Y* and *x* can be characterized through the model:

$$Y = f(x;\theta) + \varepsilon \qquad (9.8)$$

where $f(x;\theta)$ is a mathematical function, θ are model parameters, and ε are measurement errors.

Below we briefly describe how design space is determined using both methods.

9.4.2.1 *Overlapping Mean*

The design space per the overlapping mean surface method is defined as a set of *x* such that the predicted mean values of the CQAs are within their acceptable limits:

$$\Omega = \left\{ x : \hat{E}[Y \mid x] \in A \right\} \qquad (9.9)$$

where $\hat{E}[Y \mid x] = f(x;\hat{\theta})$ are the predicted of mean values when CQAs are *x* and $\hat{\theta}$ is the estimate of the model parameters.

The idea of the overlapping mean approach was graphically illustrated by Zhang and Yang (2018), as shown in Figure 9.3. The two response surfaces are predicted mean values of the yield and cell viability of a cell culture system. Temperature and pH are process parameters that were found to have significant impact on the two CQAs. The design space normalized with respect to the nominal condition is the joint shaded region of temperature and cell density in which both the yield and cell viability meet their respective specifications.

9.4.2.2 *Desirability Method*

Although the desirability method is normally utilized to find the optimum condition of a system with multiple outputs such as cell culture system, with slight modification it can also be employed to determine the design space. The method utilizes a composite desirability function to define the design space. The desirability function needs to reflect divergent needs and allow

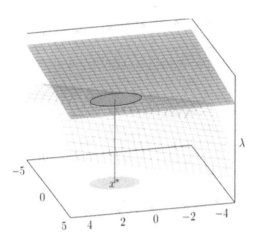

FIGURE 9.3
Operation region determined based on two overlapping mean response surfaces (adopted from Zhang and Yang 2018).

for trade-off. For example, the design space that is most suitable for producing high yield might not be optimum for reducing impurities. One way to meet these multiple goals is to construct a composite score based on a collection of desirability functions commensurate with the objectives for individual CQAs. Specifically, for each predicted mean response Y_i, $i = 1, \ldots, p$, the desirability function $d(Y)$ assumes values in the range of 0 and 1, with 0 and 1 respectively corresponding to the least and most desirable values. These functions are then combined to form an overall desirability function, using a geometric mean (Harrington 1965):

$$D(Y) = \left[\prod_{i=1}^{p} d(Y_i) \right]^{\frac{1}{p}}.$$

Several desirability functions were proposed by Derringer and Suich (1980). Denote L_i, U_i, and T_i as the lower, upper, and target values, respectively, for the quality attribute Y_i such that $L_i \leq T_i \leq U_i$. The following desirability functions $d_T(Y_i)$, $d_U(Y_i)$, or $d_L(Y_i)$ may be used to achieve target, maximization, or minimization, respectively:

$$d_T(Y_i) = \begin{cases} 0 & \text{if } Y_i < L_i \\ \left(\dfrac{Y_i - L_i}{T_i - L_i} \right)^s & \text{if } L_i \leq Y_i \leq T_i \\ \left(\dfrac{Y_i - U_i}{T_i - U_i} \right)^t & \text{if } T_i < Y_i \leq U_i \\ 0 & \text{if } Y_i > U_i \end{cases}$$

with the parameters s and t being chosen to reflect the importance to meet the target;

$$d_U(Y_i) = \begin{cases} 0 & \text{if } Y_i < L_i \\ \left(\dfrac{Y_i - L_i}{T_i - L_i}\right)^s & \text{if } L_i \leq Y_i \leq T_i \\ 1 & \text{if } Y_i > T_i \end{cases}$$

with T_i being a value deemed to be large enough;

$$d_L(Y_i) = \begin{cases} 1 & \text{if } Y_i < T_i \\ \left(\dfrac{Y_i - L_i}{T_i - L_i}\right)^s & \text{if } L_i \leq Y_i \leq U_i \\ 0 & \text{if } Y_i > U_i \end{cases}$$

with T_i being a value deemed to be small enough.

The design space can then be determined as

$$DS = \{D(\mathbf{Y}) \geq d_0\}$$

where d_0 is a prespecified threshold.

9.4.2.3 Criticisms of Current Methods

As pointed out by Peterson (2008), these traditional methods do not take into account correlations among CQAs, nor do they account for variability in the model prediction. An appropriately constructed design space needs to account for measurement uncertainties, uncertainty about the parameters of the statistical models, and correlations among the measurements in order to provide high assurance of product quality. In recent years, significant advances have been made in developing design spaces using Bayesian multivariate analysis techniques (Peterson 2008, 2009; Peterson and Lief 2010; Peterson and Yahyah 2010) and further statistical opportunities for design space development still exist. For example, so far, the concept of design space is by and large applied to input materials and process parameters. In addition, a design space is usually developed based on experiments and data from small-scale processes. How to update such design spaces, based on data from pilot and full-scale data, remains to be further researched. It will also be of great benefit to bring these statistical methods into common practice through software development (Hofer 2009).

9.4.3 Bayesian Design Space

Let $Y = (Y_1, \ldots, Y_p)'$ be a $p \times 1$ vector of measures of p CQAs, A the set of jointly acceptable ranges of the CQAs, and x a $k \times 1$ vector of process parameters and other controllable inputs, such as material attributes. As an alternative approach, and to address the deficiencies of the overlapping mean contours and desirability function methods, Peterson (2008) suggested a Bayesian approach to establishing a design space. An application of the method was demonstrated by Stockdale and Cheng (2009) through two case studies. A Bayesian design space and various extensions were also explored by LeBrun (2012). In general terms, a Bayesian design space is defined as (Peterson 2008; Stockdale and Cheng 2009):

$$\left\{ x : \Pr[\tilde{Y} \in A \mid x, \text{data}] \geq R \right\} \tag{9.10}$$

where A and x are defined as before, $\tilde{Y}$ is the $p \times 1$ vector of future CQA measurements, *data* is the data set from a controlled experiment, which includes measured values of the CQA(s) and various settings of the process parameters, and R is a pre-selected level of reliability that must be met.

Because the posterior predictive probability in Design Space (9.10) takes into account the uncertainty in the model parameters and correlation among the response variables, it overcomes the drawbacks of the overlapping mean response surface method. In addition, the Bayesian method can be easily extended to accommodate many different types of experiments such as split-plot (Peterson et al. 2009) as well as experiments involving mixed effects (LeBrun 2012). The Bayesian design space can be determined by estimating the probability $\Pr[Y \in A \mid x, \text{data}]$ over a grid of x values. The posterior predictive probability can be estimated either through a closed-form solution or by MCMC simulations.

9.4.3.1 Regression Model

Several regression models can be used to describe the measured responses of the CQAs (**Y**). For example, the following model was used by Peterson (2008) and Stockdale and Cheng (2009):

$$Y = Bz(x) + e \tag{9.11}$$

where **B** is a $p \times q$ matrix of regression coefficients, $\mathbf{z}(x)$ is a $q \times 1$ vector function of x, and **e** is a $p \times 1$ vector of measurement errors having a multivariate normal distribution with mean **0** and covariance–variance matrix Σ.

It is assumed that $\mathbf{z}(x)$ is the same for each CQA, though the method described in this section can be extended to the seemingly unrelated regressions (SUR) model (Peterson 2004), in which each response Y_j ($j=1, ..., p$) has a different function $z_j(x)$. Under such circumstances, the SUR model provides greater flexibility and accuracy in modeling the CQAs (Peterson 2007). A SUR model takes the form:

$$Y_j = z_j(x)'\beta_j + e_j, \quad j = 1,...,p.$$

The SUR model includes the standard multivariate regression model as a special case where $z_j(x) = z(x)$. A design space based on the SUR model and posterior predictive probability can be similarly obtained (Peterson 2007).

9.4.3.2 Prior Information

Use of prior information (regarding process/method parameters, CQAs, etc.) is a critical step in Bayesian inference. Peterson (2008) discussed various ways in which prior information can be determined for a design space model. For example, an informative prior distribution may be established from experiments done at the pilot scale, with the intention of using it for developing a design space for commercial-scale manufacturing. Oftentimes, however, data from pilot-scale experiments alone may not be sufficient for constructing informative priors. In Chapter 10, for example, in the context of shelf life estimation and comparison of stability design, we use historical batch data to develop priors that account for both intro- and intra-batch variations. Peterson (2008) discussed three additional sources of information that can be potentially used for specifying informative prior distributions. Please refer to Peterson (2008) for details.

9.4.3.3 Posterior Predictive Probability and Design Space

Let $Y_{obs} = (Y_1,...,Y_n)'$ be an $n \times p$ matrix consisting of n observations of the $1 \times p$ response vector Y. Let $Z_{exp} = (Z_1,...,Z_n)'$ be an $n \times q$ matrix with $Z_i = z(x_i)$, $i = 1, ..., n$, and let x_i be the ith condition of the controllable input variables and process parameters. Assume that a non-informative prior is used to describe the parameters (B, Σ):

$$\pi(B,\Sigma) \propto |\Sigma|^{-(p+1)/2} \tag{9.12}$$

It is well known (Press 1972) that the posterior predictive distribution of a future observation $\tilde{Y}$ in this case is a multivariate T with degrees of freedom $v = n - p - q + 1$:

$$\tilde{Y}|x, \text{data} \sim t_v\left(\hat{B}z(x), H\right) \tag{9.13}$$

where $H = \left[1 + z(x)'D^{-1}z(x)\right]\hat{\Sigma}$ is the scale matrix for the multivariate t distribution, $D = \sum_{i=1}^{n} Z_i Z_i'$, and $\hat{B}$ and $\hat{\Sigma}$ are the least-squares estimates of B and Σ given by

$$\hat{B} = \left(Z_{\exp}' Z_{\exp}\right)^{-1} Z_{\exp}' Y_{obs}$$

$$\hat{\Sigma} = \left[Y_{obs} - \left(\hat{B}Z\right)'\right]\left[Y_{obs} - \left(\hat{B}Z\right)'\right]/v, \text{ with } v = n - p - q + 1.$$

Because the posterior predictive distribution is a multivariate T distribution, it can be simulated as follows (Peterson 2007):

1. Draw W from the multivariate normal distribution $N(0, H)$; note that H is the variance–covariance matrix.
2. Draw U from the chi-square distribution χ_v^2.
3. Calculate $Y_j = (\sqrt{v}W_j / \sqrt{U}) + \hat{\mu}_j$, for $j = 1, \ldots, p$, where Y_j, W_j, and $\hat{\mu}_j$ are the jth elements of Y, W, and $\hat{B}z(x)$, respectively.

As suggested by Peterson (2009), the posterior predictive probability can be approximated using Monte Carlo simulation:

$$p(x) = \Pr[Y \in A | x, \text{data}] \approx \frac{1}{N} \sum_{s=1}^{N} I\left(Y^{(s)} \in A\right),$$

where $Y^{(s)}$, $s = 1, \ldots, N$, are independent random multivariate T variables simulated from the above-mentioned procedure, and $I(.)$ is an indicator function taking values of either 0 or 1. The design space defined in Design Space (9.10) can be obtained by estimating the posterior predictive probability $p(x)$ over a grid of x values and comparing it to the reliability threshold R.

Alternatively, as discussed previously, informative prior distributions may be used in the derivation of the posterior predictive probability. For example, one may use conjugate prior distributions for $p(B|\Sigma)$ and $p(\Sigma)$ (Lebrun 2012):

$$B|\Sigma \sim N(B_0, \Sigma\Sigma_0)$$

$$\Sigma \sim \text{IW}(\Omega, v_0),$$

where B_0 is the mean vector and Σ and Σ_0 are the covariance matrices of the columns and rows of B respectively; Σ follows an inverse Wishart distribution with Ω being an *a priori* response scale matrix, and v_0 the degrees of freedom.

TABLE 9.2

Liquid Chromatography Data from LeBlond (2015)

x_1	x_2	x_3	y_1	y_2	y_3	y_4
65	30	0.175	2.14	22	172	0.76
65	50	0.175	1.73	12	311	0.88
65	40	0.05	1.93	16	251	0.8
65	40	0.3	1.95	16	241	0.8
70	40	0.175	2.17	14	278	0.79
70	50	0.05	1.97	11	371	0.86
70	30	0.3	2.38	19	194	0.74
70	50	0.3	1.98	11	360	0.86
70	30	0.05	2.37	18	204	0.74
70	40	0.175	2.2	14	280	0.78
75	40	0.3	2.42	13	314	0.78
75	30	0.175	2.61	17	223	0.73
75	50	0.175	2.14	10	410	0.85
75	40	0.05	2.42	12	324	0.78
70	40	0.175	2.2	14	281	0.79

It was shown by LeBrun (2012) that the posterior predictive probability in this case is also a multivariate t-distribution. Thus, using the Monte Carlo simulation procedure previously described, the Bayesian design space can be constructed.

9.4.4 Example

For the liquid chromatography method example previously discussed, LeBlond (2015) presented a design space calculation. Data are shown in Table 9.2.

The design space is $\{x : \Pr[Y \in A \mid x, \text{data}] \geq 0.99\}$. To calculate the posterior predictive probability, let $x = (x_1, x_2, x_3)$, $y = (y_1, y_2, y_3, y_4)$, and $\beta = \{\beta_0^{(k)}, \beta_i^{(k)}, \beta_{ii}^{(k)}, \beta_{12}^{(k)}, \beta_{13}^{(k)}, \beta_{23}^{(k)}, i = 1, 2, 3\}$. The following model was fitted to the data.

$$y \mid \beta, \Sigma, x, \text{data} \sim N\big(\mu(x), \Sigma\big)$$

where

$$\mu^{(k)}(x) = \beta_0^{(k)} + \sum_{i=1}^{3} \beta_i^{(k)} x_i + \sum_{i=1}^{3} \beta_{ii}^{(k)} x_i^2 + \beta_{12}^{(k)} x_1 x_2 + \beta_{13}^{(k)} x_1 x_3 + \beta_{23}^{(k)} x_2 x_3$$

is the kth element of $\mu(x)$, $k = 1, \ldots, 4$.

Minimally informative priors $\beta \sim N(0, 30^2 I)$ are used for the 40 regression coefficients (10×4) and a scaled inverse Wishart prior is used for the variance–covariance matrix (Hofer 2009). The prior for the variance–covariance matrix is assigned based on a method suggested by Gelman and Hill (2007), who show that the simpler inverse Wishart prior often carries information. To begin, the variance–covariance matrix is first expressed as

$$\Sigma = \text{Diag}(\xi) Q \text{Diag}(\xi)$$

where $\text{Diag}(\xi)$ is a diagonal matrix with diagonal elements $\xi = (\xi_1, \xi_2, \xi_3, \xi_4)$ and Q is a correlation matrix given by

$$Q = \begin{pmatrix} 1 & \rho_{12} & \rho_{13} & \rho_{14} \\ & 1 & \rho_{23} & \rho_{24} \\ & & 1 & \rho_{34} \\ & & & 1 \end{pmatrix}.$$

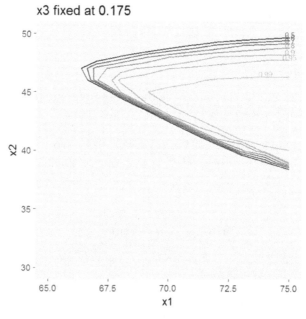

FIGURE 9.4
Contour plot of posterior predictive probabilities to meet criteria for design space.

For $i = 1, \ldots, 4$, in practice, the parameters $\xi = (\xi_1, \xi_2, \xi_3, \xi_4)$ are chosen as half-Cauchy(0, 1) for the ith diagonal element of Σ and Q is distributed according to an inserse-Wishart IW(I, 5), where I is a 4×4 identity matrix. Although $Q \sim$ IW(I, 5) is not a correlation matrix, the philosophy for building Σ with the inverse Wishart core is functionally equivalent and the distribution for Σ is called the scaled inverse Wishart. The Stan MCMC software manual (Stan 2018) suggests using a true correlation distribution for Q, setting $Q \sim$ LKJ(ν), where $\nu \geq 1$ is a shape parameter. Using MCMC methods, the posterior predictive probability for a future CQA response is estimated and the resulting design space is depicted, along with the overlapping mean contours for comparison, in Figure 9.4.

Computer code for sampling from the posterior of (β, Σ) follows.

```
require(rjags); require(runjags)

## Create the JAGS model
model.txt = "
model{

  ## Scaled-inverse Wishart prior
  for ( i in 1:4 )
  {
      D[i]  ~  dt(0., 1., 1)T(0., )
  }
  Omega  ~  dscaled.wishart( D, 5 )
  Sigma <- inverse(Omega)

  ## Prior for theta
  for ( i in 1:p )
  {
    theta1[i]  ~  dnorm( 0, 0.001 )   ## SD = 30
    theta2[i]  ~  dnorm( 0, 0.001 )
    theta3[i]  ~  dnorm( 0, 0.001 )
    theta4[i]  ~  dnorm( 0, 0.001 )
  }

  ## Likelihood
  for ( j in 1:N )
  {
    mu[j,1]  =  X[j,]%*%theta1  ## Linear model means 1-4
    mu[j,2]  =  X[j,]%*%theta2
    mu[j,3]  =  X[j,]%*%theta3
    mu[j,4]  =  X[j,]%*%theta4
    Y[j,1:4]  ~  dmnorm( mu[j,1:4], Omega )
  }
```

```
        }"


        d = read.csv("Design Space.csv")    ## Load the data

        ## Center the levels of x
        x.centers = c(x1=70, x2=40, x3=0.175)
        for ( x in names(x.centers) )
          d[,x] = d[,x] - x.centers[x]

        ## Scale the responses for better performance
        y.mult = c(y1=1, y2=0.1, y3=0.01, y4=1)
        for ( y in names(y.mult) )
          d[,y] = d[,y]*y.mult[y]

        ## Get the design matrix
        f.x = ~(x1+x2+x3)^2+I(x1^2)+I(x2^2)+I(x3^2)
        X = matrix( model.matrix(f.x, data=d), ncol=10 )

        ## Prepare data for JAGS
        data = list( N=nrow(d), p=10, X=X,
                     Y=as.matrix(d[,c("y1", "y2", "y3",
                       "y4")]) )
        dimnames(data$Y) = list(NULL, NULL)

        ## Call JAGS
        fitb = run.jags(model.txt, data=data, n.chains=3,
                    monitor=c("theta1", "theta2", "theta3",
                         "theta4", "Sigma"),
                    burnin=10000, thin=10, sample=20000,
                    modules="glm", method="parallel" )
```

The posterior predictive distribution and posterior predictive probability are calculated in R with the following code:

```
        require(ggplot2) ## Graphics library
        require(directlabels) ## For labeling contour plot

        th.post = as.matrix( as.mcmc.list(fitb) )

        ## Explore the post. pred. distribution of Y for
            (x1, x2) with x3=0.
        ## Note: x values are centered
        set.seed(822)
        d.grid = expand.grid( x1=-5:5, x2=-10:10, x3=0 )
```

```
for ( v in c("pr1", "pr2", "pr3", "pr4", "prTotal",
                     "mu1", "mu2", "mu3", "mu4") )
{
  d.grid[,v] = NA
}
## Design matrix for d.grid
X.grid = model.matrix(f.x, data=d.grid)

for ( i in 1:nrow(d.grid) )
{
  ## Get post draw for mean(Y | x1, x2, x3, data)
     for ith row of d.grid
  mu1 = th.post[,paste("theta1[", 1:10, "]",
        sep="")]%*%X.grid[i,]
  mu2 = th.post[,paste("theta2[", 1:10, "]",
        sep="")]%*%X.grid[i,]
  mu3 = th.post[,paste("theta3[", 1:10, "]",
        sep="")]%*%X.grid[i,]
  mu4 = th.post[,paste("theta4[", 1:10, "]",
        sep="")]%*%X.grid[i,]

    ## Generate posterior predictive multivariate
       errors for each draw
    # Note: rnorm(4)%*%chol(Sigma) same as
    #        rmvnorm(1, mean=rep(0, 4), sigma=Sigma)
   E = t(sapply(1:nrow(th.post), function(b){
              Sigma = matrix(th.post[b,grep("Sigma",
                colnames(th.post), value=TRUE)], 4, 4 )
              rnorm(4)%*%chol(Sigma)
              }))

    ## Posterior predictive distribution for Y | x1,
       x2, x3, data
  Ypred = cbind(mu1, mu2, mu3, mu4) + E

    ## Determine which rows of Ypred meet the
       acceptance criteria
 index = cbind(Ypred[,1] >= 1.8*y.mult[1],
            Ypred[,2] <= 15*y.mult[2],
            Ypred[,3] >= 300*y.mult[3],
            Ypred[,4] >= 0.75*y.mult[4] & Ypred[,4]
                   <= 0.85*y.mult[4])
```

```
     ## Calculate Monte Carlo probability
 d.grid[i,c("pr1", "pr2", "pr3", "pr4", "prTotal")] =
             c( colMeans(index),
             mean(apply(index, 1, all)) )

 d.grid[i,c("mu1", "mu2", "mu3", "mu4")] =
             c( median(mu1), median(mu2),
             median(mu3), median(mu4)  )
}

## Create contour plot
p=ggplot( d.grid ) +
        geom_contour(aes(x=x1+70, y=x2+40, z=prTotal,
                     color=..level..),
                 breaks=c(0.5, 0.6, 0.7, 0.8, 0.9,
                         0.95, 0.99), size=1) +
    xlab("x1") + ylab("x2") + ggtitle("x3 fixed at
        0.175") +
    theme_grey(base_size=18) + xlim( 65, 75 ) + ylim(
        30, 50 )

direct.label(p, method="top.pieces")
```

Such a design space provides over 99% confidence that movement within the design space has no impact on the assay's ability to meet its specification.

9.5 Process Validation

9.5.1 Risk-Based Lifecycle Approach

Process validation is a regulatory requirement, intended to demonstrate that a process can consistently produce batches meeting quality standards (FDA 1987a). Traditionally, validation was viewed as a one-time exercise, in which three consecutive batches of the finished product were produced and tested. In such a set-up, the process is deemed to be validated if all three lots meet the acceptance criteria. In 2011, the FDA issued updated guidance on process validation (FDA 2011a), ushering in a lifecycle approach to process validation. In the new regulatory framework, process validation is a continued effort, starting from process design through process performance quantification (PPQ) and then continuing into process monitoring. The new process validation aligns activities at each of the aforesaid three stages with the other existing regulatory guidelines, including ICH Q8(R2) and Q9-11 (ICH 2006,

2007a, 2007b, 2011), with increasing understanding of both the product and process. The use of modern pharmaceutical development concepts, quality risk management, quality systems, and statistical tools is recommended throughout the lifecycle of the product. The primary focus of the remainder of this chapter is on PPQ.

For PPQ, the new guidance no longer endorses the three-batch validation rule. The number of PPQ batches should be chosen in view of the underlying process. Adoption of Bayesian concepts can facilitate the use of knowledge acquired from the early process development. In the following, we introduce two Bayesian methods, one based on the posterior probability of process capability and the other related to the predictive probability for future commercial batches to meet specifications.

9.5.2 Method Based on Process Capability

A process that consistently produces quality products is a capable process. In literature, process capability is measured by a quantity called process capability index C_{pk} such that

$$C_{pk} = \min\left[\frac{USL - \mu}{3\sigma}, \frac{\mu - LSL}{3\sigma}\right], \tag{9.14}$$

where LSL, USL, μ, and σ are the lower and upper specification limits, mean, and variability of the CQA, respectively.

There are variants of C_{pk}. For the sake of simplicity, however, our discussion is centered on the C_{pk} given in Model (9.13). Let $\bar{X}$ and s be the sample mean and standard deviation of the CQA based on test results $\{X_1, \ldots, X_n\}$ of n PPQ batches, respectively. Assume that the CQA is normally distributed. The maximum likelihood estimate of C_{pk} is given by:

$$\hat{C}_{pk} = \min\left[\frac{USL - \bar{X}}{3s}, \frac{\bar{X} - LSL}{3s}\right].$$

An approximate one-sided $100(1 - \alpha)\%$ lower confidence limit for C_{pk} can be obtained (Bissell 1990):

$$\hat{C}_{pk} - z_{1-\alpha}\sqrt{\frac{1}{9n} + \frac{\hat{C}_{pk}^2}{2(n-1)}} \tag{9.15}$$

where $z_{1-\alpha}$ is the $100(1 - \alpha)$ percentile of the standard normal distribution.

9.5.2.1 Frequentist Acceptance Criterion

One frequentist acceptance criterion to claim that the process is validated may be given by

$$\hat{C}_{pk} - z_{1-\alpha}\sqrt{\frac{1}{9n} + \frac{\hat{C}_{pk}^2}{2(n-1)}} \geq c_0 \tag{9.16}$$

where c_0 is a pre-selected cut point representing the smallest capability index a process needs in order to be deemed capable.

The method, however, is not in keeping with the risk-based paradigm recommended in the FDA guidance (2011) because it does not incorporate any historical knowledge about the process.

9.5.2.2 Bayesian Acceptance Criterion

When the process understanding is formulated in terms of a prior distribution μ and σ, the posterior distribution of C_{pk} can be obtained through MCMC and used to declare a process validated. For example, the left side of Inequality (9.16) may be replaced with a lower 95% credible limit for C_{pk}.

To illustrate the concept, consider a process for measuring relative potency with specification limits USL $= 70\%$ and LSL $= 130\%$. Suppose that $n = 5$ test results are available from the PPQ batches that follow a normal distribution such that

$$X_i \mid \mu, \tau \sim N(\mu, \tau),$$

where τ is the precision parameter.

Further, assume a conjugate prior distribution for (μ, τ) such that $\mu \sim N(\mu_0, n_0\tau)$ and $\tau \sim Ga(\alpha, \beta)$. Letting $\mathbf{X} = \{X_1, X_2, \ldots, X_5\}$, as shown in Distributions (9.5), the marginal posterior distributions are

$$\mu \mid \mathbf{X}, \tau \sim N\left(\frac{n}{n+n_0}\bar{X} + \frac{n_0}{n+n_0}\mu_0, n\tau + n_0\tau\right) \text{ and}$$

$$\tau \mid \mathbf{X} \sim Ga\left(\alpha + \frac{n}{2}, \beta + \frac{1}{2}\sum_{i=1}^{n}(X_i - \bar{X})^2 + \frac{nn_0}{2(n+n_0)}(\bar{X} - \mu_0)^2\right).$$

The PPQ testing resulted in $\bar{X} = 102$ and $s = 4.2$ with $n = 5$. Based on development data, assume that prior parameters were assigned with hyperparameters $\mu_0 = 98$, $n_0 = 2$, $\alpha = 1.5$, and $\beta = 78$. For validation declaration purposes, let $c_0 = 2$ denote an acceptable lower limit for C_{pk}. Computer code in R is given below. From the computer code, the lower 95% posterior C_{pk} credible limit is $2.8 > c_0 = 2$ and so the process meets with the validation criterion.

```
## Priors
mu0=98; n0=2; alpha=1.5; beta = 78
```

```
## Data
n = 5
xbar = 102
s = 4.2

## Posterior distribution of (mu, tau)
set.seed(148)
B = 10000
tau = rgamma(B, shape=alpha+n/2, rate=beta+0.5*
      (n-1)*s^2 +
            0.5*((n*n0)/(n+n0))*(xbar-mu0)^2 )
mu = rnorm(B, mean=(n/(n+n0))*xbar+(n0/(n+n0))*mu0,
            sd=1/sqrt(n*tau+n0*tau))

sigma = 1/sqrt(tau)  ## Posterior distribution of
         standard deviation

## Validation test
LSL = 70; USL = 130
c0 = 2
p0=0.95

## Posterior distribution of Cpk
Cpk =apply( cbind( (USL-mu)/sigma, (mu-LSL)/sigma ),
      1, min )
Cpk.05 = quantile(Cpk, 0.05) ## Lower 95% credible
         limit
Cpk.05 >= c0
```

9.5.3 Method Based on Predictive Performance

Alternatively, the acceptance criterion can be defined based on the predictive probability for the future batches to meet specification. For the purpose of illustration, suppose the CQA is potency. Define

$$Y_i = \begin{cases} 1 & X_i \in [\text{LSL}, \text{USL}] \\ 0 & X_i \text{ not} \in [\text{LSL}, \text{USL}] \end{cases}$$

where [LSL, USL] are the specification limits.

Thus $Y_i, i = 1, \ldots n$ are independently identically distributed according to Bernoulli distribution Bernoulli(p), where p is the probability for a batch to pass the potency specification. It follows that

$$Y = \sum_{i=1}^{n} Y_i \sim \text{binomial}(n, p).$$

Let $\tilde{x}$ be the potency test outcome of a future batch after the PPQ study is conducted. Let $\tilde{Y} = 1$ if the test outcome falls inside [LSL, USL] and $\tilde{Y} = 0$ otherwise. The PPQ is considered successful and the process validated if

$$\Pr(\tilde{Y} = 1 | Y) \geq p_0 \qquad (9.17)$$

where p_0 is a prespecified probability.

Suppose that p has a conjugate beta prior distribution Beta(α, β). From Chapter 2, the posterior probability of $p|Y$ follows a beta distribution Beta$(\alpha + Y, \beta + n - Y)$. Let $f(p|Y)$ denote the beta distribution PDF. Consequently,

$$\Pr(\tilde{Y} = 1 | Y) = \int_0^1 \Pr(\tilde{Y} = 1 | p) f(p | Y) dp$$

$$= \int_0^1 pf(p | Y) dp \qquad (9.18)$$

$$= \frac{\alpha + Y}{\alpha + \beta + n}$$

Combining Inequality (9.17) and Equation (9.18), the process is validated if

$$\frac{\alpha + Y}{\alpha + \beta + n} \geq p_0. \qquad (9.19)$$

Note that the parameters α and β may be respectively interpreted as the number of successful and failed batches and $\alpha + \beta$ may be given as the total number of batches produced during the process development. As the quantity on the left-hand side of Inequality (9.19) is an increasing function of α, the more successful batches are produced, the higher the chance is to meet the PPQ testing criteria. As a simple example, suppose that $n = 16$ PPQ batches are tested with $Y = 15$ batches falling inside [LSL, USL]. Further, suppose that four out of five development batches met the specification limits so that $\alpha = 4$ and $\beta = 1$. Thus,

$$\Pr(\tilde{Y} = 1 | Y) = \frac{\alpha + Y}{\alpha + \beta + n} = \frac{4 + 15}{5 + 16} = 0.904.$$

Given a prespecified value $p_0 = 0.95$, because $0.904 < 0.95$, the PPQ batches would not meet with the validation criterion based on the posterior predictive distribution.

9.5.4 Determination of Number of PPQ Batches

Both of the above Bayesian methods can be used to determine the number of PPQ batches, n, through the concept of predictive assurance outlined in Section 6.3 and O'Hagan et al. (2005). In the first example, the predictive distribution of C_{pk} may be generated for various sample sizes. The sample size calculation is illustrated with hyperparameter values $\mu_0 = 102$, $n_0 = 4$, $\alpha = 2.5$, and $\beta = 60$. The sample size n may be determined, for example, such that the statistical assurance of Inequality (9.16) is at least p_0 (e.g., $p_0 = 0.8$). The steps to calculate assurance are

1. Sample from the prior distribution for (μ, τ).

2. Generate B (e.g., $B = 10,000$) prior predictive samples $(\bar{X}, s)$ for a given sample size n.

3. From each prior predictive sample, calculate the lower 95% confidence limit for C_{pk}.

4. Assurance is approximated by the proportion of times (out of B) such that the lower 95% confidence limit for $C_{pk} \geq c_0$.

Computer code is given below to calculate assurance for the C_{pk} example. By running the code, it can be seen that at least $n = 9$ PPQ batches will be needed to meet or exceed an assurance of 0.8.

```
## Specification Limits
LSL=70; USL=130
## Priors
mu0=102; n0=4; alpha=2.5; beta = 60
   ## Cpk criterion
c0 = 2
p0 = 0.8
set.seed(842)
B = 10000
   ## prior distribution (mu, tau)
tau = rgamma(B, shape=alpha, rate=beta)
mu = rnorm(B, mean=mu0, 1/sqrt(n0*tau))
sigma = 1/sqrt(tau)
stats = data.frame(n=3:10, assurance=NA)
for (i in 1:nrow(stats))
{

    n = stats$n[i]
```

```
## Predictive distribution
xbar = rnorm(B, mean=mu, sd=sigma/sqrt(n))
s = sigma*sqrt( rchisq(B, n-1)/(n-1) )
Cpk.hat = apply( cbind( (USL-xbar)/s, (xbar-LSL)/s
           ), 1, min )

## Lower 95% Confidence interval
Cpk.95 = Cpk.hat - qnorm(0.95)*sqrt( 1/(9*n) +
           Cpk.hat^2/(2*(n-1)) )
stats$assurance[i] = mean(Cpk.95 >= c0)
                          ## Statistical assurance
}
```

Similarly, statistical assurance may be calculated for the second example for which we tested $\Pr\left(\tilde{Y} = 1 \mid Y\right) \geq p_0$. Given hyperparameters (α, β), the sample size n may be determined such that

$$E\left[\Pr\left(\tilde{Y} = 1 \mid Y\right) \geq p_0\right] \geq 0.8.$$

The steps to calculate assurance are

1. Sample from the prior distribution for $p \sim \text{Beta}(\alpha, \beta)$.
2. Generate B (e.g., $B = 10{,}000$) prior predictive samples $Y \sim \text{binomial}(n, p)$ for a given sample size n.
3. From each prior predictive sample, calculate $\Pr\left(\tilde{Y} = 1 \mid Y\right) = \dfrac{\alpha + Y}{\alpha + \beta + n}$.
4. Assurance is approximated by the proportion of times (out of B) such that $\dfrac{\alpha + Y}{\alpha + \beta + n} \geq p_0$.

Computer code is given below to calculate assurance with $\alpha = 19$, $\beta = 1$, and $p_0 = 0.95$. By running the code up to $n = 100$ PPQ batches, it can be seen that assurance never reaches 0.8 so that validating the process through this statistical method is risky.

```
## Priors
alpha = 19; beta = 1

## Posterior predictive probability criterion
p0 = 0.95

set.seed(277)
B = 10000
```

```
## prior distribution p
p = rbeta(B, alpha, beta)

stats = data.frame(n=seq(5, 100, by=5), assurance=NA)
for (i in 1:nrow(stats))
{

  n = stats$n[i]
  ## Predictive distribution
  Y = rbinom(B, size=n, prob=p)

  ## Posterior predictive probability that Y.tilde ==1
  prob = (alpha+Y)/(alpha+beta+n)
  stats$assurance[i] = mean(prob >= p0) ## Statistical
                            assurance
}
```

9.6 Concluding Remarks

The launch of the FDA initiative "Pharmaceutical cGMPs for the 21st Century" (FDA 2004a) has spurred significant interest and advances in using QbD principles in drug process development. At the heart of the development is the design space, which renders better manufacturing control and regulatory flexibility when an improvement to the process is implemented. Greater use of available data and understanding of the manufacturing process is the key to successful development of design space. Bayesian methods bring about new opportunities for applying QbD principles in design space determination. In addition, process validation is also a very important component of process development. As drug product development and manufacturing has become more complex, the traditional one-time, three-batch validation can hardly provide sufficient assurance that future batches will meet quality standards. The establishment of a robust design space and determination of the right number of batches for process performance quantification argues for the use of statistical methods capable of synthesizing information from disparate sources. In this chapter, we discussed three Bayesian approaches in the identification of CQAs, development of design space, and process validation. Many other aspects of process development can also benefit from the use of Bayesian thinking and principles.

10

Stability

10.1 Introduction

Stability testing is a key component in all stages of drug development. It is used to ensure that a drug product continues to meet standards for quality, safety, and efficacy over its shelf life. Along with release time, shelf life is a key product quality attribute. Since 1984, several regulatory guidelines on stability testing for new drugs, biological substances, and products have been issued (FDA 1987b; ICH 1993, 1995b, 2003a; WHO 2006). A common thread among the guidance documents is how to use stability data to justify shelf life in registration applications. In ICH Q1A (R2) (ICH 2003a), shelf life is formally defined as "[t]he time period during which a drug product is expected to remain within the approved shelf life specification, provided that it is stored under the conditions defined on the container label." A method based on at least three batches of drug product and regression analysis is recommended in ICH Q1E (ICH 2003b) for shelf-life determination. Shelf life is defined as the time at which the lower or upper bound (whichever comes first) of the 95% confidence interval intersects with its respective specification limit. Various other regression-based methods for shelf-life calculation were suggested to include random effects in the model or use a prediction or tolerance interval in lieu of the confidence interval. Sponsors are often also interested in the probability that a future batch will remain in specification throughout the shelf life of the product. In addition, since stability design may have significant impact on the accuracy and precision of the shelf life, selection of appropriate time points for stability testing is a key consideration in developing a stability program. In this chapter, through several case examples, we discuss Bayesian methods for stability design and analysis.

10.2 Stability Study

Since both drug substance and drug product often degrade over time, it is mandated by regulatory guidelines to set an expiration date or shelf life on the immediate container label (FDA 1987) for all marketed pharmaceutical products. The requirement is meant to ensure that the product remains safe and efficacious within its shelf life. As noted by Riley and Yang (2019), in practice, a shelf life between 18 and 24 months with storage at room temperature will likely ensure manageable inventories and supply chains for traditional (small molecule) pharmaceuticals. Many biopharmaceuticals have refrigerated or frozen storage requirements. Many of the newer biopharmaceuticals, such as cell therapies, have extremely short shelf lives, often shorter than two weeks. Shorter shelf lives at refrigerated temperature are generally reserved for special cases or for situations in which the stability of the product does not allow room-temperature storage for 18–24 months. To estimate the shelf life, a well-designed stability study is conducted in which the degradation of the drug is evaluated through various analytical methods. The shelf life of a drug product is the time period during which the average characteristics such as identity, potency, and purity of the drug product remain within their respective specifications. In the literature, the mean drug characteristic is usually described using a linear regression model (Shao and Chow 2001). When the degradation curve appears to be nonlinear, the data might be linearized through a proper transformation. Alternatively, nonlinear models may be used. For example, Yang (2017) used a piecewise regression model to describe stability data. To ensure that the variability of the manufacturing process is fully accounted for in shelf-life estimation, ICH Q1E (2003b) further suggests that at least three batches of the drug product or substance be observed over time. In the following, we assume that the relationship between the stability attribute Y_{ij} and time t_{ij} ($i = 1, ..., n$ batches; $j = 1, ..., m$ time points) can be fully described through the following linear model:

$$Y_{ij} = a_i + b_i t_{ij} + \varepsilon_{ij} \tag{10.1}$$

where a_i and b_i are the intercept and slope parameters for the ith batch. The (a_i, b_i) can be viewed either as fixed or random effects. In the latter case, a_i and b_i, which characterize the batch effect, are assumed to be bivariate normally distributed with mean vector (a, b) and variance–covariance matrix V. The ε_{ij} are measurement errors, which are assumed to be independently and identically distributed (*iid*) according to a normal distribution $N(0, \sigma^2)$.

Stability studies are also conducted for other purposes. For example, stability studies can be used to support manufacturing process changes, including site, scale, formulation, storage, shipping conditions, and delivery device. To ensure accurate and precise characterization of a product stability and shelf life, considerations should be given to the selection of time points at which stability samples are collected and tested, the statistical model used to analyze the data, and historical data and knowledge that may be used to construct prior distributions in the event that a Bayesian analysis is intended.

10.3 Shelf-Life Estimation

10.3.1 Current Methods

Various methods have been suggested for shelf-life estimation. For example, ICH Q1E (2003b) recommends that the shelf life be estimated as the time point at which the lower limit of the one-sided 95% confidence interval (CI) for the mean predicted value intersects with the approved lower specification. The ICH guidance further requires that three batches of the product be used for establishing the shelf life to account for variability due to batch. For illustration, Figure 10.1 shows how the shelf life of one batch of product is calculated.

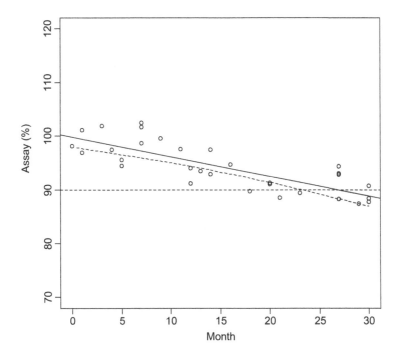

FIGURE 10.1
Plot of stability data, linear regression, and the associated 95% lower confidence limit. The shelf life is determined to be 23 months, the point where the lower 95% confidence interval of mean response intersects the lower specification limit.

As shown by Shao and Chow (2001), the ICH-recommended method gives rise to a biased underestimate of the theoretical mean shelf life with the intent to provide consumers with greater assurance that the estimated (labeled) expiration date is smaller than the theoretical mean shelf life. In addition, the shelf life based on ICH Q1E only provides quality assurance as measured against the batch mean as opposed to individual units. As a result, it may not provide adequate protection from the consumer risk (Kiermeier et al. 2004; Yang and Zhang 2012). Alternate methods based on a prediction interval (Carstensen and Nelson 1976) and a tolerance interval (Kiermeier et al. 2004 and Komka et al. 2010) were also proposed. Yang and Zhang (2012) suggested a unified risk-based approach for evaluating the above three shelf life estimation methods. A collective effort was made by a stability working group to examine existing statistical methods to develop improved procedures (Capen et al. 2012; Quinlan et al. 2013; Stroup and Quinlan 2010, 2016).

10.3.2 Bayesian Approaches

Determination of shelf life based on the frequentist methods mentioned above usually involves estimation of the parameters of the random effects Model (10.1). These estimates allow for construction of the 95% confidence interval for the mean response value at any time of a future batch. The shelf life can be determined as the time point at which the mean response is below the lower specification limits or above the upper specification limits, whichever comes first. Alternatively, a Bayesian analysis can be performed to estimate model parameters and shelf life. Describe a Bayesian procedure for shelf-life estimation based on MCMC sampling. A similar method was proposed by Yu et al. (2017) for comparing degradation slopes to demonstrate comparability before and after a progress change. A simple example using Bayesian analysis to predict the performance of an annual stability batch, which is typically required for vaccines, is presented by Yang (2012). From the Bayesian perspective, a mixed model is viewed as a hierarchical model. For example, Model (10.1) can be hierarchically formulated as:

$$Y_{ij} \mid a_i, b_i \sim N\left(a_i + b_i t, \sigma_e^2\right)$$

$$a_i \sim N\left(a, \sigma_a^2\right)$$

$$b_i \sim N\left(b, \sigma_b^2\right)$$

$$\frac{1}{\sigma_a^2} \sim \text{gamma}\left(\alpha_{0a}, \beta_{0a}\right)$$

$$\frac{1}{\sigma_b^2} \sim \text{gamma}\left(\alpha_{0b}, \beta_{0b}\right)$$

$$\frac{1}{\sigma_e^2} \sim \text{gamma}(\alpha_{0e}, \beta_{0e}),$$

where $(\alpha_{0k}, \beta_{0k})$, $k = a, b, e$ are prespecified hyperparameters. The hierarchical distributions and hyperparameters are chosen according to whether the priors are informative or not.

As noted by Yu et al. (2017), one advantage of the Bayesian method is that the scientific knowledge or expert opinion accumulated during the previous pharmaceutical development can be incorporated into the analysis through informative priors. For example, prior knowledge of the analytical method variability σ_e can be provided as the intermediate precision estimate from the analytical method validation study or robustness study. For a typical bioassay that measures relative potency, the %CV of intermediate precision has a range of (5%, 30%), meaning that either a truncated log-normal or uniform distribution might be selected for σ_e.

In general, the following procedure can be used to generate a posterior sample of the model parameters and predictive sample for the response. Let (a', b', σ') denote a posterior draw from the posterior distribution of of (a, b, σ). Given a stability design with time points $\{t_j\}$, a predictive data set may be generated as $\tilde{Y}_j = a' + b' t_j + \tilde{e}_j$ where $\tilde{e}_j \sim N(0, \sigma'^2)$. By fitting a straight line via ordinary least squares to the set $\{t_j, \tilde{Y}_j\}$, the shelf life $\tilde{sl}$ may be determined. By repeatedly drawing new posterior samples (a', b', σ'), each producing a posterior data set $\{(a_j, b_j, \sigma_j)\}$ and a predictive data set $\{t_j, \tilde{Y}_j\}$, the posterior predictive distribution of the shelf life may be generated. The shelf life might, for example, be set to the lower 5%-ile of the distribution of $\tilde{sl}$. In this manner, estimation and inference of both model parameters and shelf life can be made.

It is important to note that Bayesian approaches to shelf-life estimation rely on an objective function based on either the posterior distribution of the stability characteristics such as mean potency at the time of lot expiration or the posterior predictive distribution of the observations of the future lot(s) at times of interest such as time of lot release or shelf life. One way to define the objective function is to directly relate it to the probability of success. Suppose the stability characteristic degrades over time. Let LSL be the associated lower specification limit. Below are two examples of the objective functions:

$$\Pr[a + bt_{\text{SL}} \geq \text{LSL} \mid Y] \geq p_0 \tag{10.2a}$$

$$\Pr\left[\tilde{Y}_{\text{SL}} \geq \text{LSL} \mid Y\right] \geq p_0 \tag{10.2b}$$

where is t_{SL} is the shelf life, $a + bt_{\text{SL}}$ represents the mean response at the end of the shelf life, Y are the data from the current stability study, $\tilde{Y}_{\text{SL}}$ is the response at the end of the shelf life of a future lot, and p_0 is a pre-selected cutoff value, such as 95%.

There are several advantages of using Bayesian methods for stability evaluation. First, the quality assurance of the shelf life is quantified through a probability. Second, estimation of the shelf life does not require a closed-form analytical solution as objective functions can be evaluated using the MCMC methods discussed in Chapter 2. Last, as previously mentioned, they provide a means to combine historical data or prior knowledge of the product with the current data in making statistical inferences about the shelf life. The last is especially important as stability testing is an on-going regulatory commitment and cumulative stability data are available at any stage of drug development.

10.3.3 Examples

Two applications of the above Bayesian analysis for stability studies are presented in this section. The first is to show shelf-life estimation through a real example. The second is concerned with prediction of the performance of an annual stability lot of a vaccine product.

10.3.3.1 Shelf Life of Influenza Vaccine

10.3.3.1.1 Study Design

A stability study was conducted to determine the shelf life of an influenza vaccine based on a potency assay, which measures log10 focus-forming units (FFU) per dose. Six consecutive daily samples are collected for each of 21 weeks for a total of 132 observations. The product's lower and upper specification limits (LSL and USL) are LSL = 6.5 and USL = 7.5 log10 FFU/dose. Four lots of stability data, which are shown in Figure 10.2, contain about 120 measurements per lot, sampled nearly every day over 21 weeks.

10.3.3.1.2 Shelf Life of Individual Lots

To gain some understanding of the product stability, we first determined shelf life for each of the four lots, using the standard CI approach (ICH Q1E; Shao and Chow 2001). Basically, the shelf life of an individual lot is determined by fitting a straight line by OLS to the stability data and determining the largest time point for which a 95% confidence interval of the mean value from the line is contained within LSL and USL. Before comparison to LSL and USL, the 95% confidence interval is rounded to the nearest single decimal to match with the specification limits. For simplicity, we did not attempt to pool slopes/intercepts, as suggested by ICH Q1E. Summary statistics for each lot, including the shelf lives, are given in Table 10.1. Whether or not a linear model is appropriate for the potency stability data shown in Figure 10.2 is beyond the scope of this chapter.

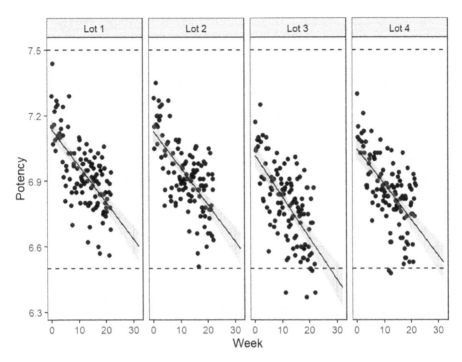

FIGURE 10.2
The black circles show potency stability data from four lots. The black line and grey area respectively show linear fits with unrounded 95% confidence bands. The dashed lines show specification limits.

TABLE 10.1

Summary Statistics for Each of Four Historical Stability Lots

Lot	Intercept	Slope	SD	Shelf Life
1	7.13	−0.0167	0.118	35.9
2	7.13	−0.0168	0.123	35.2
3	7.02	−0.0189	0.137	26.5
4	7.05	−0.0162	0.126	31.9

10.3.3.1.3 Product Shelf Life

To apply the above Bayesian procedure to determine the overall product shelf life, we need to obtain the posterior distribution of (a, b, σ). This can be accomplished by fitting a linear model to the stability data from Lot 1 via Bayesian methods with a flat prior. In R, the MCMCregress() function of the *MCMCpack* library in R (Martin et al. 2011) may be called by

fit = MCMCregress(*Potency* ~ *Week*, data=subset(*d*, *Lot*=="*Lot 1*"), mcmc=*B*)

The object d is a data.frame containing the Lot 1 stability data with columns Lot, Week (the time variable), and Potency, and the object *fit* contains B posterior draws with column names "(Intercept)", "Week", and "sigma2", representing parameters a, b, and σ^2. The posterior predictive distribution of shelf life was determined using both Equation (10.2a) and Equation (10.b) with $p_0 = 95\%$.

Let $\mu'_t = a' + b't$ denote the posterior distribution of mean potency at time t and let $\tilde{Y}_t$ denote the posterior predictive distribution of Potency at time t generated from $\tilde{Y}_t = \mu'_t + \tilde{e}_t$, where $\tilde{e}_t \sim N(0,\sigma'^2)$ for each posterior sample (a',b',σ'^2) in *fit*. The probability $\Pr[a+bt_{SL} \geq LSL \mid Y]$ from Equation (10.2a) is the percent of posterior samples μ'_t out of B that meet the criteria $\mu'_t \geq LSL$ and the probability $\Pr[\tilde{Y}_{SL} \geq LSL \mid Y]$ from Equation (10.2b) is the percent of predictive posterior sample $\tilde{Y}_t$ out of B that meet the criterion $\tilde{Y}_t \geq LSL$. The associated R code with $B = 100{,}000$ MCMC draws is given below. The simulation result shows that the shelf life is 36.7 weeks using Equation (10.2a) and 28.9 weeks using Equation (10.2b). Although the shelf-life calculation of 28.9 weeks based on Equation (10.2b) produced a result smaller than that given by Equation (10.2a) and the ICH-based estimate in Table 10.1, it provides greater consumer protection because Equation (10.2b) is based on individual units in Lot 1 and not the mean result across units.

```
d = read.csv("Stability Data.csv")   ## Load the data
LSL = 6.5  ## Lower specification limit

set.seed(820)
   ## Fit linear model to Lot-1 data with flat priors
fit = MCMCregress( Potency~Week, data=subset(d,
                   Lot=="Lot 1"),
                   mcmc=100000 )
t.seq = seq(0, 50, length=1000) ## Sequence of times
                                (weeks)
## Calculate posterior predictive probability
prob.pp = sapply( t.seq, function(t0){
               ## Posterior predictive distribution of Y
                  at time t0
               mu = fit[,"(Intercept)"] + fit[,"Week"]*t0
               ytilde = mu + rnorm(nrow(fit), mean=0,
                                   sd=sqrt(fit[,"sigma2"]))
               prob.in.speca = mean( round(mu, 1) >= LSL )
               prob.in.specb = mean( round(ytilde, 1) >= LSL )
               return(c(prob.in.speca, prob.in.specb))
               })
## Get the time point at which the probability = 0.95.
shelf.lifea = t.seq[ which.min( abs(prob.pp[1,]-0.95) ) ]
shelf.lifeb = t.seq[ which.min( abs(prob.pp[2,]-0.95) ) ]
```

A potential flaw in the analysis (so far) is that Lot 1 alone may not be representative of all future lots, meaning that the calculated shelf life could be anti-conservative. By examining Figure 10.1 and Table 10.1, it appears that there are clear lot-to-lot differences that should be captured in order to predict the potency activity of a random future lot. The entire shelf-life exercise is reprised through consideration of both lot-to-lot and within-lot variability. The posterior distribution of (a, b, σ) may be obtained by fitting a hierarchical (i.e., mixed-effects) linear model to the stability data across all lots Model (10.1) with $i = 1, 2, 3, 4$ lots. Whereas flat priors were used for fitting a linear model to Lot 1 alone, the use of a completely vague prior for V may result in an improper posterior distribution (Gelman 2006). The prior distributions for a, b, and σ are created to be proper, but flat in the regions of their respective point estimates. They are given by

$$a \sim N\left(\hat{a}, 5SE(\hat{a})\right),$$

$$b \sim N\left(\hat{b}, 5SE(\hat{b})\right),$$

$$\sigma \sim \text{half-Cauchy}(0,1),$$

where $(\hat{a}, \hat{b})$ are the restricted maximum likelihood (REML) estimates and $SE(\hat{a})$ and $SE(\hat{b})$ are their respective standard errors. As suggested by Gelman and Hill (2007, Chapter 13), a vague, but proper prior for the covariance–variance matrix V of y_{ij} may be constructed as a scaled inverse Wishart distribution with scale parameter $D = \text{diag}\{d_1, d_2\}$ and three degrees of freedom. That is, re-express V as

$$V = DV_0D$$

where V_0 is the correlation matrix and $d_i \sim$ half-Cauchy(0, 1). The hierarchical linear model was fitted to the full data set using JAGS (Plummer 2003) with the following code.

```
require(rjags); require(runjags)
model.txt = "
model{
  ## SigmaLot ~ scaled inverse Wishart
  for ( i in 1:2 )
  {
    D[i] ~ dt(0., 1., 1)T(0.,)
  }
  OmegaLot ~ dscaled.wishart(D, 3)
  SigmaLot <- inverse(OmegaLot)

  theta[1] ~ dnorm( Est[1], tauML[1] ) ## Population
                                            intercept
```

```
  theta[2] ~ dnorm( Est[2], tauML[2] ) ## Population
                                              slope

  sigmaErr ~ dt(0., 1., 1)T(0., )    # Residual standard
                                              deviation
  tauErr <- 1/(sigmaErr*sigmaErr)

  ## Likelihood terms for Lots
  for ( j in 1:nLot )
  {
    thetaLot[j,1:2] ~ dmnorm( theta, OmegaLot )
  }

  ## Likelihood terms for samples within lots
  for ( k in 1:N )
  {
    mu[k] <- thetaLot[ lot[k], 1]
           + thetaLot[ lot[k],2 ]*Time[k]
    y[k] ~ dnorm( mu[k], tauErr )
  }
}"

## REML model fit (from "lme4" library)
fit0 = lmer( Potency~Week+(1+Week|Lot), data=d )

## Prepare data for JAGS
data = list( N=nrow(d), nLot=nlevels(d$Lot),
             lot=as.vector(unclass(d$Lot)),
             y = d$Potency, Time=d$Week,
             Est=as.vector(fixef(fit0)), ## MLE Est
             tauML=0.04/diag(summary(fit0)$vcov)
                                     ## 5x(MLE SE)
           )

## JAGS code (3 CPUs, run in parallel)
fitb = run.jags(model.txt, data=data, n.chains=n.chains
         monitor=c("theta", "SigmaLot", "sigmaErr"),
         burnin=10000, thin=10, sample=20000,
         modules="glm", method="parallel" )

th.post = as.matrix( as.mcmc.list(fitb) )
```

A summary of posterior distributions from the linear model fit to Lot 1 via MCMCregress() and the hierarchical linear model fit across the four lots via JAGS is shown in Table 10.2.

TABLE 10.2

Posterior Medians and, in Parentheses, 95% Credible Intervals
for Linear Model Parameters

	Lot 1 (MCMCregress)	Lots 1 – 4 (JAGS)
a	7.14 (7.09, 7.18)	7.08 (6.98, 7.18)
b	−0.0167 (−0.0202, −0.01327)	−0.0172 (−0.0201, −0.0143)
σ	0.119 (0.105, 0.136)	0.126 (0.119, 0.135)
SD(a_i)		0.079 (0.032, 0.273)
SD(b_i)		0.001 (0, 0.008)
Corr(a_i, b_i)		0.09 (−0.74, 0.82)

It is clear from the results in Table 10.2 that there are significant lot-to-lot intercept differences and to a much lesser extent some slope differences as well. Instead of basing the shelf life on individual units from a single batch, the posterior predictive distribution of future units will include a variance component for a random batch. The shelf-life calculation based on Equation (10.2b), paired with the 60,000 posterior draws from the linear hierarchical modeling performed in JAGS, is shown below. By predicting the potency of a random batch, the new estimated shelf life is 19.4 weeks.

```
LSL = 6.5  ## Lower specification limit

t.seq = seq(0, 50, length=1000)  ## Sequence of times
                                          (weeks)

## Get posterior predictive distribution of
   (a=intercept, b=slope)
th.lot = apply(th.post[,1:6], 1, function(th){
            Sigma = matrix( th[3:6], 2, 2 )
            return( rmvnorm( 1, mean=th[1:2],
                 sigma=Sigma ) )
            })

prob.pp = sapply( t.seq, function(t0){
       ## Posterior predictive distribution of Y
       ##    for a future batch at time t0
          mu = th.lot[1,] + th.lot[2,]*t0
          ytilde = mu + rnorm(nrow(th.post), mean=0,
                           sd=th.post[,"sigmaErr"])
          prob.in.spec = mean( round(ytilde, 1) >= LSL )
          return(prob.in.spec)
             })
## Get the time point at which the probability = 0.95.
shelf.life = t.seq[ which.min( abs(prob.pp-0.95) ) ]
```

10.3.3.1.4 Prediction of Lot Performance

For many drug products such as vaccines, it is a regulatory requirement to place the first lot of product on stability for the annual manufacturing campaign. The goal is to verify the product shelf life and ensure the manufacturing process continues to produce quality products, as intended. In addition, it is also of interest to determine the sampling points and amount of testing that are needed. Since stability testing is carried out sequentially, it is of interest to predict the outcome of the stability study as data become available. This on-going update allows for a timely response to any unexpected result. Yang (2012) described an example demonstrating the utility of Bayesian stability analysis in predicting the performance of the lot of an influenza vaccine, which was placed on the annual stability study. For the purposes of discussion, suppose that the key stability indicator is the degradation rate. The acceptance criterion is that the rate of decrease is no more than $0.025 \log_{10}$ titer/month, which confirms a 20-month shelf life when the lot is released at an acceptable potency level of $7.0 \log_{10}$ titer. Potency measurements are taken at 0, 3, 6, 9, 12, 18, and 24 months. For the single lot, assume the model

$$Y_i = a + b t_i + e_i$$

where Y_i = the potency measurement from time point t_i and the independent errors are $e_i \sim N(0, \sigma^2)$, $i = 1, 2, \ldots, m$. Let $\hat{b}$ be the OLS estimate of slope based on the collected data up to k months ($k < 24$). The posterior probability $\Pr[b \geq -0.025 \mid \hat{b}]$ provides a level of confidence that the stability of the lot will behave as expected. The prior distribution for the slope b of commercial lots is assumed to follow a normal distribution $N(b_0, \sigma_0^2)$. Because $\hat{b} \mid b$ also follows a normal distribution with mean b and variance $\sigma_b^2 = \sigma^2 / S_{tt}(k)$, where $S_{tt}(m) = \sum_{i=1}^{m} (t_i - \bar{t}(k))^2$, with $\bar{t}(k) = \frac{1}{m} \sum_{i=1}^{m} t_i$ denoting the average time point up to k months, it can be easily verified that the posterior distribution of b is

$$b \mid \hat{b} \sim N\left(\frac{\sigma_b^2}{\sigma_b^2 + \sigma_0^2} b_0 + \frac{\sigma_0^2}{\sigma_b^2 + \sigma_0^2} \hat{b}, \frac{\sigma_b^2 \sigma_0^2}{\sigma_b^2 + \sigma_0^2} \right).$$

Consequently,

$$\Pr[b \geq -0.025 \mid \hat{b}] = 1 - \Phi\left(\left[-0.025 - \frac{\sigma_b^2}{\sigma_b^2 + \sigma_0^2} b_0 - \frac{\sigma_0^2}{\sigma_b^2 + \sigma_0^2} \hat{b} \right] \middle/ \sqrt{\frac{\sigma_b^2 \sigma_0^2}{\sigma_b^2 + \sigma_0^2}} \right),$$

where Φ is CDF of the standard normal distribution.

As an illustration, suppose that $\hat{b} = -0.027$ and $S_{tt}(9) = 45$ based on data collected up to nine months. It is further assumed that the mean and variance in the prior distribution are $b_0 = -0.01$ and $\sigma_0^2 = 0.01^2$, implying a very stable product. Under these assumptions and assay variability of $\sigma^2 = 0.04$, it can be calculated that $\Pr[b \geq -0.025 \mid \hat{b}] = 91.2\%$.

Therefore, there is a 91% probability that the product will have a desirable stability profile, even though the partial data seemingly suggest a faster degradation rate. The simple R code for the calculation is given here.

```
## Hyperparameters
b0 = -0.01; sigSq0 = 0.01^2
  ## Data
b.hat = -0.027; Stt = 45
  ## True error variance
sigSq = 0.04
  ## Variance of slope
sigSqb = sigSq/Stt
  ## Posterior parameters
Mean = (sigSqb*b0 + sigSq0*b.hat)/(sigSqb+sigSq0)
SD = sqrt( sigSqb*sigSq0/(sigSqb+sigSq0) )
  ## Posterior probability
1 - pnorm( -0.025, Mean, SD )
```

10.3.4 Selection of Stability Design

Stability testing can be very costly particularly when the drug product is intended for the global markets. Although regulatory authorities in Europe, Japan, and the United States generally recommend that a stability program be developed in accordance with ICH guidelines, many other countries may have their own requirements. The expense can become even more prohibitive for drug products with multiple strengths and packages, further stressing analytical resources. It is of great interest for the drug manufacturer to reduce the amount of stability testing without compromising the consumer's confidence in the product quality, safety, and efficacy within its shelf life. One way to achieve this is to explore so-called "reduced" designs, in which stability testing is carried out only for a subset of time points of the full designs. Per the ICH guidance (2002), a full study design is one in which samples for every combination of all design factors are tested at all time points. A reduced design is one in which samples for every factor combination are not all tested at all time points. Although the ICH guideline allows the use of a reduced design when multiple design factors are involved, its suitability needs to be justified. It stresses that "Any reduced design should have the ability to adequately predict the retest period or shelf life. Before a reduced design is considered, certain assumptions should be assessed and justified. The potential risk should be considered of establishing a shorter retest period or shelf life than could be derived from a full design due to the reduced amount of data collected." (ICH 2002).

In literature, various reduced designs including matrixing and bracketing designs have been proposed (Barron 1994; Nordbrock and Valvani 1995; Lin and Fairweather 1997; ICH 2002; Chow 2007). Also suggested were many criteria for selecting suitable stability designs (Nordbrock 1992; Murphy 1996; DeWoody and Raghavarao 1997; Pong and Raghavarao 2000). Chow (2007) provides an excellent review of these selection methods. One clear drawback of these selection criteria, however, is that they do not provide a direct link between a selected design and its impact on the shelf life. Yang and Zhang (2012) developed a method using simulation to select an appropriate design based on its impact on the accuracy and precision of the shelf-life estimate.

10.3.5 Bayesian Criterion

Note that the predictive posterior distribution of the objective functions in Equations (10.2a) and (10.2b) is dependent on the stability design. Thus, either Equation (10.2a) or Equation (10.2b) can be used to choose, among many options, a design that has a greater probability for the future lot to meet the predefined shelf life. In the following, we demonstrate how the above Bayesian method can be applied to compare two reduced designs with the full design for the influenza vaccine described in Section 10.3.3.

10.3.5.1 Design Options

Three designs, each with sampling from 0 to 22 weeks, are examined with the goal to choose the smallest (fewest number of samples) design such that the probability for a future lot to meet or exceed an 18-week shelf life is at least 95%. A future lot will be modeled by Model (10.1).

Design 1: Six consecutive daily samples are collected for each of 21 weeks for a total of 132 observations. This is considered to be the full design.

Design 2: Six consecutive daily samples are collected every other week for each of 20 weeks and also on the 21st week, for a total of 72 observations.

Design 3: Six consecutive daily samples are collected across 21 weeks, starting on weeks 0, 1, 2, 5, 10, 16, and 21, for a total of 42 observations.

Design 1 is most similar to the historical data and will represent the gold standard. Relative to Design 1, Designs 2 and 3 represent substantial savings in time and sampling costs. The three proposed designs are illustrated in Figure 10.3.

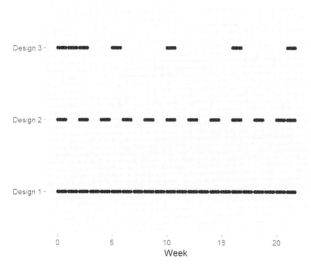

FIGURE 10.3
Three stability study designs under consideration.

10.3.5.2 Results

The three proposed designs were evaluated using Bayesian predictive modeling and simulation (BPMS). The posterior predictive distribution of potency stability data for a new lot measured with time points from Design k (k=1, 2, 3) was generated using the method in Section 10.3.3. With the posterior predictive distribution, the probability that a future lot will meet or exceed the shelf-life goal of 18 weeks may be calculated.

The three designs under consideration are given in R code by

```
Design = list(
            t1 = as.vector(sapply(0:21, function(wk)
                { wk + (0:5)/7 })),
            t2 = as.vector(sapply(c(seq(0, 20, by=2), 21),
                            function(wk){ wk + (0:5)/7 })),
            t3 = as.vector(sapply(c(0, 1, 2, 5, 10, 16, 21),
                            function(wk){ wk + (0:5)/7 }))
            )
```

As with the previous example, the posterior distribution of (a, b, σ) was generated by fitting a hierarchical linear model to the full stability data set via Bayesian methods. Using the 60,000 posterior draws from the JAGS call in Section 10.3.3 (summarized in Table 10.2), computer code is given to generate the posterior predictive distribution of shelf life using the ICH Q1E calculation under the three designs. To keep our computer code simple, we do not test for pooled slopes/intercepts as suggested by ICH Q1E. To speed

up computations, the posterior predictive distribution of summary statistics
for linear fits was generated.

```
require(mvtnorm)   ## library for multivariate normal
                          distribution

th.post = as.matrix( as.mcmc.list(fitb) )
B = nrow(th.post)  ## Number of MCMC posterior samples
## Specification limits
LSL = 6.5
USL = 7.5
t.seq = seq(0, 50, length=1000)  ## Sequence of time
                                       points (weeks)
sl.mat = matrix(NA, B, 3)

  ## Generate posterior predictive distribution
  ##  for (a=intercept, b=slope) for future lots
th.lot = apply(th.post[,1:6], 1, function(th){
               Sigma = matrix( th[3:6], 2, 2 )
               return( rmvnorm( 1, mean=th[1:2],
                   sigma=Sigma ) )
               })
for ( k in 1:3 ) ## Cycle through the designs
{

  tj = Design[[k]]   ## Time points for Design k
  X = model.matrix(~Week, data=data.frame(Week=tj))
                                     ## Design matrix
  xTx.inv = solve( t(X)%*%X )
  degFree = nrow(X) - 2

    ## Posterior predictive distribution of OLS
        estimate for sigma
  sigma.hat = th.post[,"sigmaErr"] *
              sqrt( rchisq(nrow(th.post), degFree)/
                  degFree )

    ## Posterior predictive distribution of OLS estimate
    ## for (a=intercept, b=slope)
  beta.errors = rmvnorm( B, mean=c(0, 0), sigma=xTx.inv )
  beta.hat = t(th.lot) + sigma.hat*beta.errors

  for ( b in 1:B )
  {
      ## 95% confidence interval for the bth posterior
         draw
```

```
mu.hat = beta.hat[b,1]+beta.hat[b,2]*t.seq
SE = sigma.hat[b]*sqrt( sapply( t.seq,
        function(t0){ c(1, t0)%*%xTx.inv%*%c(1, t0)
                    } ) )
pred = cbind( lwr=mu.hat - qt(0.975, degFree)*SE,
              upr=mu.hat + qt(0.975, degFree)*SE )

## Get shelf life
sl.tilde = max( t.seq[ round(pred[,"lwr"],1) >= LSL &
                    round(pred[,"upr"],1) <= USL ] )
if ( is.infinite(sl.tilde) )
  sl.tilde = 0
sl.mat[b,k] = sl.tilde
}
}
## Posterior predictive probability that shelf life > 18
prob18 = colMeans( sl.mat >= 18 )

## Lower 95% credible interval for shelf life (for
    each design)
apply(sl.mat, 2, quantile, p=c(0.5, 0.05))
```

The posterior predictive probability for a new lot to meet or exceed 18 weeks of shelf life is 0.98, 0.97, and 0.97, respectively for the three designs. Posterior medians with lower 95% credible limits for shelf life for the three designs are 32.4 (21.3), 31.5 (20.8) and 29.9 (19.5) weeks. Although there is not much differentiation among the three designs, Design 3 may be less attractive than the other two considering its greater potential to miss the target of 18 weeks. Figure 10.4 shows the predictive posterior density of shelf life for each design. Note that for all three designs, in roughly 0.3% of cases (out of 60,000), the hierarchical model BPMS resulted in some shelf life values of 0 weeks (the intercept was too low or high), and in approximately 3% of cases, the BPMS shelf life values were truncated to 50 weeks.

10.4 Setting Release Limit

10.4.1 Background

Release limits are the bounds of critical quality attributes at the time of product release. They are established to provide greater assurance that the product meets specifications before the end of its shelf life. As such, they are narrower than the specification limits. It is conceivable that tightening the release specification decreases the likelihood that the product will fail

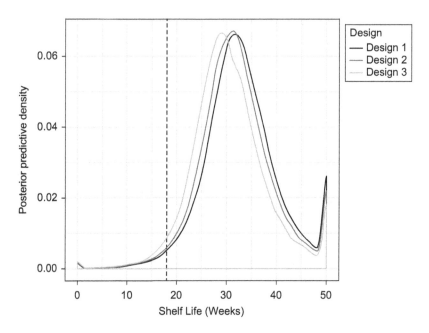

FIGURE 10.4
Posterior predictive distribution of shelf life. A dashed vertical line is drawn at 18 weeks.

the specification during its shelf life. However, too tight a release specification will result in more batches failing at release. Therefore, the release limits need to be constructed to maintain a balanced control of both the consumer's risk and producer's risk. As pointed out by Riley and Yang (2019), the use of release and stability specifications is one area in ICH Q6A that is not harmonized. In the United States, a product must meet a single specification at release and throughout the shelf life (this is also generally true for a pharmacopeial monograph). By contrast, in the EU, separate specifications are required at release and on stability.

Various statistical methods have been proposed to determine the release limits (Allen et al. 1991; Shao and Chow 1991; Wei 1998, 2003). Allen et al. (1991) used the least-squares regression to estimate the expected degradation from batch release to the end of shelf life. For a stability-indicating attribute that decreases over time, the release limit (RL) is calculated as

$$RL = LSL - bt_{SL} + t_{1-\alpha,df}\sqrt{t_{SL}^2\sigma^2 + \sigma_e^2/n} \qquad (10.4)$$

where LSL is the lower specification limit, t_{SL} is the shelf life, $b < 0$ is the average degradation rate, σ^2 is the variance of the slope estimate, and σ_e^2/n is the variability associated with the testing of n samples at release. The value $|b|t_{SL}$ represents the total loss due to degradation over the shelf life. Equation (10.4) may be understood as the determination of the intercept of Model (10.1) such that a $100(1 - \alpha)\%$ prediction interval for the mean of n samples touches the LSL at $t = t_{SL}$.

The relationship among the lower release limit (LRL), LSL, and other elements in Equation (10.4) is illustrated in Figure 10.5.

The method by Allen et al. (1991) controls the risk of out-of-speciation (OOS) results and is very simple to implement. A similar but statistically more rigorous method was proposed by Wei (1998, 2003). Even though these methods control the failure rate at the end of the product shelf life (i.e., the consumer risk), they do not take into account the loss due to rejecting a lot at release even though the lot has the desired shelf life (i.e., the producer risk). As a remedy, Shao and Chow (1991) introduced a Bayesian decision theory approach to construct the release limits. The advantage of using a Bayesian formulation is to quantify the risks of consumers and manufacturers as the OOS probabilities. More recently, Manola (2012) extended the method devised by Allen et al. using mixed-effects models with additional variance terms for batch-to-batch variability. Yu et al. (2018) suggested a Bayesian approach for estimating the release limit for a general setting in which the product has gone through several storage conditions before its use. Common to methods by Manola (2012) and Yu et al. (2018) is the determination of the release limit, RL, such that the best trade-off between the consumer risk (CR) and producer risk (PR) can be achieved:

$$CR = \Pr(y_{SL} < LSL \mid y_0 > RL)$$

$$PR = \Pr(y_0 < RL \mid y_{SL} > LSL) \tag{10.5}$$

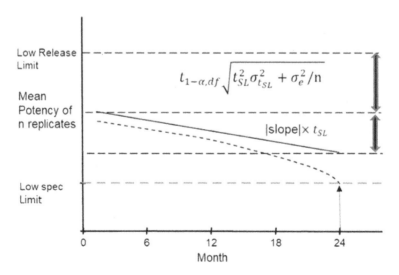

FIGURE 10.5
Release limit based on lower specification, total loss of potency over shelf life of 24 months, variability in release potency and estimated slope.

where y_0 and y_{SL} are measured values of the stability characteristic of a future lot at time 0 and the product shelf life, respectively, and can be simulated from the method described below.

There are alternate ways that such trade-off can be defined. For example, (1) both CR and PR meet pre-selected acceptance criteria; (2) the minimum or maximum of CR and PR is below a prespecified limit; and (3) the total cost associated with the two types of risk is minimized. The selection of RL can be achieved through simulation. It is assumed that the stability characteristic follows the hierarchical linear Model (10.1). Given a prior distribution for model parameters, the probabilities in Equation (10.5) are estimated via the posterior predictive distribution derived from Model (10.1). For different choices of *RL*, CR and PR in Equation (10.5) may be estimated. The final choice of RL may be constructed as a trade-off of the two criteria.

An Example

Consider the data shown in Figure 10.2. Model (10.1) was fitted to the data by Bayesian methods in Section 10.3.3 and summarized in Table 10.2. The R variable *fitb* holds 60,000 posterior samples of the model parameters. To illustrate the concept of Equation (10.5), y_0 will be the average of six units evaluated at time t = 0 and y_{SL} will be the average of six units evaluated at time $t = t_{SL} = 20$ weeks. The lower specification limit is *LSL* = 6.5 log10 FFU/dose. We will consider a range of values for *RL* from 6.6 to 7.4 log10 FFU/dose. The computer code to evaluate CR and PR is given below with the variable *results* shown in Table 10.3. Based on Table 10.3, while the CR is fairly low, it is clear that the PR is too high unless $RL \leq 6.9$. To minimize CR and PR about equally, it is reasonable to set $RL = 6.8$.

```
require(mvtnorm)  ## library for multivariate normal
                     distribution
th.post = as.matrix( as.mcmc.list(fitb) )
B = nrow(th.post)  ## Number of MCMC posterior samples
## Specification limits
LSL = 6.5
USL = 7.5

tSL = 18 ## Shelf life = 18 weeks

RL = seq(6.6, 7.4, by=0.1)

## Get posterior predictive distribution of (a=intercept,
    b=slope)
th.lot = apply(th.post[,1:6], 1, function(th){
               Sigma = matrix( th[3:6], 2, 2 )
               return( rmvnorm( 1, mean=th[1:2],
                       sigma=Sigma ) )
             })

    ## Post. Pred. distribution of mean of six units at t=0
        and t=tSL
```

```
ytilde = cbind( th.lot[1,] + rnorm(B, mean=0,
                         sd=th.post[,"sigmaErr"]/sqrt(6)),
                th.lot[1,]+th.lot[2,]*tSL + rnorm(B, mean=0,
                         sd=th.post[,"sigmaErr"]/sqrt(6))
                )
## CR = P( ySL < LSL | y0 > RL )
CR = sapply(RL, function(rl){
        mean(ifelse(ytilde[,1] > rl, ytilde[,2] < LSL, NA ),
                                     na.rm=TRUE) })

## PR = P( y0 < RL | ySL > LSL )
PR = sapply(RL, function(rl){
        mean(ifelse(ytilde[,2] > LSL, ytilde[,1] < rl, NA ),
                                     na.rm=TRUE) })

results = round(rbind( RL, CR, PR ), 3)
```

TABLE 10.3

Posterior Predictive Probabilities for CR and PR for Select Values of RL

RL	6.6	6.7	6.8	6.9	7.0	7.1	7.2	7.3	7.4
CR	0.028	0.023	0.016	0.008	0.004	0.002	0.001	0.001	0.001
PR	0.000	0.000	0.006	0.042	0.198	0.549	0.851	0.955	0.983

10.5 Concluding Remarks

Stability testing and establishment of robust release limit are integral parts of the lifecycle of drug development. They are broadly utilized to ensure product safety and efficacy before the product expiration date and to mitigate manufacturing risk. Well-designed stability studies not only provide a reliable estimation of shelf life and release limits but also reduce stability testing costs. Various Bayesian methods for stability study design and analysis are discussed in this chapter. Through several case examples, we demonstrate the utility of these Bayesian solutions. The methods presented in this chapter can be easily extended to other applications where stability studies are used to optimize formulation and demonstrate comparability of manufacturing process before and after changes.

11

Process Control

11.1 Introduction

The manufacture of drug substance and drug product is a very complex process. There are many factors that impact the quality of the product, such as starting materials, environmental conditions, equipment setting control, analytical methods, and operator capability. Statistical process control ensures product quality by monitoring and controlling critical quality attributes and helps to identify and solve manufacturing issues before product release. In the past decade, the launch of several regulatory quality initiatives has brought to bear the concepts of QbD to drug product development. The quality of a product is achieved through the development of a manufacturing process based on robust understanding and effective control of the process. In pharmaceutical manufacturing, *process* is a broader concept. It may refer to the well-defined unit operations through which the drug is produced. It may also relate to analytical testing procedures used to measure quality attributes, environmental conditions under which the product is made, or the detailed steps with which an out-of-specification result is investigated. Continuous confirmation and verification that the said processes are in a state of control provides quality assurance to the consumers and lends competitiveness to the manufacturer. It is well known that processes and analytical methods are affected by "common cause" variations such as measurement errors and "special cause" variations such as operator errors. The common cause variations are inherent in critical quality attributes due to differences in starting materials, environmental conditions, equipment control setting, and uncontrolled sources of variability at both the batch and dosage unit levels (Stand and Strickland 2016). The sources of special cause variations are often associated with unknown factors and characterized by a shift in output, which may push the process out of control. It is imperative to provide on-going assurance that the process/method remains in a state of control in order to furnish a quality product fit for its intended use. Control charts are an effective tool for monitoring the performance of a process or analytical method throughout. They are also instrumental in ensuring that the manufacturing environment is in a state of control, and the post-release product continues to be of high quality. The recently updated regulatory guidelines (FDA 2011a; USP 2015) call for continued validation and verification of both the manufacturing process and the analytical methods during commercial manufacturing. When coupled with other tools in the quality systems, such as specification, stability testing, and acceptance sampling, control charts enable the manufacturer to correct, anticipate, and prevent issues before the process can fall out of control. This chapter starts with an introduction of the most commonly used control charts, followed by a discussion of the construction of control charts based on Bayesian methods. Process control methods are introduced in various contexts, including the setting control limits in the presence of censored data, an OOS investigation, and a situation in which an excess of zeros is observed.

11.2 Quality Control and Improvement

The concept of quality control and improvement was introduced as early as the 19th century. It was not until 1924, however, when Walter Shewhart first introduced the control chart concept, that it began to be rapidly adopted by manufacturers (Shewhart 1980). In the past decades, many companies have striven to develop quality products, propelled by increasing public demand for products to be free of defects and the publication of the ISO 9000 series of standards in 1987 for quality management and quality assurance by the international organization for standardization. The ISO 9000 standards provide guidance for manufacturers to implement effective quality systems. They are also widely used by customers as a yardstick to measure the adequacy of the producer's quality system. Manufacturers are motivated to be certified by registrars accredited by the ISO to enhance potential customer confidence in the quality of their products. In modern-day industry, product quality control and improvement have become key components of business strategies. Successful utilization of statistical tools for process control and improvement lends the manufacturers the ability to increase productivity, enhance their market penetration, and achieve greater profitability and a strong competitive edge (Montgomery 2013).

Despite the advances in the field of quality control and the wide adoption of its principles in other industries, the uptake of statistical process control has been slow in the pharmaceutical industry before the United States Congress passed the cGMP Act in 1994 (FDA 1995). The cGMP stipulates that modern standards and technologies be adopted in the design, monitoring, and control of manufacturing processes and facilities to ensure a consistent supply of high-quality drug products to the patient. Violations of cGMP may result in costly recalls and lost sales and also, in some cases, closure of manufacturing facilities and denial of access to the US market. Therefore, non-compliance findings may also lead to severe shortages of drug supplies, causing serious public health concerns. After the publication of the cGMP, in the mid- to late 1990s, several lawsuits were filed by the FDA against a few pharmaceutical companies for failing to appropriately implement cGMP guidelines in their product release. By the early 2000s, however, the FDA had uncovered a number of widespread issues, including uneven quality, substandard practices in manufacturing, insufficient understanding of manufacturing breakdowns, and low manufacturing efficiencies (Yang 2017). Companies, burdened by extensive testing and required to comply with regulations, were wary of improving manufacturing processes because any change to the manufacturing process would require a post-approval filing. Consequently, companies were slow to adopt new technologies. Realizing that there was a clear need to modernize the manufacturing processes and that overly stringent regulatory oversight might impede pharmaceutical innovation, in August 2012 the FDA launched a significant initiative entitled "Pharmaceutical cGMPs for the 21st Century: A Risk-Based Approach" (FDA 2004a). Together with several ICH guidance documents (ICH Q8 (R2), 9, 10, and 11) related to pharmaceutical development, quality risk management, and pharmaceutical quality systems (ICH 2006, 2007a, 2007b, 2011), these regulatory documents stress the importance of manufacturing process development based on systematic product and process understanding, control of risk, and implementation of quality management systems. The 2011 publication of the FDA guidance on process validation further aligns process validation activities with a risk-based product lifecycle approach. The extensive regulatory discussion on product quality, risk management, quality by design, and holistic lifecycle approach entails the needs of statistical principles and techniques for product quality control and improvement.

11.3 Control Charts

The performance of manufacturing processes can be influenced by unforeseen variability. It is required by regulatory guidance (FDA 2011a) that the manufacturer provide on-going assurance that the process remains in a state of control. This continued validation is meant to provide assurance that the processes and analytical methods remain fit for use through the product lifecycle. To this end, data from various sources collected over time are used to understand additional sources of variations, detect and quantify their impact, and develop control strategies commensurate with the risk to consumers. Over the years, various statistical methods have been developed and used for trending analysis. Control charts are perhaps the simplest and most effective graphical tools for such an analysis to detect issues related to special cause variations. There are many types of control charts that can

TABLE 11.1

Nelson Rules Applied to a Control Chart for Detecting an Unusual Shift or Trend

Rule	Description	Indication
1	One point exceeds three standard deviations from the centerline	One sample is out of control
2	Nine or more points in a row on the same side of the centerline	There is a mean shift in performance
3	Six or more points in a row continuously increasing or decreasing	A trend exists
4	Fourteen or more points in a row, alternating in direction	There is a negative correlation between neighboring points
5	Two out of three data points on the same side and more than two standard deviations away from the centerline	A possible increase in process/assay variability
6	Four out of five points on the same side and more than one standard deviation away from the centerline	A possible increase in process/assay variability
7	Fifteen points in a row within one standard deviation of the centerline	A possible decrease in process/assay variability
8	Eight points in a row on both sides of the centerline but none within one standard deviation of the centerline	Non-random sample

be used for routine monitoring of analytical method performance. These include the Shewhart individual control chart, also known as individual/ moving range (I-MR) control chart, exponentially weighted moving average (EWMA) chart, cumulative sum (CUSUM) chart, and J-chart. A typical control chart consists of a centerline and lower and upper warning and control limits, also known as alert and action limits. The centerline and limits can be established based on historical data collected when the analytical method is in a state of control. The chart provides a visual means for identifying out-of-trend observations, unusual shifts, and variability indicative of potential performance issues. The data are assumed to follow a statistical distribution such as normal distribution. This allows for the quantification of the magnitude of trend or shift that qualifies as a rare event. From example, under the normality assumption of the data, the probability for nine points in a row to be greater than the population mean is 0.12%. Several well-established rules have been suggested to detect out-of-control results, based on control charts. Notable are the rules developed by WECO (Montgomery 2013) and Nelson (1984). Table 11.1 lists the Nelson Rules.

11.4 Types of Control Charts

In the following, we discuss a few control charts commonly used in drug manufacturing. A common issue with these charting methods, however, is that the variability in the parameters used to describe the distribution of the sample test results is not counted in setting the control limits. Bayesian methods provide natural alternatives.

11.4.1 Shewhart I-MR Charts

The construction of the Shewhart control charts for individual measurements or I-charts relies on the underlying assumption that the observed values X_i $i = 1,\ldots,n$ are normally distributed. When the normality assumption does not hold, data may be transformed to achieve normality. For the I-chart, which is used to trend individual observations, the centerline is estimated by the sample mean $\bar{X} = \sum_{i=1}^{n} X_i / n$ and the UCL and LCL are obtained as

$$UCL = \bar{X} + k\hat{\sigma}$$

$$LCL = \bar{X} + k\hat{\sigma}.$$

where k is a constant, e.g., $k = 3$, and

$$\hat{\sigma} = \sqrt{\frac{\sum_{i=1}^{n} (X_i - \bar{X})^2}{n-1}}.$$

The I-chart is obtained by plotting the observed values X_i against the sample number i, along with the UCL and LCL. The chart allows for the detection of a shift that is characterized by one or more points above either a prespecified alert or action limit. Alert and action limits are control limits that, when crossed, respectively trigger a small and large response by investigators. Control limits are typically set using "good" data; however, such data may inadvertently contain trends and shifts. In such a case, the standard deviation is inflated relative to the true controlled state. As a consequence, the control limits may be overly broad, thus decreasing the chance of detecting unexpected trends of shifts. To address this issue, in lieu of standard deviation to estimate the variability, Shewhart I-MR control charts use the average moving range of successive control observations. Specifically, the moving range, $M_i = |X_i - X_{i-1}|$, $i = 2, \ldots, n$, is calculated. The average of M_i is given by $\overline{MR} = \sum_{i=2}^{n} M_i/(n-1)$. Accordingly, the UCL and LCL are determined to be

$$LCL = \bar{Y} - k \times \frac{\overline{MR}}{d_2}$$

$$UCL = \bar{Y} + k \times \frac{\overline{MR}}{d_2}$$

where k is a constant associated with a predicted percentage of coverage and d_2 is a constant that depends on the number of observations associated with the moving range calculation. For example, $k=3$ is used to cover approximately 99.7% of the data. If a moving range of two observations is used to compute $\overline{MR}$, then $d_2 = 1.128$.

Likewise, the MR chart can be constructed using the following formulas:

$$LCL_{MR} = d_3 \overline{MR}$$

$$UCL_{MR} = d_4 \overline{MR}$$

where d_3 and d_4 are dependent on the size of the moving range. For $n=2$, $d_3 = 0$ and $d_4 = 3.267$.

Consider an example where the I-MR is constructed based on potency data from 20 lots of product which have been released. The test results are given in Table 11.2.

From the table, the control limits of the I-chart are calculated to be

$$LCL = 99.6 - 3 \times \frac{10.2}{1.128} = 72.5$$

TABLE 11.2

Potency Values of 20 Lots

Day	Potency	Moving Range
1	99.4	
2	94.7	4.7
3	112.2	17.5
4	95.7	16.4
5	100.5	4.7
6	103.5	3.0
7	101.7	1.8
8	89.7	12.0
9	100.2	10.5
10	102.0	1.7
11	97.8	4.1
12	101.8	4.0
13	124.0	22.2
14	90.4	33.6
15	89.4	1.0
16	109.3	19.9
17	96.9	12.4
18	97.7	0.9
19	101.9	4.2
20	83.3	18.6
Mean	99.6	10.2

$$UCL = 99.6 + 3 \times \frac{10.2}{1.128} = 126.7.$$

The control limits of the MR chart are:

$$LCL_{MR} = 0 \times 10.2 = 0$$

$$UCL_{MR} = 3.267 \times 10.2 = 33.3.$$

The I-MR charts are plotted in Figures 11.1 and 11.2.

11.4.2 EWMA Control Chart

The EWMA control chart was first introduced by Roberts (1959) and is known to be able to detect small changes. The chart is constructed using the average values:

$$Z_i = \lambda X_i + (1 - \lambda) X_{i-1}$$

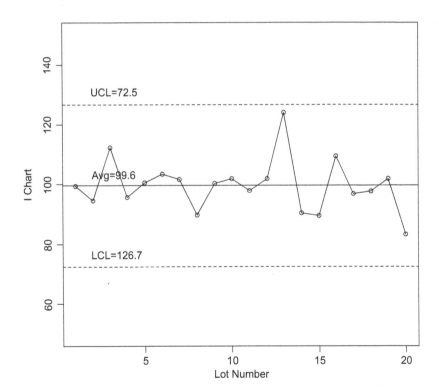

FIGURE 11.1
I-chart for 20 lots.

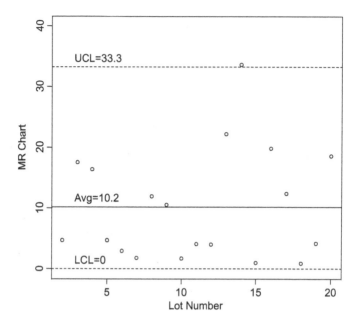

FIGURE 11.2
MR chart for 20 lots.

where Z_i $i = 1, ..., n$ is a value calculated as a weighted average of two adjacent observations X_{i-1} and X_i and $0 < \lambda \leq 1$ is a constant. Let $z_0 = \mu_0$ denote a starting point, where μ_0 could be either the target value or the average of historical data if the process target is unknown.

It can be shown that Z_i is a weighted average of previous sample means (Montgomery 2013). Because of this property, it is not sensitive to the normality assumption and is thus suitable to use when the underlying distribution of the data is not normal. Like for Shewhart I-MR charts, the construction of EWMA is also based on the premise that the observations X_i are independently and normally distributed. The UCL and LCL are given by

$$\text{UCL}_i = z_0 + k\hat{\sigma}\sqrt{\left(\frac{\lambda}{2-\lambda}\right)\left\{1-(1-\lambda)^{2i}\right\}}$$

$$\text{LCL}_i = z_0 - k\hat{\sigma}\sqrt{\left(\frac{\lambda}{2-\lambda}\right)\left\{1-(1-\lambda)^{2i}\right\}}$$

There is no theoretical guidance concerning the choice of the weighting constant λ. Using the data from the previous example, the centerline was determined to be $z_0 = 30$ and control limits were calculated using the above two formulas with $\lambda = 0.2$. For example, for the first sample

$$UCL_1 = 30 + 3 \times 1.93 \sqrt{\left(\frac{0.2}{2-0.2}\right)\left\{1-(1-0.2)^{2 \times 1}\right\}} = 31.1,$$

$$LCL_1 = 30 - 3 \times 1.93 \sqrt{\left(\frac{0.2}{2-0.2}\right)\left\{1-(1-0.2)^{2 \times 1}\right\}} = 28.9.$$

The EWMA is shown in Figure 11.3.

11.4.3 CUSUM Chart

CUSUM stands for cumulative sum. Originally proposed by Page (1954), CUSUM charts are more efficient than Shewhart control charts in detecting small process change. The CUSUM can be defined in various ways. One method is to calculate the high-side and low-side CUSUMs by

$$C_i^+ = \max\left[0, x_i - (\mu_0 + K) + C_{i-1}^+\right]$$

$$C_i^- = \max\left[0, (\mu_0 - K) - x_i + C_{i-1}^-\right]$$

Here μ_0 is the target value, which is either known or estimated, and K is the slack factor. It is often chosen to be a fraction, say 50%, of the difference between the target value and the out-of-control value mean. The process is out of control if either C_i^+ or C_i^- exceeds the decision interval H.

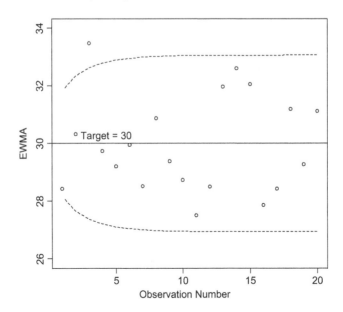

FIGURE 11.3
EWMA Chart.

11.4.4 J-Chart

More recently, another type of control chart, the J-chart, has been used for monitoring control samples (AMC 2003). The J-chart, also called "zone control chart", combines characteristics of both Shewhart and CUSUM charts and is straightforward to construct. It begins by estimating the mean μ and standard deviation σ from the control sample, and then constructs the chart based on these estimates. The J-chart consists of eight zones defined by the horizontal lines $y = -\infty, \mu - 3\sigma, \mu - 2\sigma, \mu - \sigma, \mu, \mu + \sigma, \mu + 2\sigma, \mu + 3\sigma, + \infty$. The x-axis is time. Each observed value is assigned a weight according to the rules listed in Table 11.3.

Finally, the cumulative sum is calculated as follows:

$$S_i = \begin{cases} 0, & \text{if } X_{i-1} \text{ and } X_i \text{ are on opposite sides of the centerline} \\ w_i + S_{i-1}, & \text{otherwise} \end{cases}$$

A J-chart is displayed in Figure 11.4.

TABLE 11.3

Conversion of Observed Values to Weight

Observed Value (X)	Weight (w)
$X \in (\mu - \sigma, \mu, \mu + \sigma)$	0
$X \in (\mu - 2\sigma, \mu)$ or $(\mu, \mu + 2\sigma)$	2
$X \in (\mu - 3\sigma, \mu - 2\sigma)$ or $(\mu + 2\sigma, \mu + 3\sigma)$	4
$X \in (-\infty, \mu - 3\sigma)$ or $(\mu + 3\sigma, +\infty)$	8

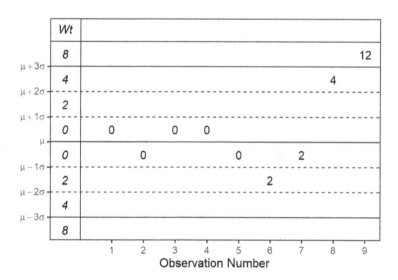

FIGURE 11.4
J-Chart with weights shown by the column *Wt* (adapted from AMC 2013).

11.4.5 Multivariate Control Chart

Statistical process control charts discussed in the previous section are well-established procedures for monitoring univariate processes. The Hotelling's T^2 chart (Montgomery 2013) represents a natural extension of the univariate Shewhart chart to multivariate situations. Multivariate process control techniques reduce the dimensionality of data generated from process development, optimization, and monitoring down to one or two metrics through the application of multivariate statistical modeling. For this purpose, statistical procedures such as principal component analysis (PCA) and partial least squares regression can be used. A detailed discussion of this topic can be found in Zhang and Yang (2018)

11.5 Bayesian Control Charts

One deficiency of many frequentist control charts is that they do not account for the uncertainty in the statistics used for constructing the control charts. To overcome this issue, more sophisticated methods include the use of a statistical interval, such as a prediction or tolerance interval. Calculating statistical intervals becomes tricky for the frequentist when data are not strictly Gaussian. Such data, however, present no difficulty for the Bayesian. As discussed previously, Bayesian methods provide a flexible framework that blends prior knowledge of a process with current data. Operationally, it begins with choosing a prior distribution of the unknown parameters. The prior is then combined with the likelihood to obtain the posterior distribution, based on which the predictive distribution of a future observation can be obtained. The predictive distribution is used to obtain control limits. The recent literature contains a considerable amount of research on Bayesian methods for control charting, particularly in the field of industrial engineering (Colosimo and Castillo 2007). The Bayesian approaches, however, are unfamiliar to quality engineers and statisticians in pharmaceutical manufacturing. In the following, through several examples in pharmaceutical quality control, we demonstrate the applicability and computational ease of Bayesian methods.

11.5.1 Control Chart for Data with Censoring

Data censoring is a common issue in quality attribute measurements, either due to rounding or limits of qualification of the analytical methods. The censored data impose technical challenges to the traditional frequentist methods used for control charts. Failure to account for the censoring may lead to an inappropriate control chart. In the following, we use a simple example with modified Gaussian data to illustrate the concept and provide a Bayesian alternative. Consider a manufacturing process that produces an inhaled product with acceptance limits 90% and 110% for data that follow a normal distribution with mean $\mu = 105\%$ and standard deviation $\sigma = 2.5\%$. Using the common 3-sigma rule, it is expected that 99.7% of values from this system will fall between 97.5 and 112.5, meaning that some of the larger values will not meet with the acceptance limits. Suppose that the process is monitored with respect to percent of drug delivery relative to the expected amount. One value from each of 25 lots is observed. After rounding to the nearest integer, the values are $\{x_i\} = \{100, 101, 102, 103, 103, 104, 104, 104, 105,$ 105, 105, 105, 105, 106, 106, 106, 106, 107, 107, 107, 108, 108, 108, 109, 110\}, result- ing in a sample mean of $\bar{x} = 105.4$ and sample standard deviation $s = 2.4$. The $\bar{x} \pm 3s$ rule yields the control limits (98, 113), which would be sensible in the absence of acceptance limits. Unfortunately, the upper control limit falls above the upper acceptance limit, meaning that the $\bar{x} \pm 3s$ cannot be used for this example without modification.

Though originally Gaussian, the x_i are rounded to the nearest integer, meaning that the statistical model should accommodate the interval censor- ing $(x_i - \frac{1}{2}, x_i + \frac{1}{2})$. Further, to recognize that control limits can only be built from data that meet the acceptance limits (90, 110), the x_i are assumed to stem from a truncated normal distribution. Fortunately, the Bayesian para- digm makes it easy to sample from the posterior distribution of (μ, σ) when the model for the x_i includes both interval censoring and truncation. The R/JAGS code to calculate the control limits is given below.

```
model.txt = "
model{

  ## Priors
  mu   ~ dnorm(100., 0.01)   ## SD = 10
  sigma ~ dt(0., 1., 1)T(0., )
  tau  <- 1/(sigma*sigma)

  ## Data distribution
  for ( i in 1:N )
  {
    ## Interval censoring
      ## x.censored[i] = 0, then x[i] < Lim[i,1]
      ## x.censored[i] = 1, then Lim[i,1] < x[i] <
                        Lim[i,2]
      ## x.censored[i] = 2, then x[i] > Lim[i,2]
    x.censored[i] ~ dinterval( x[i], Lim[i,] )

    x[i] ~ dnorm(mu, tau)T(90., 110.)   ## Truncated
                                  normal distribution
```

```
    }
  } "


data = list(N=length(x), x=x, x.censored=rep(1,
        length(x)), Lim=cbind(x-0.5, x+0.5))

fitb = run.jags( model.txt, data=data, n.chains=3,
            monitor=c("mu", "sigma"),
            burnin=10000, thin=10, sample=20000,
            method="parallel" )

th.post = as.matrix( as.mcmc.list(fitb) )

## A function for generating truncated normal random
   variables
rtnorm = function(n, mu, sigma, a=-Inf, b=Inf)
{
  U = runif(n, 0, 1)
  x.inner = pnorm((a-mu)/sigma) + U*( pnorm((b-mu)/
                           sigma) - pnorm((a-mu)/sigma) )
  x = mu + sigma*qnorm(x.inner)
  return(x)
}

## xpp = posterior predictive distribution of x
xpp = rtnorm(nrow(th.post), mu=th.post[,"mu"],
                sigma=th.post[,"sigma"], a=90, b=110)

## Control limits are 99.5% beta-expectation tolerance
   limits
control.lims = HPDinterval( as.mcmc(xpp), prob=0.995 )
```

In the computer code, the R object *xpp* contains 60,000 random draws from the posterior predictive distribution of *x*, shown in Figure 11.5. The distribution is left-skewed, meaning that setting the control limits with the symmetric $\bar{x} \pm 3s$ is inappropriate. For control limits, we opted to use a 99.5% β-expectation tolerance interval, which is equivalent to Bayesian 99.5% prediction interval. The resulting control limits are (97, 110), which provides a suitable range for good-quality data.

11.5.2 Control Chart for Discrete Data

As discussed by Yu, Ren, and Yang (2017), discrete quality attributes are abundant in pharmaceutical manufacturing and quality control. While

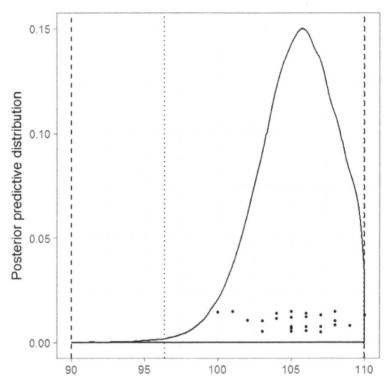

FIGURE 11.5
The density shows the posterior predictive distribution of x. The filled circles show the data. The dashed vertical lines show the acceptance limits and the dotted vertical lines show the control limits.

some discrete attributes, such as microbial count in raw materials, number of complaints, or number of non-conforming items during the product quality monitoring, are intrinsic to count data, other discrete attributes may arise from the discretization of continuous measures due to rounding and limit of quantitation. For example, the antibody titer value in the enzyme-linked immunosorbent assay (ELISA), which is the reciprocal of the highest dilution where the readout occurs, is usually recorded as the fold of dilution 8, 16, 32, 64, etc. As with continuous CQAs, it is necessary to establish set control limits for discrete CQAs. A typical example is the establishment of control limits for bioburden levels in cleanrooms where sterile drug products are manufactured. In fact, environmental cleanliness of aseptic manufacturing operations is a regulatory requirement (FDA 2004c; 21 CFR 211). Sterile drug products are manufactured in facilities where airborne particles are controlled. Although a sterile manufacturing environment consists of rooms which are designed, maintained, and controlled to minimize the introduction and retention of airborne particles and microbial excursions, opportunistic contaminations are unavoidable. Therefore, it is essential to establish an environmental monitoring (EM) program to assess the cleanliness of the manufacturing areas and to ensure a state of environmental control. Establishment of an EM program is required both by regulatory guidance and by law (FDA 2004c; 21 CFR 211). To monitor the performance of the cleanrooms, samples are routinely collected and the level of bioburden is determined. The data are compared to alert and action limits. Potential corrective steps may be taken if there are microbial excursions outside the limits.

The bioburden level is typically characterized through the number of colony forming units (CFUs) of bacteria on a manufacturing surface. A CFUs number is a non-negative integer with no upper bound and so modeling the data with a Poisson distribution may be reasonable. When the variability in the data exceeds its mean, which is also the variability under the Poisson assumption, the data are deemed to be overdispersed. For data with overdispersion, the negative binomial (a.k.a., gamma-Poisson) distribution is more suitable. Assume that X follows a negative binomial distribution $NB(\mu, r)$, with density function given by

$$f(x \mid \mu, r) = \frac{\Gamma(x+r)}{\Gamma(r)x!}(r/(r+\mu))^r (\mu/(r+\mu))^x$$

where $\mu > 0$ and $r > 0$. The distribution of X has a mean μ and variance $\mu(1+\mu/r)$. Whereas the mean and variance are equal for the Poisson distribution, it is evident that the variance is greater than the mean for the NB distribution.

In the following, using data from a real environmental monitoring program, we show how to set 95/99.5 Bayesian upper tolerance limit for CFUs. The data, which are shown in Table 11.4, are measured against an upper acceptance limit of 100 CFUs.

Let μ_0 and r_0 be the ML estimates of the model parameters μ and r, respectively. The following priors are used

$$\ln(\mu) \sim N\left(\ln(\mu_0), 1\right)$$

TABLE 11.4

Data for 430 Bioburden Measurements. Table Shows the Number of Times (out of 430) that Yielded the Given CFU Value

CFUs	0	1	2	3	4	5	6	7
# times	366	40	2	4	1	2	7	1
CFUs	15	24	26	28	29	38	91	
# times	1	1	1	1	1	1	1	

$$\ln(r) \sim N\big(\ln(r_0), 1\big).$$

A negative binomial model was fitted to the data using R/JAGS with the following computer code.

```
model.txt = "
model{

  ## Prior distribution
          ## mu0 and phi0 are ln-scaled maximum
            likelihood estimates
  mu ~ dlnorm( mu0, 1. )
  r ~ dlnorm( phi0, 1. )
  p <- r/(r+mu)

  ## data distribution
  for ( i in 1:N )
  {
    y[i] ~ dnegbin(p, r)
  }
}"

## Bioburden data
y = rep( c(0, 1, 2, 3, 4, 5, 6, 7, 15, 24, 26, 28, 29,
          38, 91),
         c(366, 40, 2, 4, 1, 2, 7, 1, 1, 1, 1, 1, 1,
           1, 1)
         )


## Maximize the negative binomial likelihood

nlogLik.nb = function( theta, y )
{
    L = -sum( dnbinom(y, mu = exp(theta[1]),
                      size = exp(theta[2]), log=TRUE) )

  return(L)
}
fit0 = optim( c(0, 0), nlogLik.nb, y=y )

data = list(N=length(y), y=y, mu0=fit0$par[1],
       phi0=fit0$par[2])
```

```
fitb = run.jags(model.txt, data=data, monitor=c("mu",
      "r", "p"),
         burnin = 10000, sample = 10000, thin=5,
         n.chains=3, method="parallel")

th.post = as.matrix( as.mcmc.list(fitb) )

## 95/99.5 upper tolerance limit for CFUs
control.lim = quantile( qnbinom(0.995,
            size=th.post[,"r"],
                             mu=th.post[,"mu"]), 0.95 )
```

The R variable *control.lim* is the 95/99.5 Bayesian upper tolerance limit for CFUs, with *control.lim* = 39 CFUs, serving as a satisfactory control limit for bioburden.

In some bioburden data sets, an event with CFUs > 0 may be quite rare. A second real bioburden set of data with 388 measurements contains 382 events with 0 CFUs and two events each with 1, 2, and 4 CFUs. The upper acceptance limit associated with this data set is 10 CFUs. Suppose the laboratory wishes for an upper control limit to contain 95% of future data. Because, in this case, 98% of the CFU values are equal to 0, even a 95/95 Bayesian upper tolerance interval yields a value of 0. Instead, we considered the distribution of CFU values, conditioned on CFU > 0. To calculate the conditional $100q\%$ quantile, consider solving for c: $q = \Pr(X \le c | X > 0) = \Pr(1 \le X \le c) / \{1 - \Pr(X = 0)\}$. The solution is $c = F^{-1}\{q + (1 - q)\Pr(X = 0)\}$, where $F^{-1}(.)$ is the inverse probability mass function (pmf) for the negative binomial distribution. In the computer code below, a 95% β-expectation tolerance interval (a.k.a., Bayesian 95% prediction interval) for CFUs, conditioned on CFU > 0, is calculated.

```
y = rep( c(0, 1, 2, 4), c(382, 2, 2, 2) )


## Maximize the negative binomial likelihood
fit0 = optim( c(0, 0), nlogLik.nb, y=y )

data = list(N=length(y), y=y, mu0=fit0$par[1],
        phi0=fit0$par[2])

fitb = run.jags(model.txt, data=data,
        monitor=c("mu", "r", "p"),
            burnin = 10000, sample = 10000, thin=5,
            n.chains=3, method="parallel")

th.post = as.matrix( as.mcmc.list(fitb) )
```

```
## Pr( X==0 | data ) = 0.98
mean( rnbinom(nrow(th.post), size=th.post[,"r"],
                    mu=th.post[,"mu"]) == 0)

## 95/95 tolerance limit (= 0)
control.lim = quantile( qnbinom(0.95, size=th.post[,"r"],
                    mu=th.post[,"mu"]), 0.95 )

## 95% beta-expectation tolerance interval, conditioned
   on CFU > 0
U = runif(nrow(th.post), 0, 1)
xpp.c = qnbinom( U +
            (1-U)*pnbinom(1, size=th.post[,"r"],
            mu=th.post[,"mu"]),
            size=th.post[,"r"], mu=th.post[,"mu"] )
control.lim.c = quantile(xpp.c, p=0.95)
```

Whereas the value of the 95%/95% β-content unconditional tolerance limit in the R variable *control.lim* is 0, the 95% β-expectation conditional tolerance limit in the R variable *control.lim.c* yields a control limit of 9 CFUs. In effect, because 98% of the CFU values equal zero, the control limit is $98\% + 0.95 \times 2\% = 99.9\%$ quantile. Indeed, calculating the unconditional 99.9% β-expectation tolerance limit

```
quantile( rnbinom(nrow(th.post), size=th.post[,"r"],
                    mu=th.post[,"mu"]), 0.999 )
```

provides a similar control limit of 7 CFUs.

11.5.3 Control Limit for Aberrant Data

11.5.3.1 Background

Atypical or OOS results may occur during the production of drug substance and final product, as well as in stability testing. Since these results may have a significant impact on the disposition of a drug product lot, investigation of OOS results is an important component of the manufacturing quality system. To mitigate the risk of releasing a lot of substandard quality or rejecting a good lot, regulatory guidance (FDA 2006) requires that a root cause investigation be carried out when faced with an OOS result. In the past, failure to conduct adequate OOS investigations resulted in numerous (≥483) citations as well as legal proceedings by the FDA for more severe cases. In the FDA guidance (FDA 2006), a stepwise approach of laboratory assessment is recommended. If no assignable cause is identified, statistical methods may be used to assess if the OOS result is a statistical outlier, thus justifying additional resampling and retesting to aid disposition of the lot in question. The historical data of the manufacturing process that operated in a state of control provide a useful canvas for evaluating the OOS result and deciding on the disposition of the batch under evaluation. Bayesian methods provide a means to make full use of the historical data. In addition, a Bayesian approach also results in a probabilistic statement of how likely an OOS result is to be a true outlier.

11.5.3.2 Methods

Let $\tilde{X}$ and X_{OOS} be a future observation and the observed OOS result, respectively. Let p_0 denote a pre-determined small number such as 1%. To simplify the discussion, assume that X_{OOS} exceeds the upper specification limit, U. One way to judge if X_{OOS} is a statistical outlier or not is to calculate the predictive probability $P(\tilde{X} > X_{OOS} \mid X)$, where X denotes the collected data. The observation X_{OOS} is declared to be an outlier if

$$P(\tilde{X} > X_{OOS} \mid X) < p_0.$$

For a simple example, suppose

$$X_i \sim N\left(\mu, \sigma^2\right) \quad (i = 1, 2, \ldots, n)$$

are independent historical data collected from analytical testing. Assume that priors

$$\mu \mid \sigma^2 \sim N\left(\mu_0, \frac{\sigma^2}{\kappa_0}\right)$$

$$\sigma^2 \sim \text{inverse-Gamma}\left(\frac{\gamma_0}{2}, \frac{\gamma_0 \sigma_0^2}{2}\right),$$

where $\mu_0, \kappa_0, \sigma_0^2$, and γ_0 are the hyperparameters, the predictive probability distribution of $\tilde{X}$ can be derived (Colosimo and Castillo 2007).

The joint normal inverse gamma prior is

$$\left(\mu, \sigma^2\right) \sim \text{NIG}\left(\mu_0, \kappa_0, \gamma_0, \sigma_0^2\right).$$

It can be shown that the joint posterior distribution is

$$\left(\mu, \sigma^2\right) \mid \bar{X}, s^2 \sim \text{NIG}\left(\mu_n, \kappa_n, \gamma_n, \sigma_n^2\right),$$

where

$$\mu_n = \frac{\kappa_0}{\kappa_0 + n}\mu_0 + \frac{n}{\kappa_0 + n}\bar{X},$$

$$\kappa_n = \kappa_0 + n, \quad \gamma_n = \gamma_0 + n,$$

$$\gamma_n\sigma_n^2 = \gamma_0\sigma_0^2 + (n-1)s^2 + \frac{\kappa_0}{\kappa_0 + n}\left(\bar{X} - \mu_0\right)^2.$$

Further, the marginal posterior distributions are

$$\sigma^2 \mid \bar{X}, s^2 \sim \text{inverse-Gamma}\left(\frac{\gamma_n}{2}, \frac{\gamma_n\sigma_n^2}{2}\right)$$

$$\mu \mid \bar{X}, s^2 \sim t\left(\mu_n, \frac{\sigma_n^2}{\kappa_n}, \gamma_n\right).$$

The posterior predictive distribution of $\tilde{X}$ can be obtained through the following integration:

$$p\left(\tilde{X} \mid X\right) = \iint p\left(\tilde{X} \mid \mu, \sigma^2\right) p(\mu, \sigma^2 \mid X) d\mu d\sigma^2 \qquad (11.1)$$

which yields

$$\tilde{X} \mid X \sim t\left(\mu_n, \frac{\sigma_n^2(\kappa_n + 1)}{\kappa_n}, \gamma_n\right).$$

Thus, the probability $\Pr(\tilde{X} > X_{OOS} \mid X)$ can be estimated either through numerical or Monte Carlo integration.

For an illustration, consider the summary statistics from $n=25$ independent historical analytical test samples: $\bar{X} = 99.8$ and $s^2 = 22.3$ and an OOS observation of $X_{OOS} = 117$. With hyperparameters $\mu_0 = 100$, $\sigma_0^2 = 32$, $\kappa_0 = 2$, and $\gamma_0 = 3$, the posterior predictive probability $\Pr(\tilde{X} > X_{OOS} \mid X)$ may be estimated in a number of ways. The direct method is given by the code below.

```
## Prior hyper parameters
mu0 = 100;  kappa0 = 2;  gamma0 = 3;  sigmaSq0 = 32

## Data
xbar = 99.8;  sSq = 22.3; N = 25
x.oos = 109

## Posterior hyper parameters
mu.n = (kappa0*mu0+N*xbar)/(kappa0+N)
```

```
kappa.n = kappa0 + N
gamma.n = gamma0 + N
sigmaSq.n = (gamma0*sigmaSq0 + (N-1)*sSq +
                    (kappa0/(kappa0+N))*(xbar-mu0)^2)/
                                        gamma.n
```

The posterior predictive probability is directly calculated through the T distribution as

```
pt( (x.oos-mu.n)/sqrt(sigmaSq.n), gamma.n,
                                lower.tail=FALSE)
```

Alternatively, the Monte Carlo integral is derived by sampling from the posterior predictive distribution of $\tilde{X}$ with

```
sigmaSq.post = 1/rgamma(10000, shape=0.5*gamma.n,
                        rate=(gamma.n*sigmaSq.n)/2)
mu.post = rnorm(10000, mean=mu.n,
            sd=sqrt(sigmaSq.post/kappa.n))
xtilde = rnorm( 10000, mean=mu.post,
            sd=sqrt(sigmaSq.post) )
mean( xtilde > x.oos )   ## Monte Carlo integral
```

In both cases, the posterior predictive probability is about 3%. With a decision-making cutoff of 1%, we cannot call X_{OOS} a statistical outlier.

While the Gaussian data conjugate prior provides a simple solution, it is possible that historical information is better represented by a non-conjugate prior. In such a case, the posterior predictive distribution for $\tilde{X}$ cannot be written in a closed form and so, generally, sampling of (μ, σ^2) allows estimation of Distribution (11.1). An illustration is provided with the non-conjugate priors $\mu \sim T(100, 1.5^2, 4)$ and $\ln(\sigma) \sim N(\ln(5), SD=0.6)$.

```
model.txt="
model{
  ## Priors
  mu  ~ dt(100, 1.5, 4)
  lsigma  ~ dnorm( 1.609, 0.6 )

  sigmaSq <- exp(2*lsigma)
  tau <- 1/sigmaSq

  ## Likelihood
  xbar  ~ dnorm(mu, N*tau)
  sSq  ~ dgamma( 0.5*(N-1), 0.5*(N-1)*tau )
}"
```

```
data = list( N=25, xbar=99.8, sSq=22.3 )
fitb = run.jags( model=model.txt,
        monitor=c("mu", "sigmaSq"),
            data=data, n.chains=3,
            burnin=20000, sample=10000, thin=5,
            method="parallel" )
th.post = as.matrix( as.mcmc.list(fitb) )
```

Just like with the conjugate Monte Carlo integration code, we write

```
x.tilde = rnorm( nrow(th.post), mean=th.post[,"mu"],
                    sd=sqrt(th.post[,"sigmaSq"]) )
mean( xtilde > x.oos )   ## Monte Carlo integral
```

The posterior predictive probability is again about 3%.

Next, consider the non-Gaussian bioburden example in Section 11.4.2 with data shown in Table 11.4. The bioburden upper acceptance limit is 100 CFUs. Suppose a value of $X_{OSS} = 101$ CFUs is observed. Although must bioburden values in Table 11.4 are small, there is one value of 91 CFUs, so it may be possible to achieve a bioburden value of 101 CFUs. Recall that the data follow a negative binomial distribution and the R variable "th.post" contains the sampled posterior distribution of parameters (μ, r, p). The posterior predictive distribution of new bioburden samples is generated by

```
xtilde = rnbinom(nrow(th.post), size=th.post[,"r"],
        mu=th.post[,"mu"])
```

The posterior predictive probability $\Pr(\tilde{X} > X_{OOS} \mid X)$ is estimated by

```
x.oos = 101
mean( xtilde > x.oos )
```

Since the posterior predictive probability is essentially zero, $X_{OOS} = 101$ CFUs is declared a statistical outlier.

Alternatively, one may determine an upper limit, U, of the $(1 - p_0) \times 100\%$ Bayesian prediction interval. The suspected OOS, X_{OOS}, is confirmed as a true OOS result if it exceeds the limit U. For example, with $p_0 = 0.9999$, the value U is 91 and is calculated from the following code.

```
p0 = 0.9999
U = quantile( rnbinom(nrow(th.jags), size=th.jags[,"r"],
                    mu=th.jags[,"mu"]), p0 )
```

Again, the value $X_{OOS} = 101$ CFUs is declared a statistical outlier.

11.5.4 Product Quality Control Based on Safety Data from Surveillance

11.5.4.1 Background

In drug clinical development, the cumulative safety data from early Phase I/II and late-stage Phase III trials allow for general characterization of drug safety profile. The occurrences of rare adverse events (AEs) cannot be fully determined due to drug exposure of a limited number of patients. As part of post-marketing regulatory requirements, manufacturers are mandated to monitor and report serious AEs stemming from the use of the marketed drug. Post-marketing approval, AEs are continuously collected from patients receiving the drug. Further assessment of this safety data might lead to a change in the product label as well as revision of the risks and benefits of the product.

Although the post-marketing safety data are primarily used to characterize rare AEs, unexpected increasing trends of AEs can be indicative of quality issues with commercial lots of the drug, particularly when no other clinical causes can be prescribed. Some researchers suggest the monitoring and evaluation of such a trend to identify defective product lots. Aquilina et al. (2006) developed a pharmacovigilance procedure for timely detection of suspicious AE trends. The procedure consists of the on-going review of alert events such as severe hypersensitivity (anaphylaxis), acute major organ failure (renal, hepatic, pulmonary, or cardiac failure), or cases of possible bacterial contamination (sepsis), and monthly and annual determination of the frequency of AEs by product lot. The occurrences of alert events or increase in AE frequency trigger further investigation of a product lot. If effectively utilized, such a procedure can greatly facilitate detection of product defects and minimize the resources spent on investigating those issues unlikely to involve bona-fide safety concerns.

11.5.4.2 Current Methods

In recent years, several statistical methods have been developed to detect changes in the reporting rate of a specific AE using post-marketing adverse event reports. Tsong (1992, 1999) proposed a confidence interval (CI) approach. Based on both the frequency of the AE and the number of sales of the drug product in two reporting periods, Tsong (1992) derived the 95% CI for the expected AE frequency of the current reporting period, conditioned on the observed frequency of the previous period. The rate of AE is believed to be significantly increased if the observed AE frequency of the current period exceeds the upper limit of the CI. Chuang-Stein (1993) suggested a Bayesian approach to model adverse events. As pointed out by Chuang-Stein et al. (1998), even though the method by Chuang-Stein (1993) was proposed for clinical trials, it can be generalized to evaluate post-marketing AEs under the assumption that both the number of patients receiving the drug product and the number of individuals experiencing the event of interest are known. The method by Chuang-Stein (1993) uses a binomial distribution to model the number of patients experiencing the AEs, and a β prior for the event rates in different reporting periods. Let n and X be the total numbers of patients who were followed in the previous reporting periods and who had experienced AEs, respectively. It is assumed that

$$X \sim \text{binomial}(n, p)$$

with a prior

$$p \sim \text{Beta}(\alpha, \beta).$$

Denote n' and X' as the numbers of patients who are to be followed in the next reporting period and who will experience AEs, respectively. Hence, X' event follows Beta-binomial distribution

$$X' \mid X \sim \text{Beta-binomial}(n', \alpha + X', \beta + n - X').$$

From the above distribution, the probability of as many as the observed number of individuals experiencing the event can be calculated and compared to a cutoff value p_0:

$$\Pr(X' \geq x_0' \mid X).$$

If this probability turns out to be low, one can reasonably conclude that the event rate has increased.

However, there is an apparent drawback with this method in that it requires the number of patients receiving the drug be known. In reality, patients who do not experience the event are usually not included in the safety reports. As a remedy, Chuang-Stein et al. (1998) suggested another Bayesian model to describe the mean number of AE per 1,000 prescriptions, which are typically available through mandatary post-marketing surveillance AE reporting programs. The method assumes this mean value follows a Poisson distribution. By assigning a gamma prior to the mean of the Poisson distribution, the posterior mean number of AEs per 1,000 follows a negative binomial distribution. Similar to the Beta-binomial model, the density may be used to calculate the predictive probability of observing at least as many AEs as are being detected in the next reporting period to assess whether or not there is an increase in the event rate.

In pharmacovigilance safety data monitoring, reviewers are primarily searching for signals of alert AEs, for which the potential for a product quality defect cannot be reasonably ruled out, based on clinical data such as medical history. Such AEs are singled out for further investigation. Because of the rarity of the events, an excess of zero AEs is often observed for each reporting period. This is especially true for serious AEs. The high occurrence of zero observations often invalidates the assumption that the data follow an underlying distribution such as normal or Poisson distribution, as used by Tsong (1992, 1999), Chuang-Stein (1993), and Chuang-Stein et al. (1998).

11.5.4.3 Zero-Inflated Models

An alternative method based on a zero-inflated Poisson (ZIP) model was proposed by Yang et al. (2007). A zero-inflated model is often used to describe random observations, each of which stems from one of two populations. The first population places all its mass at zero with probability p while the second population assumes non-zero integers according to a probability distribution, such as Poisson, with probability $1 - p$.

Let $X_i, i = 1,\ldots,n$ denote the numbers of AEs per dose in the previous n report periods. Yang et al. (2007) modeled X_i through the following ZIP model:

$$X_i = WY + (1-W)Z, \tag{11.2}$$

where W is Bernoulli random variable with $\Pr[W=1]=p$, Y is a degenerated random variable with $\Pr(Y=0)=1$, $Z \sim \text{Poisson}(\lambda)$, and W, Y, and Z are independent. It can be readily verified that

$$\Pr[X_i = x] = \begin{cases} p + (1-p)e^{-\lambda} & \text{if } x = 0 \\ (1-p)\dfrac{\lambda^x e^{-\lambda}}{x!} & \text{else} \end{cases} \tag{11.3}$$

Supposed that $(x_1,\ldots,x_n)$ are observed values of $(X_1,\ldots X_n)$. Without loss of generality, we assume that $x_i = 0, i = 1,\ldots,n_1$, and $n_2 = n - n_1$. Then the likelihood function of x_i is given by

$$L = \left[p + (1-p)e^{-\lambda} \right]^{n_1} \prod_{i=n_1+1}^{n} \left[(1-p)\frac{\lambda^{x_i} e^{-\lambda}}{x_i!} \right]$$

$$= \left[p + (1-p)e^{-\lambda} \right]^{n_1} (1-p)^{n_2} \frac{\lambda^{\sum_{i=n_1+1}^{n} x_i}}{\prod_{i=n_1+1}^{n} x_i!} e^{-\lambda n_2}. \tag{11.4}$$

We assume that the parameters p and λ have a prior distribution of Beta(a, b) and gamma(α,β) respectively. Hence,

$$f(p) \propto p^{\alpha-1}(1-p)^{\beta-1}$$

$$f(\lambda) \propto \frac{\lambda^{\alpha-1}e^{-\lambda/\beta}}{\beta^{\alpha}}. \tag{11.5}$$

Combining Functions (11.4) and (11.5), it can be shown that the posterior distribution of $\theta = (p, \lambda)$ is given by

$$f(\theta \mid x_1, \ldots x_n) = C_2^{-1} \sum_{j=1}^{n_1} p^{j+a-1} (1-p)^{n-j+b-1} \lambda^{\sum_{i=n_1+1}^{n} x_i + \alpha - 1} e^{-\lambda(n-j+1/\beta)} \qquad (11.6)$$

where C_2 is a normalization factor having an expression:

$$C_2 = \sum_{j=1}^{n_1} \binom{n_1}{j} \text{Beta}(j+a, n-j+b) \frac{\Gamma\left(\lambda^{\sum_{i=n_1+1}^{n} x_i + \alpha}\right)}{\left(n-j+\dfrac{1}{\beta}\right)^{\sum_{i=n_1+1}^{n} x_i + \alpha}}. \qquad (11.7)$$

From Distributions (11.3) and (11.6), given a fixed value x_0, the predictive posterior probability for the number of AEs of a future reporting period can be calculated as:

$$p(x_0) = \Pr[X \geq x_0] = \int_0^1 \int_0^{\infty} \sum_{x=x_0}^{\infty} (1-p) \frac{\lambda^x e^{-\lambda}}{x!} f(\theta \mid x_1, \ldots x_n) d\lambda \, dp.$$

Carrying out the above integration, we obtain

$$p(x_0) = C_2^{-1} \sum_{k=x_0}^{\infty} \sum_{j=1}^{n_1} \frac{\binom{n_1}{j} \text{Beta}(j+a, n-j+b)\Gamma(s)}{\left(n-j+\dfrac{1}{\beta}\right)^s} \qquad (11.8)$$

with $s = \sum_{i=n_1+1}^{n} x_i + \alpha + x_0$.

11.5.4.4 Alert Limit for AEs

The alert limit for future report periods can be defined as a cutoff point such that

$$p(x_0) \geq p_0, \qquad (11.9)$$

where p_0 is a prespecified small positive number, say, 0.05.

Although Equation (11.8) provides a closed form for the predictive posterior probability, the calculation is not straightforward. Fortunately, we can use the MCMC method to determine the cut point, using the R code below. It is worth noting that to simulate the random variable from the ZIP distribution, one may use the mixed Bernoulli-Poisson representation, where

$$X \mid W \sim \text{Poisson}(\lambda(1-D)) \text{ with } D \sim \text{Bernoulli}(p)$$

An Example

To illustrate the concept, consider an example data set in which zero AEs were reported in 14 of the last 20 report periods with the remaining six report periods yielding the set {2, 3, 3, 2, 3, 1} out of 1,000 doses prescribed. JAGS code is provided to calculate the posterior predictive probability that $X \geq x_0$, where $x_0 = 5$ in a future period is considered a large number of AEs per 1,000 doses. JAGS does not permit the mixture of different distribution families, so there is no straightforward method to write the ZIP distribution. Instead, we programmed a near-ZIP equivalent so that, with probability p, $X_i \sim \text{Poisson}(10^{(-10)})$ and, with probability $1 - p$, $X_i \sim \text{Poisson}(\lambda)$. Informative priors were applied to this problem with $p \sim \text{Beta}(10, 3)$ and $\lambda \sim \gamma(5, 1)$. Most of the mass for the prior distribution for p is above 0.5 and the prior for λ was set so that the mean and variance are both equal to 5. The ensuing posterior predictive probability $p(x_0 = 5) = 3.5\%$ means that the risk of a large number of AEs in a future period is non-zero, but low.

```
model.txt = "
model{

  ## Prior distributions
  p ~ dbeta(10, 3)    ## Skewed to the left. 99% of values
                         are > 0.45.
  lam ~ dgamma(5, 1)  ## Mean = variance = 5

## Likelihood
  for ( i in 1:N )
  {
    ## lambda[i] = 1e-10 with probability p
    ##        and = lam with probability (1-p).
    lambda[i] <- lam*(1-zero[i]) + 1e-10*zero[i]

    zero[i] ~ dbern(p)
    x[i] ~ dpois(lambda[i])
  }
}"
data = list(N=20, x=c(rep(0, 14), 2, 3, 3, 2, 3, 1))

fitb = run.jags(model.txt, data=data,
       monitor=c("lam", "p"),
           n.chains=3, burnin=10000, sample=10000, thin=5,
           method="parallel")

th.post = as.matrix(as.mcmc.list(fitb))

## Get posterior predictive distribution of ZIP data
w.tilde = rbinom(nrow(th.post), size=1,
             prob=th.post[,"p"])
x.tilde = ifelse( w.tilde==1, 0,
             rpois(nrow(th.post), lambda=th.post[,"lam"]) )

## Estimate p(x0=5)
mean(x.tilde >= 5)
```

When applied to safety data from surveillance data, the ZIP may not be adequate. This is primarily due to the fact that the actual variability in the data is often larger than that expected under the Poisson assumption. This phenomenon is often referred to as overdispersion. For the surveillance data collected at different times and locations, although at each fixed time or location the number of AEs may exhibit behavior that can be described through a Poisson distribution, the collective data as a whole may not follow any Poisson distribution. The negative binomial (NB) distribution is a variant of Poisson distribution that has increased flexibility to address the issue of overdispersion. Mathematically it can be formulated as a mixture of Poisson distributions (Hoffman 2004). The zero-inflated negative binomial (ZINB) is suitable for modeling the safety surveillance data when both excessive numbers of zero observation and overdispersion issues are expected. The probability function of the negative binomial variable is given by:

$$f(x \mid \pi, \tau) = \frac{\Gamma(x+\tau)}{x!\Gamma(\tau)} \pi^{\tau}(1-\pi)^{x}.$$

By a reparameterization $\lambda = \frac{\tau(1-\pi)}{\pi}$, the ZINB model can also be derived from a mixed representation (Ghosh et al. 2006):

$$X \mid W \sim \text{NB}(x \mid \pi, \tau) \text{ with } \pi = \frac{\tau}{[\tau + »(1-D)]}, D \sim \text{Bernoulli}(p).$$

With this representation, the sampling of the ZINB random variable can be easily implemented in JAGS or Stan.

11.6 Concluding Remarks

As the pharmaceutical industry entered the 21st century, there has been a significant shift in regulatory thinking from "testing into compliance" to QbD. Increasingly, a risk-based lifecycle approach to product development, based on a sound quality system, has become the dominant business and governance paradigm. From this perspective, a consistent supply of quality pharmaceutical products is a key to a company's success. In the past decades, while statistical quality control techniques have been developed and become part of core quality management systems in many fields, the uptake of this philosophy has been slow in the pharmaceutical industry. In keeping with the recent regulatory guidelines concerning QbD and the use of holistic risk-based lifecycle development paradigms, it is imperative to use statistical tools such as control charts to monitor, control, and optimize the manufacturing process. Bayesian control charts take full advantage of knowledge gained from the early development of the process to set control charts that are better suited for ensuring product quality and regulatory compliance. In this chapter, we discussed several Bayesian methods that allow for incorporation of prior knowledge. They are particularly suitable for situations in which a large amount of historical data is available.

Appendix: Stan Computer Code

In this appendix, Stan computer code is provided for all of the MCMC statements for which JAGS was called. The Stan library is called through the statement *require(rstan)*, after which the following message is printed to the screen.

For execution on a local, multicore CPU with excess RAM we recommend calling

options(mc.cores = parallel::detectCores()).

To avoid recompilation of unchanged Stan programs, we recommend calling

rstan_options(auto_write = TRUE)

Throughout this appendix, to run Stan in parallel on three CPUs, we start each program in R with

```
options(mc.cores=3); rstan_options(auto_write=TRUE)
```

As shown in Section 2.4 (Table 2.4–1), the Stan program requires separate sections with the heading *data*, *parameters*, and the *model*. A Stan program often also contains a section with the header *transformed parameters*, which allows new parameters to be declared as functions of the variables declared in the *parameters* section. The reader is referred to Stan (2017, 2018) for the inner workings of the MCMC algorithm and for the language manual.

Unlike JAGS, Stan requires a compilation step. We prefer the method in which the compilation is performed using the function *stan_model()* so that the compiled object may be saved or reused in the future. For this chapter, assume that the results from *stan_model()* are placed in the R object *model*. MCMC sampling is performed with the function *sampling()*. With little or no modification, the list() object used by JAGS may also be used with Stan. For this chapter, the results from *sampling()* are stored in the R object *fitb*. Graphical diagnostics with Stan may be performed on *fitb* with the built-in plotting functions in the "rstan" library, including *stan_trace()* and *stan_dens()*. To place *fitb* into a matrix, use the command

```
th.post = as.matrix(fitb)
```

The remaining R code from Chapters 2–11 may then be used with little alteration.

Section 2.4: Univariate Normal Distribution

```
data{
  int<lower=0> n; // number of observations
  real y[n];   // the data
// hyperparameters
  real mu0;
  real k0;
  real nu0;
  real sigSq0;
}
parameters{
  real mu;
  real tau;
}
transformed parameters{
  real sigma;
  sigma = 1/sqrt(tau);
}
model{

  // Prior
  mu ~ normal( mu0, sigma/sqrt(k0) );
  tau ~ gamma( 0.5*nu0, 0.5*nu0*sigSq0 );

  // Likelihood
  for ( i in 1:n )
  {
    y[i] ~ normal( mu, sigma );
  }
}


## Data for Stan
data = list(n=length(y), y=y, mu0=100, k0=1.5,
       nu0=2, sigSq0=64 )

## Collect MCMC samples
fitb = sampling( model, data=data, pars=c("mu", "sigma",
       "lambda"), chains=3,
                 warmup=5000, thin=5, iter=5000+5*10000 )
```

Section 3.2.2: Batch Defects

[3.1]

```
data{
  int<lower=0> nBatch; // number of batches
  int<lower=0, upper=10> X[nBatch];  // # units before
                                        defect found
    // rightCens: = 0 if defect found, = 1 if no defect
                                        found in 10
  int<lower=0, upper=1> rightCens[nBatch];
}
parameters{
  real<lower=0, upper=1> p;  // probability of a
                                defective unit
}
transformed parameters{
  real<lower=0, upper=1> pRel; // probability to
                                  release a batch
  real<lower=0> bta;  // Parameter used in the Stan
                         negative binomial

  pRel = (1-p)^10;
  bta = p/(1-p);
}
model{

  // prior
  p ~ beta(2, 198);

  for ( i in 1:nBatch )
  {
    if ( rightCens[i]==1 )
    {
      // right-censoring with negative binomial dist
      target += neg_binomial_lccdf( X[i] | 1, bta );
    }
    else
    {
      X[i] ~ neg_binomial( 1, bta );
    }
  }
}
```

```
data = list( nBatch=5, X=c(10, 10, 10, 10, 6),
             rightCens=c(1, 1, 1, 1, 0) )
fitb = sampling(model, data=data, warmup = 5000,
     iter = 5000+10000,
              thin=1, chains = 3 )
```

[3.2]

```
data{
  int<lower=0, upper=5> Y;    // number of released
                                  batches out of 5
}
parameters{
  real<lower=0, upper=1> p;   // probability of a
                                  defective unit
}
transformed parameters{
  real<lower=0, upper=1> pRel; // probability to
                                  release a batch

  pRel = (1-p)^10;

}
model{

  // log-prior for p, explicitly written
  p ~ beta(2, 198);

  // likelihood based on probability to release a batch
  Y ~ binomial( 5, pRel );
}

data = list( Y=4 )   ## Four batches out of five are
                        released
fitb = sampling(model, data=data, warmup = 5000,
     iter = 5000+10000,
              thin=1, chains = 3 )
```

Section 3.3: Phase II Study

```
data{
  real ybar;      // Mean result
  real N;         // number of observations
  }
parameters{
  real delta;
}
model{

  // Prior for delta
  delta ~ student_t( 3, 2.0, 0.6 );

  // Likelihood: ybar ~ N( delta, 2/N )
  ybar ~ normal( delta, sqrt(2/N) );
}

pr = rep(NA, 100)
for ( i in 1:100 )
{
  delta.design = rnorm(1, mean=2.4, sd=sqrt(0.028))
                  ## Design prior
    ## ybar: Virtual patient summary statistic
  ybar = rnorm(1, mean=delta.design, sd=sqrt(2/N))
  data = list(N=N, ybar=ybar)
  fitb = sampling(model, data=data, warmup = 4000,
         iter = 4000+8000,
                  thin=1, chains=3 )
  th.stan = as.matrix(fitb)   ## Put the Stan output into
                                      a matrix
    ## Posterior probability that p > 1.5
  pr[b] = mean(th.stan[,"delta"] > 1.5)
}
mean(pr > 0.95)  ## Statistical power
```

Section 3.4.3: Futility Analysis

One of the advantages of the Stan language is its flexibility when it comes to censored values. For those who survived beyond 18 months, the JAGS code in Section 3.4.3 requires (1) setting the observed value *surv* to NA; (2)

denoting the distribution of *surv* as exponential; and (3) setting an indicator variable *rightCens* to the value 1 to show that the *surv* > 18. In Stan, we accomplish this in one line of code with the probability function *exponential_lccdf*() multiplied by the number of subjects who survived beyond the final study time point.

```
data{
   real Tsum[2];    // Sum of times for those who are dead
   real m[2];       // Number of dead patients (out of 100)
   real n[2];       // Number of alive patients = 100 - m
   real est[2];     // Maximum likelihood estimates for theta
   }
parameters{
   real theta[2];
}
model{

   for ( i in 1:2 )
   {
     // Prior for theta ~ N( MLE, 4*SE )
     theta[i] ~ normal(est[i], 0.5);

     // Likelihood: Tsum ~ gamma( m, exp(theta) )
     Tsum[i] ~ gamma( m[i], exp(theta[i]) );

     // Likelihood term for those alive (> 18 months)
     target += n[i]*exponential_lccdf(18. | exp(theta[i]) );
   }
}
```

```
data = list(Tsum=c(450, 540), est=c(ln(1/12), ln(1/18)),
            m=c(75, 65), n=c(25, 35))

fitb = sampling(model, data=data, warmup=10000,
        iter = 10000+5000*10,
                              thin=10, chains = 3)
```

Section 4.2.3: Drug Combination Bliss

```
d = read.csv("Drug Combo Data.csv")   ## Load the data

data{

    int<lower = 0> m1;   // number of monotherapy doses,
                               drug 1
    int<lower = 0> m2;   // number of monotherapy dose,
                               drug 2
    int<lower = 0> mc;   // number of combination doses

    int<lower=1> N0;   // number of control observations
    int<lower=1> N1[m1];   // number of monotherapy obs,
                                 drug 1, per dose
    int<lower=1> N2[m2];   // number of monotherapy obs,
                                 drug 2, per dose
    int<lower=1> Nc[mc];  // number of combination obs,
                                 per dose

    real y1[m1];       // monotherapy observations, drug 1
    real y2[m2];       // monotherapy observations, drug 2
    real yc[mc];       // combination observations
    real y0;             // control observations

    real<lower=0> degFree;        // Estimated pooled var
                                     and degrees of freedom
    real<lower=0> SigSqHat;

    real logX1[m1];   // log doses, drug 1
    real logX2[m2];   // log doses, drug 2

}
parameters{

    real<lower=0.5, upper=1.> yMax;   // The yMax parameter=
                                         mean of control
    real<lower=0., upper=0.5> yMin1; // parameters for
                                         monotherapy drug 1
    real theta1;
    real<lower=0.> s1;

    real<lower=0., upper=0.5> yMin2;   // parameters for
                                         monotherapy drug 1
```

```
   real theta2;
   real<lower=0.> s2;

   real<lower=0., upper=1.> muC[mc];   // mean parameter
                                       //        for combinations

   real<lower=0> sigma;
}
model{

   // declarations
   real mu1[m1];
   real mu2[m2];

   // Priors
   yMax ~ normal(0.9, 10.);

   // Compound 1
   yMin1 ~ normal(0.1, 10.);
   theta1 ~ normal(0.5, 10.);
   s1 ~ normal(1., 2.);

   // Compound 2
   yMin2 ~ normal(0.1, 10.);
   theta2 ~ normal(0.5, 10.);
   s2 ~ normal(1., 2.);

   sigma ~ cauchy(0., 0.1); // Half-cauchy with scale=0.1

   // Likelihood
   SigSqHat ~ gamma( 0.5*degFree, 0.5*degFree/(sigma*sigma) );

   // Negative control
   y0 ~ normal( yMax, sigma/sqrt(N0) );

   // Monotherapy for Cpd 1
   for ( i in 1:m1 )
   {
     mu1[i] = yMin1 + (yMax-yMin1)/( 1 + exp( s1*logX1[i]
                                       - s1*theta1 ) );
     y1[i] ~ normal( mu1[i], sigma/sqrt(N1[i]) );
   }
```

```
  // Monotherapy for Cpd 2
  for ( j in 1:m2 )
  {
    mu2[j] = yMin2 + (yMax-yMin2)/( 1 + exp( s2*logX2[j]
                                      - s2*theta2 ) );
    y2[j] ~ normal( mu2[j], sigma/sqrt(N2[j]));
  }

  // Combinations
  for ( k in 1:mc )
  {
    muC[k] ~ normal(0.5, 10.);        // Prior for muC
    yc[k] ~ normal( muC[k], sigma/sqrt(Nc[k]));
                                      // Likelihood for yc
  }

}
## For this data/model, Stan needs help with the
   starting values
inits = list(
        list( yMax=0.7, yMin1=0.1, theta1=0, s1=1,
              yMin2=0.1,
                        theta2=0,s2=1, muC=rep(0.5, 49),
                        sigma=0.1 ),
        list( yMax=0.8, yMin1=0.05, theta1=0, s1=1.1,
              yMin2=0.15,
                        theta2=0, s2=1,muC=rep(0.5, 49),
                        sigma=0.1 ),
        list( yMax=0.9, yMin1=0.1, theta1=0, s1=1,
              yMin2=0.08,
                        theta2=0, s2=1.1,
                        muC=rep(0.5, 49), sigma=0.1 )
            )
fitb = sampling( model, data=data,
           pars=c("yMax", "yMin1", "theta1", "s1",
                "yMin2", "theta2", "s2", "muC", "sigma"),
          chains=3, init=inits, warmup=10000, thin=10,
          iter=10000+10*20000 )
```

Section 4.2.3: 2 × 2 *In-vivo* Follow-up Study (Vague Prior)

```
data{

    int<lower=0> nTrt;          // number of treatments
    int<lower=0> nStudy;        // number of studies
    int<lower=0> nObs;          // total number of observations

    int<lower=1> trt[nObs];     // categories for treatment
    int<lower=1> study[nObs];   // categories for study
    int<lower=1> N[nObs];       // Number of obs for each
                                //   study/treatment

    real ybar[nObs];            // Observed mean from each
                                //   study/treatment
    real<lower=0> degFree;      // Pooled variance and
                                //   degrees of freedom
    real<lower=0> SigSqHat;

}
parameters{
    real eta[nTrt];             // treatment mean
    real<lower=0> sigmaS;       // Study standard deviation
    real<lower=0> sigmaE;       // Within-study standard deviation

    real thetaS[nStudy];
}
model{

    real mu[nObs];

    // Priors
    for ( i in 1:nTrt )
    {
        eta[i] ~ normal(5, 2.);
    }
    sigmaS ~ cauchy(0., 0.1);
    sigmaE ~ cauchy(0., 0.1);


    // Likelihood
    SigSqHat ~ gamma( 0.5*degFree, 0.5*degFree/
                                    (sigmaE*sigmaE) );
```

```
  // Hierarchical likelihood for mean
  for ( j in 1:nStudy )
  {
    thetaS[j] ~ normal(0., sigmaS);
  }

  for ( k in 1:nObs )
  {
    mu[k] = eta[ trt[k] ] + thetaS[ study[k] ];
    ybar[k] ~ normal( mu[k], sigmaE/sqrt(N[k]) );
  }
}

fitb = sampling( model, data=data, chains=3,
                 warmup=10000, thin=20,
                 iter=10000+20*20000 )
```

Section 4.3.4: Survival Analysis

The parameterization of the Weibull distribution in Stan differs from that of JAGS. In addition, the manner in which Stan handles right-censored values differs from that of JAGS. See Stan (2018) for details.

```
data{
  int<lower=1> nObs;   // number of uncensored observations
  int<lower=1> nCens;  // number of right-censored
                              observations
  int<lower=1> nTrt;   // number of treatment groups

  int trtObs[nObs];         // treatment group category for
                              uncensored subjects
  real xObs[nObs];       // covariate for uncensored subjects
  real<lower=0> timeObs[nObs];  // observed time for
                                  uncensored subjects

  int trtCens[nCens];    // treatment group category for
                              right-censored subjects
  real xCens[nCens];   // covariate for right-censored
                          subjects
  real<lower=0> timeCens[nCens];  // time var for
                                     right-censored subjects
```

```
   real InterEst[nTrt];      // estimated intercept terms
   real SlopeEst[nTrt];      // estimated slope terms
}
parameters{

   real Inter[nTrt];
   real Slope[nTrt];
   real<lower=0> eta;      // Weibull shape parameter
}
model
{
   real mu[nObs];
   real nu[nCens];

   // Prior distribution
   for ( i in 1:nTrt )
   {
     Inter[i] ~ normal(InterEst[i], 5.);
     Slope[i] ~ normal(SlopeEst[i], 5.);
   }
   eta ~ exponential(0.02);   // Same as rgamma(1, 0.02).
                                  Mean=5, range: 0-45

   // Likelihood for observations
   for ( j in 1:nObs )
   {
     mu[j] = Inter[ trtObs[j] ] + Slope[ trtObs[j]
                                  ]*xObs[j];
     timeObs[j] ~ weibull(eta, exp(mu[j]));
   }
   // Likelihood for right-censored time points
   for ( k in 1:nCens )
   {
     nu[k] = Inter[ trtCens[k] ] + Slope[ trtCens[k]
                                  ]*xCens[k];
     target += weibull_lccdf(timeCens[k] | eta, exp(nu[k]));
   }
}


## Weibull survival model fitted by maximum likelihood
fit0 = survreg( Surv(Time, !Censor)~Trt + Trt:x - 1,
       data = d, dist="weibull" )
```

```
  ## Prepare data for Stan
data = list( nObs=sum(!d$Censor),
        timeObs=d$Time[!d$Censor],
            xObs=d$x[!d$Censor],
            trtObs=as.vector(unclass(d$Trt))[!d$Censor],
            nTrt=nlevels(d$Trt),
            nCens=sum(d$Censor), xCens=d$x[d$Censor],
            trtCens=as.vector(unclass(d$Trt))[d$Censor],
            timeCens=d$Time[d$Censor],
            InterEst=as.vector(summary(fit0)$coef[1:3]),
            SlopeEst=as.vector(summary(fit0)$coef[4:6]) )


fitb = sampling( model, data=data,
            warmup = 10000, iter = 20000*5+10000, thin=5,
                    chains = 3 )
```

Section 5.3.2: CRM Study Design for Phase I Cancer Trials

```
data{

  int<lower=1> nDose;   // number of doses
  int<lower=1> nObs;    // number of observations

  real a0;                  // A constant = -4.5
  real dose[nDose];    // Doses
  int Y[nObs];         // Observed Bernoulli responses
  int<lower=1> index[nObs];     // index for the doses
                                    for each observations
}
parameters{

  real<lower=0> theta;
}
transformed parameters{
  real<lower=0, upper=1> p[nDose];

  for ( i in 1:nDose )
  {
    p[i] = 1./(1. + exp(-( a0+theta*dose[i] )));
  }
}
```

```
model{

  // Prior
  theta ~ exponential(500);

  // Likelihood
  for ( j in 1:nObs )
  {
    Y[j] ~ bernoulli( p[index[j]] );
  }

}

for ( i in 1:30 )
{
    ## Response of ith patient
  Y[i] = rbinom( 1, size=1, prob=p.true[index[i]] )

  data = list(nDose=length(doses), dose=doses, a0=-4.5,
        nObs=i,
              Y=array(Y[1:i], i),
              index=array(index[1:i], i))




  ## Update posterior distribution of p[j]
  ## Note that Stan needed initial values so that chains
     would converge.
  fitb = sampling(stan.compiled, data=data, pars="p",
            init=lapply(1:3, function(j){
            list(theta=rexp(1, 500)) }),
            warmup = 10000, iter = 20000*5+10000,
                    thin=5, chains = 3 )
  print(fitb)
  th.post = as.matrix(fitb)

  ## Get posterior mean of p[j]
  pj[i,] = colMeans(th.post[,1:6])
  if ( i < 30 )
  {
      ## As noted in Chapter 5, the following line may
         be changed to:
      ##                    index[i+1] = max( which( pj[i,]
                    <= p0 ) )
```

```
    index[i+1] = which.min( abs(pj[i,]-p0) )
    x[i+1] = doses[ index[i+1]   ]
  }
}
```

Section 5.5.3: Escalation with Overdose Control

```
data{

  int<lower=1> N;        // number of observations
  int<lower=0> Y[N];     // Bernoulli responses
  real x[N];             // Assigned doses

  real<lower=0, upper=1> theta;      // probability of
                                        DLT when x=MDT
  real xmin;                         // smallest possible
                                        dose
  real xmax;                         // largest possible
                                        dose

}
parameters{
  real<lower=xmin, upper=xmax> lgamma;       // log MDT
  real<lower=0, upper=1> rho0;  // probability of DLT
                                   when x=xmin
}
transformed parameters{
  real beta0;
  real beta1;
  real<lower=0, upper=1> p[N];

 beta0 = (1./(lgamma-xmin))*( lgamma*log(rho0/(1.-rho0)) -
                              xmin*log(theta/(1.-theta)));
  beta1 = (1./lgamma)*( log(theta/(1.-theta)) - beta0 );

  for ( i in 1:N )
  {
    p[i] = 1./(1.+exp(-(beta0+beta1*x[i])));
  }
}
```

```
model{

  // Priors for rho0 and log(gamma)
     // Mean = center of log-scaled (xmin, xmax)
        with SD = 1.,
     //            truncated between xmin and xmax
  lgamma ~ normal(6.1, 1.)T[xmin, xmax];
    // Mean of the distribution is about 0.05 with 95%
       range: 0.01-0.13.
  rho0 ~ beta(3, 50);

  // Likelihood
  for ( i in 1:N )
  {
    Y[i] ~ bernoulli( p[i] );
  }
}



for ( i in 1:30 )
{
    ## Generate data for ith patient with true DLT
       probability
  Y[i] = rbinom( 1, size=1, prob=prob.dlt(x[i]) )

  data = list(N=i, x=array(x[1:i], i), Y=array(Y[1:i], i),
              xmin=log(100), xmax=log(2000), theta=0.3)

  ## Update posterior distribution
  fitb = sampling(stan.compiled, data=data,
            pars=c("rho0", "lgamma", "beta0", "beta1"),
            warmup = 10000, iter = 20000*25+10000,
                    thin=25, chains = 3 )
  th.post = as.matrix( fitb )

    ## Lower 90% credible limit of log-scaled gamma
  if ( i < 30 )
    x[i+1] = quantile(th.post[,"lgamma"], 0.10)
}
```

Section 6.3.2: Historical Placebo Data

In this example, after initially calling Stan with the defaults in *sampling()*, the output indicated that an increase in "adapt_delta" over 0.8 would improve sampling. We increased adapt_delta to 0.9, which raises confidence in the MCMC results, but slows sampling.

```
data{
  int<lower=1> nStudy;

  int<lower=1> N[nStudy];
  real ybar[nStudy];
  real<lower=0> degFree[nStudy];
  real<lower=0> sigSqHat[nStudy];
}
parameters{
  real mu0;
  real<lower=0> sigmaS;
  real<lower=0> sigmaE;

  real mu[nStudy];

}
model
{

  // Priors
  mu0 ~ normal( 0., 1. );              // Placebo mean
  sigmaS ~ cauchy(0., 0.1)T[0.,];      // Study-to-study
                                       //   variability
  sigmaE ~ cauchy(0., 0.1)T[0., ];     // Within-study
                                       //   variability

  // Likelihood
  for ( i in 1:nStudy )
  {
    mu[i] ~ normal( mu0, sigmaS );
    ybar[i] ~ normal( mu[i], sigmaE/sqrt(N[i]));
    sigSqHat[i] ~ gamma( 0.5*degFree[i], 0.5*degFree[i]/
                (sigmaE*sigmaE) );
  }

}
```

```
fitb = sampling( model, data=data, chains=3,
            pars=c("mu0", "sigmaS", "sigmaE"),
            warmup = 10000, iter = 20000*10+10000,
                    thin=10,
            control=list(adapt_delta = 0.9))
```

Section 7.4.2: Go/No-Go for Phase II Trial

As with the JAGS version of this exercise, looping through the Stan code
takes a very long time. Instead of three CPU cores, we again used eight cores
with the R command *options(mc.cores=8)*.

```
data{

    int<lower=1> nDose;        // number of doses
    int<lower=1> nSubject;     // number of subjects
    int<lower=1> N;            // number of observations

    int<lower=1> dose[N];      // categories for dose
    int<lower=1> subject[N];   // categories for subject

    real x[nDose];             // doses
    int<lower=0, upper=1> Y[N];        // Bernoulli responses

}
parameters{
    real E0;
    real Emax;
    real<lower=0> E50;
    real<lower=0> tau;

    real thetaSubj[nSubject];
}
transformed parameters{
    real sigma;
    real mu[nDose];

    sigma = 1/sqrt(tau);

    for ( i in 1:nDose )
    {
```

```
    mu[i] = E0 + Emax*x[i]/(E50+x[i]);
  }

}
model{

  real p[N];

  // Priors
  E0 ~ normal(-2, 0.5);
  Emax ~ normal(2, 0.5);
  E50 ~ normal(200., 50.)T[0., ];
  tau ~ gamma(2, 0.3);

  // Likelihood
  for ( j in 1:nSubject )
  {
    thetaSubj[j] ~ normal( 0., sigma );
  }

  for ( k in 1:N )
  {
    p[k] = 1/(1+exp(-( mu[dose[k]] +
            thetaSubj[subject[k]]))));
    Y[k] ~ bernoulli( p[k] );
  }

}


fitb = sampling( model, data=data, chains=8,
            pars=c("mu", "E0", "Emax", "E50", "sigma"),
            warmup = 5000, iter = 7000*15+5000, thin=15 )
```

Section 8.2.5: Method Validation with Vague Prior

```
data{
  int<lower=1> N;         // number of observations
  int<lower=1> nConc;     // number of concentrations
  int<lower=1> nRun;      // number of runs
  int<lower=1> nAnalyst;  // number of analysts
```

```
   int<lower=1> conc[N];        // category for concentration
   int<lower=1> run[N];          // category for run
   int<lower=1> analyst[N];     // category for analyst

   real y[N];              // responses
   real mu0[nConc];        // hyper parameter value
}
parameters{

   real<lower=0> sigmaA;    // analyst SD
   real<lower=0> sigmaR;    // run SD
   real<lower=0> sigmaE;    // residual SD

   real mu[nConc];     // Mean for each concentration

   real thetaR[nRun];
   real thetaA[nAnalyst];

}
transformed parameters{

   real sigmaTotal;

   sigmaTotal = sqrt( sigmaA^2 + sigmaR^2 + sigmaE^2 );
}
model{

   real Mean[N];

   // Priors
   sigmaA ~ cauchy(0., 0.1)T[0., ]; // half-Cauchy
   sigmaR ~ cauchy(0., 0.1)T[0., ];
   sigmaE ~ cauchy(0., 0.1)T[0., ];

   for ( i in 1:nConc )
   {
      mu[i] ~ normal(mu0[i], 1);     // On the ln scale,
                                      SD=1 is small
   }

   // Likelihood
   for ( j in 1:nRun )
   {
      thetaR[j] ~ normal(0., sigmaR);
   }
```

```
for ( k in 1:nAnalyst )
{
  thetaA[k] ~ normal(0, sigmaA);
}
for ( m in 1:N )
{
  Mean[m] = thetaR[ run[m] ] + thetaA[ analyst[m] ]
            + mu[ conc[m] ];
  y[m] ~ normal( Mean[m], sigmaE );
}
}

fitb = sampling( model, data=data, chains=3,
          pars=c("mu", "sigmaR", "sigmaA", "sigmaE",
            "sigmaTotal") ,
          warmup = 10000, iter = 20000*10+10000,
                thin=10 )
```

Section 8.2.5: Method Validation with Informative Prior

```
data{
  int<lower=1> N;          // number of observations
  int<lower=1> nConc;      // number of concentrations
  int<lower=1> nRun;       // number of runs
  int<lower=1> nAnalyst;   // number of analysts

  int<lower=1> conc[N];    // category for concentration
  int<lower=1> run[N];     // category for run
  int<lower=1> analyst[N]; // category for analyst

  real y[N];          // responses

  // hyper parameters
  real sEst[3];
  real<lower=0> sSD[3];
  real mu0[nConc];

}
parameters{

  real lsigmaA;  // analyst SD
```

```
    real lsigmaR;   // run SD
    real lsigmaE;   // residual SD

    real mu[nConc];    // Mean for each concentration

    real thetaR[nRun];
    real thetaA[nAnalyst];

}
transformed parameters{

    real sigmaA;
    real sigmaR;
    real sigmaE;
    real sigmaTotal;

    sigmaR = exp(lsigmaR);
    sigmaA = exp(lsigmaA);
    sigmaE = exp(lsigmaE);
    sigmaTotal = sqrt( sigmaA^2 + sigmaR^2 + sigmaE^2 );
}
model{

    real Mean[N];
    ## Prior distributions
    lsigmaR ~ normal( sEst[1], sSD[1] );
    lsigmaA ~ normal( sEst[2], sSD[2] );
    lsigmaE ~ normal( sEst[3], sSD[3] );

    for ( i in 1:nConc )
    {
      mu[i] ~ normal(mu0[i], 0.25);   // Based on prior
                                      //       data, higher prec.
    }


    // Likelihood
    for ( j in 1:nRun )
    {
      thetaR[j] ~ normal(0., sigmaR);
    }
    for ( k in 1:nAnalyst )
    {
      thetaA[k] ~ normal(0, sigmaA);
    }
```

```
for ( m in 1:N )
{
    Mean[m] = thetaR[ run[m] ] + thetaA[ analyst[m] ]
            + mu[ conc[m] ];
    y[m] ~ normal( Mean[m], sigmaE );
}
}

data = list( N=nrow(d.val), nRun=nlevels(d.val$Run),
            nAnalyst=nlevels(d.val$Analyst),
            nConc=nlevels(d.val$Conc), run=as.
            vector(unclass(d.val$Run)),
            analyst=as.vector(unclass(d.val$Analyst)),
            conc=as.vector(unclass(d.val$Conc)),
            y=log(d.val$Observed.RP),
            mu0=log(c(67, 82, 100, 122, 150)),
            sEst=c(-3.3, -3.0, -2.9), sSD=c(0.9,
            1.2, 0.2) )


fitb = sampling( stan.compiled, data=data, chains=3,
            pars=c("mu", "sigmaR", "sigmaA", "sigmaE",
                "sigmaTotal") ,
            warmup = 10000, iter = 20000*5+10000, thin=5 )
```

Section 8.3.4: Method Transfer

We made a minor change to the code when translating from JAGS to Stan. Instead of the scaled inverse Wishart distribution for SigmaRun, Stan (2018) advises to set the variance–covariance matrix to $\text{diag}(\tau)\,\Omega\,\text{diag}(\tau)$, where the τ elements are independent half-Cauchy and Ω follows an LKJ distribution. In this manner, Ω is generated as a correlation matrix and the vector τ may be interpreted as the standard deviation values. Currently, the LKJ distribution is unavailable in JAGS. If desired, a scaled inverse Wishart could be constructed in Stan by declaring Omega with type *cov_matrix[2]* and setting the prior Omega ~ inverse_wishart(3, R), where R is a 2×2 identity matrix.

```
data{

    int<lower=1> nRun;      // number of runs
    int<lower=1> N;         // number of observations
```

```
   int<lower=1> run[N];   // category for run
   real x[N];             // covariate
   real y[N];             // responses

   // hyper parameters
   real Est[2];                    // Estimated Mean for
                                   //     intercept and slope
   real<lower=0> sigmaML[2];  // Estimated 5*SD for
                                   //     intercept and slope

}
parameters{

   vector[2] theta;         //    (Intercept, Slope)
   real<lower=0> sigmaErr;
   corr_matrix[2] Omega;    // Correlation matrix for
                                   //     thetaRun
   vector<lower=0>[2] tau;  // Scale vector for thetaRun
   vector[2] thetaRun[nRun];
}
transformed parameters{

   matrix[2,2] SigmaRun;       // Variance-covariance matrix

       // SigmaRun= diag(tau)%*%Omega%*%diag(tau)
   SigmaRun = quad_form_diag(Omega, tau);
}
model{


   real mu[N];

   for ( i in 1:2 )
   {
      tau[i] ~ cauchy(0., 1.)T[0., ];
   }
   Omega ~ lkj_corr(2);


   theta[1] ~ normal( Est[1], sigmaML[1] );  // Population
                                                  //  intercept
   theta[2] ~ normal( Est[2], sigmaML[2] );  // Population
                                                  //  slope
```

```
  sigmaErr ~ cauchy(0., 1.)T[0., ];   // Residual standard
                                            deviation

  // Likelihood terms for Lots
  for ( j in 1:nRun )
  {
    thetaRun[j] ~ multi_normal( theta, SigmaRun );
  }

  // Likelihood terms for samples within lots
  for ( k in 1:N )
  {
    mu[k] = thetaRun[ run[k], 1]
          + thetaRun[ run[k],2 ]*x[k];
    y[k] ~ normal( mu[k], sigmaErr );
  }
## Model fit for Lab A
dA = subset(d, Lab=="A")
fit0 = lmer( y~x+(1+x|Run), data=dA )   ## Get REML
                                            estimates

data = list( N=nrow(dA), nRun=nlevels(dA$Run),
             run=as.vector(unclass(dA$Run)),
             y = dA$y, x=dA$x,
             Est=as.vector(fixef(fit0)),    ## REML Est
             sigmaML=5*sqrt(diag(summary(fit0)$vcov))
                                            ## 5*(REML SE)
                )
fitb.A = sampling( stan.compiled, data=data, chains=3,
             pars=c("theta", "SigmaRun", "sigmaErr"),
             warmup = 10000, iter = 20000*50+10000,
                   thin=50,
             control=list(adapt_delta=0.9) )




## Model fit for Lab B
dB = subset(d, Lab=="B")
fit0 = lmer( y~x+(1+x|Run), data=dB )   ## Get REML
                                            estimates

data = list( N=nrow(dB), nRun=nlevels(dB$Run),
             run=as.vector(unclass(dB$Run)),
             y = dB$y, x=dB$x,
```

```
        Est=as.vector(fixef(fit0)),    ## REML Est
        sigmaML=5*sqrt(diag(summary(fit0)$vcov))
                                        ## 5*(REML SE)
           )


fitb.B = sampling( stan.compiled, data=data, chains=3,
            pars=c("theta", "SigmaRun", "sigmaErr"),
            warmup = 10000, iter = 20000*50+10000,
                    thin=50,
            control=list(adapt_delta=0.9) )
```

Section 9.3.4: Oncogenic Risk

In this example, the integer value of $M = 2.41 \times 10^9$ posed a problem to Stan.
Either M is too large of an integer for Stan or the product $k*(M-1)$ was too
large in the line

```
Nmk ~ binomial(k*(M-1),p);
```

As a workaround, we imported all three of k, *Nmk*, M as real numbers
and wrote out the log binomial distribution formula using the log-gamma
function.

```
data{
  int<lower=1> nObs;
  real x[nObs];
  real y[nObs];

    // All three of k, M, and Nmk should be imported as
       integers;
    //   however, because M, as an integer, is too big
         for Stan,
    //   M is imported as real.  We imported all three
         are real and then
    //   wrote out the log binomial distribution in long
         form.
  real<lower=0> k;
  real<lower=0> Nmk;  // Nmk is a large integer.
  real<lower=0> M;    // M is actually an integer, but
                         is too big for Stan

}
```

```
parameters{
  real<lower=0> tau;
  real Om;

  real<lower=0> tau1;
  real U;

  real<lower=0, upper=1> p;
}
transformed parameters{
  real sigma;
  real sigma1;

  sigma = 1/sqrt(tau);
  sigma1 = 1/sqrt(tau1);
}
model{

  // Priors
  tau ~ gamma(0.001, 0.001);
  Om ~ normal(0., sqrt(2)*sigma);

  tau1 ~ gamma(0.001, 0.001);
  U ~ normal(0., sqrt(2)*sigma1);

  p ~ beta(0.5, 0.5);

  // Likelihood
  // This Nmk~binomial() line caused an error due to the
     size of the integer
  // Nmk ~ binomial( k*(M-1), p );
       // We wrote out the log binomial distribution
          the long way.
  target += lgamma( k*(M-1) + 1 ) - lgamma(Nmk+1) -
             lgamma( k*(M-1) -
             Nmk + 1) + Nmk*log(p) +
(k*(M-1)-Nmk)*log(1.-p);

  for ( i in 1:nObs )
  {
    x[i] ~ normal( Om, sigma );
    y[i] ~ normal( U, sigma1 );
  }

}
```

```
fitb = sampling( model, data=data, pars=c("Om", "sigma",
       "U", "sigma1", "p"),
           warmup = 10000, iter = 10000*5+10000,
                      thin=5, chains = 3 )
```

Section 9.4.4: Liquid Chromatography

As with the "method transfer" example in Section 8.3.4, we made a minor change to the code when translating from JAGS to Stan. Instead of the scaled inverse Wishart distribution for sigma, we set the variance–covariance matrix to $\mathrm{diag}(\tau)\,\Omega\,\mathrm{diag}(\tau)$, where the τ elements are independent half-Cauchy and Ω follows an LKJ distribution. If desired, a scaled inverse Wishart could be constructed in Stan by declaring omega with type *cov_matrix[4]* and setting the prior omega ~ inverse_wishart(5, R), where R is a 4×4 identity matrix.

```
data{
   int<lower=1> N;     // number of observations
   int<lower=1> p;     // number of parameters (per model)
   vector[p] X[N];     // Design matrix
   vector[4] Y[N];     // responses
}
parameters{

   corr_matrix[4] Omega;    // Correlation matrix
   vector<lower=0>[4] tau;  // Scale vector for variance
matrix

   vector[p] theta1;
   vector[p] theta2;
   vector[p] theta3;
   vector[p] theta4;
}
transformed parameters{

   matrix[4,4] Sigma;
```

```
      // Sigma = diag(tau)%*%Omega%*%diag(tau)
  Sigma = quad_form_diag(Omega, tau);
}
model{

  vector[4] mu[N];

  // Priors
  for ( i in 1:4 )
  {
     tau[i] ~ cauchy(0., 1.)T[0., ];
  }
  Omega ~ lkj_corr(2);    // Correlation matrix

  // Prior for theta
  for ( j in 1:p )
  {
    theta1[j] ~ normal( 0., 30. );
    theta2[j] ~ normal( 0., 30. );
    theta3[j] ~ normal( 0., 30. );
    theta4[j] ~ normal( 0., 30. );
  }

  // Likelihood
  for ( k in 1:N )
  {
    mu[k,1] = dot_product(X[k], theta1);    // Linear model
                                                     mean
    mu[k,2] = dot_product(X[k], theta2);
    mu[k,3] = dot_product(X[k], theta3);
    mu[k,4] = dot_product(X[k], theta4);
    Y[k] ~  multi_normal( mu[k], Sigma );
  }
}
}


fitb = sampling( model, data=data, chains=3,
            pars=c("theta1", "theta2", "theta3",
                "theta4", "Sigma"),
            warmup = 10000, iter = 20000*10+10000,
                    thin=10)
```

Section 10.4.2: Stability Data Analysis

As with the "method transfer" example in Section 8.3.4, we made a minor change to the code when translating from JAGS to Stan. Instead of the scaled inverse Wishart distribution for SigmaLot, we set the variance–covariance matrix to $\text{diag}(\tau)\,\Omega\,\text{diag}(\tau)$, where the τ elements are independent half-Cauchy and Ω follows an LKJ distribution. If desired, a scaled inverse Wishart could be constructed in Stan by declaring omega with type *cov_matrix[2]* and setting the prior omega ~ inverse_wishart(3, *R*), where *R* is a 2 × 2 identity matrix.

```
data{

    int<lower=1> nLot;       // number of lots
    int<lower=1> N;          // number of observations

    int<lower=1> lot[N];
    real Time[N];
    real y[N];

    real Est[2];             // Estimated Mean for
                             //     intercept and slope
    real<lower=0> sigmaML[2];  // Estimated SD for
                             //     intercept and slope

}
parameters{

    vector[2] theta;         //     (Intercept, Slope)
    real<lower=0> sigmaErr;
    corr_matrix[2] Omega;    // Correlation matrix for
                             //     thetaLot
    vector<lower=0>[2] tau;  // Scale vector for
                             //     thetaLot
    vector[2] thetaLot[nLot];
}
transformed parameters{

    matrix[2,2] SigmaLot;    // Lot variance-covariance
                             //     matrix

        // SigmaLot = diag(tau)%*%Omega%*%diag(tau)
    SigmaLot = quad_form_diag(Omega, tau);
}
```

```
model{

  real mu[N];

  for ( i in 1:2 )
  {
    tau[i] ~ cauchy(0., 1.)T[0., ];
  }
  Omega ~ lkj_corr(2);


  theta[1] ~ normal( Est[1], sigmaML[1] );   // Population
                                                  intercept
  theta[2] ~ normal( Est[2], sigmaML[2] );   // Population
                                                  slope

  sigmaErr ~ cauchy(0., 0.1)T[0., ]; // Residual standard
                                            deviation

  // Likelihood terms for Lots
  for ( j in 1:nLot )
  {
    thetaLot[j] ~ multi_normal( theta, SigmaLot );
  }

  // Likelihood terms for samples within lots
  for ( k in 1:N )
  {
    mu[k] = thetaLot[ lot[k], 1] + thetaLot[ lot[k],2
                                    ]*Time[k];
    y[k] ~ normal( mu[k], sigmaErr );
  }
}


data = list( N=nrow(d1), nLot=nlevels(d1$Lot),
             lot=as.vector(unclass(d1$Lot)),
             y = d1$Potency, Time=d1$Week,
             Est=as.vector(fixef(fit0)),   ## MLE Est
             sigmaML=5*sqrt(diag(summary(fit0)$vcov))
                    ## 5 x (MLE SE)
             )
```

```
fitb = sampling(model, data=data, chains=3,
          pars=c("theta", "SigmaLot", "sigmaErr"),
          warmup = 10000, iter = 20000*10+10000,
                    thin=10)
```

Section 11.2.3: Control Chart for Inhaled Product Data

```
data{
  int<lower = 1> N; // number of observations
  real xLower[N];
  real xUpper[N];
}
parameters{
  real mu;
  real<lower=0> sigma;
}
model{

  // priors
  mu ~ normal( 100., 10. );
  sigma ~ cauchy(0., 1.)T[0.,];

  // likelihood.  Truncated normal for interval-censored
data
  for ( i in 1:N )
  {
      // numerator term of truncated normal for interval-
         censored data
    target += log_diff_exp(normal_lcdf(xUpper[i]
             | mu, sigma),
                          normal_lcdf(xLower[i] | mu,
                          sigma));

      // denominator term
    target += -log_diff_exp(normal_lcdf(110 | mu, sigma),
                          normal_lcdf(90 | mu, sigma));

  }

}
```

```
data = list(N=length(x), xLower=pmax(90, x-0.5),
        xUpper=pmin(110, x+0.5))

## Initial values were useful in setting the MCMC chains
   in the right zone.
inits = lapply(1:3, function(i){
            list( mu=rnorm(1, mean=100, sd=1),
                  sigma=sd(x)*sqrt( rchisq(1, 24)/24)) })

fitb = sampling( model, data=data, chains=3, init=inits,
            warmup = 10000, iter = 20000*10+10000,
                    thin=10 )
```

Section 11.2.3: Control Chart for Bioburden Data

```
data{
  int<lower=1> N;          // Number of observations
  int<lower=0> y[N];       // Integer responses

  // hyperparameters
  real mu0;
  real phi0;
}
parameters{
  real mu;     // Mean
  real r;      // Gamma-distribution shape
}
transformed parameters{

  real beta;
  beta = r/mu;
}
model{

  // priors
  mu ~ lognormal( mu0, 1. );
  r ~ lognormal( phi0, 1. );

  // likelihood
  for ( i in 1:N )
```

```
    {
      y[i] ~ neg_binomial(r, beta);
    }
}


fitb = sampling( model, data=data, chains=3,
        pars=c("r", "mu"),
            warmup = 10000, iter = 10000*5+10000, thin=5 )
```

Section 11.3.2: Twenty-five Analytical Test Samples

```
data{
  int<lower=1> N;       // number of observations
  real xbar;            // sample mean
  real<lower=0> sSq;    // sample variance
}
parameters{
  real mu;
  real lsigma;
}
transformed parameters{
  real sigmaSq;

  sigma = exp(2*lsigma);
}
model{
  // Priors
  mu ~ student_t(4, 100., 1.5);
  lsigma ~ normal( 1.609, 0.6 );


  // Likelihood
  xbar ~ normal(mu, sqrt(sigmaSq/N));
  sSq ~ gamma( 0.5*(N-1), 0.5*(N-1)/sigmaSq );
}


fitb = sampling( model, data=data, chains=3,
        pars=c("mu", "sigmaSq"),
            warmup = 20000, iter = 10000*5+20000, thin=5 )
```

Section 11.4.5: Twenty AEs

Unlike JAGS, Stan can indirectly accommodate the ZIP model using the "target +=" paradigm for the likelihood.

```
data{
  int<lower=0> N;        // Number of observations
  int<lower=0> x[N];     // Number of AEs
}
parameters {
real<lower=0, upper=1> p;    // Probability that x = 0
real<lower=0> lambda;        // Poisson parameter
}
model {

  // Priors
  p ~ beta(10, 3);        // Skewed to the left. 99% of
                          // values are > 0.45.
  lambda ~ gamma(5, 1);   // Mean = variance = 5

  // Likelihood
  for (i in 1:N)
  {
    if ( x[i] == 0)   // If X==0, X comes from the
                      // mixture distribution.
      target += log_sum_exp( bernoulli_lpmf(1 | p),
                    bernoulli_lpmf(0 | p) + poisson_
                    lpmf(x[i] | lambda));
    else   // If X > 0, X comes from the Poisson
           // distribution
      target += bernoulli_lpmf(0 | p)+
              poisson_lpmf(x[i] | lambda);
  }
}


fitb = sampling( model, data=data, chains=3,
        pars=c("lambda", "p"),
            warmup = 10000, iter = 10000*5+10000, thin=5 )

th.post = as.matrix(fitb)
```

```
## Get posterior predictive distribution of ZIP data
w.tilde = rbinom(nrow(th.post), size=1, prob=th.post[,"p"])
x.tilde = ifelse( w.tilde==1, 0, rpois(nrow(th.post),
lambda=th.post[,"lambda"]) )

## Estimate p(x0=5)
mean(x.tilde >= 5)
```

References

Allen, P.V., Dukes, G.R., and Gerger, M.E. (1991). Determination of release limits: A general methodology. *Pharmacological Research*, 9(9), 1210–1213.

AMC (2003). The J-chart: a simple plot that combines the capabilities of Shewhart and cusum charts for use in analytical quality control. AMC Technical Brief. http://www.rsc.org/images/shewhart-cusum-charts-technical-briefs-12_tcm18-214864.pdf. Accessed on May 17, 2019.

Aquilina, T., Medelson, E., Yang, H., Cho, I., and Ynen, S. (2006). A multitiered risk-based approach to investigate for product quality defects. Poster presented at 2006 International Epidemiology and Pharmacovigilance Conference, Lisbon, Portugal.

Babb, J., Rogatko, A., and Zacks, S. (1998). Cancer phase I clinical trials: Efficient dose escalation with overdose control. *Statistics in Medicine*, 17, 1103–1120.

Barron, A.M. (1994). Use of fractional factorial (or matrix) designs in stability analysis. In: *Proceedings of Biopharmaceutical Section of American Statistical Association ASA*, Alexandria, VA.

Berenbaum, M.C. (1989). What is synergy? *Pharmacological Reviews*, 41, 93–141.

Berry, D.A., and Stangl, D.K. (1996a). Bayesian methods in health-related research. In: *Bayesian Biostatistics*, edited by Berry, D.A., and Stangl, D.K. CRC Press, Boca Raton, FL.

Berry, D.A., and Stangl, D.K. (1996b). *Bayesian Biostatistics*. CRC Press, Boca Raton, FL.

Berry, S.M., Carlin, B.P., Lee, J.J., and Muller, P. (2011). *Bayesian Adaptive Methods for Clinical Trials*. CRC Press, Boca Raton, FL.

Bissell, A.F. (1990). How reliable is your capability index? *Applied Statistics*, 39(3), 331–340.

Bliss, C.I. (1939). The toxicity of poisons applied jointly. *Annals of Applied Biology*, 26, 585–615.

Borman, P., Nethercote, P., Chaftield, M., Thompson, D., and Truman, K. (2007). The application of quality by design to analytical methods. *Pharmaceutical Technology*, 31(10), 142–152.

Boulanger, B., Chiap, P., Dewe, W. et al. (2003). An analysis of the SFSTP guide on validation of chromatographic bioanalytical methods: progresses and limitations. *Journal of Pharmaceutical and Biomedical Analysis*, 32, 753–765.

Boulanger, B., Devanaryan, V., Dewe, W., and Smith, W. (2007). Statistical considerations in analytical method validation. In *Pharmaceutical Statistics Using SAS: A Practical Guide*, edited by Dmitrienko, A., Chuang-Stein, C., and D'Agostino, R. SAS Publishing, Cary, NC.

Boulanger, B., Dewe, W., Gibert, A., Govaerts, B., and Maumy-Bertrand, M. (2007). Risk management for analytical methods based on the total error concept: concilating the objectives of the pre-study and in-study validation phases. *Chemometrics and Intelligent Laboratory Systems*, 86, 198–207.

Bretz, F., Pinheiro, J.C., and Branson, M. (2005). Combining multiple comparisons and modeling techniques in dose-response studies. *Biometrics*, 61, 738–748.

Brutti, P., and De Santis, F. (2008). Avoiding the range of equivalence in clinical trials: Robust Bayesian sample size determination for credible intervals. *Journal of Statistical Planning and Inference*, 138, 1577–1591.

Brutti, P., De Santis, F., and Gubbiotti, S. (2008). Robust Bayesian sample size determination in clinical trials. *Statistics in Medicine*, 27, 2290–2306.

Bryant, J., and Day, R. (1995). Incorporating toxicity considerations into the design of two-stage phase II clinical trials. *Biometrics*, 51(4), 1372–1383.

Bryder, M., Etling, H., Fleming, J., Hu, Y., and Levy, P. (2005). Topic 1—stage 2 process validation: determining and justifying the number of process qualification batches. ISPE discussion paper: PV stage 2, number of batches (version 2). https://www.pharmamedtechbi.com/~/media/Supporting%20Documents/The%20Gold%20Sheet/47/2/stage2processvalidation1.pdf.

Bunnage, M.E. (2011). Getting pharmaceutical R&D back on target. *Nature Chemical Biology*, 7, 335–339.

Burdick, R., LeBlond, D., Sandell, D., and Yang, H. (2013a). Acceptance criteria for method validation of accuracy and precision. *Pharmacopeial Forum*, May–June Issue, 39(3).

Burdick, R.K., LeBlond, D., Sandell, D., and Yang, H. (2013b). Statistical methods for validation of procedure accuracy and precision. *Pharmacopeial Forum*, 39(3).

Burdick, R.K., LeBlond, D.J., Pfahler, L.B., Quiroz, J., Sidor, L., Vukovinsky, K., and Zhang, L. (2017). *Statistical Applications for Chemistry, Manufacturing and Controls (CMC) in the Pharmaceutical Industry*. Springer, Cham, Switzerland.

Cai, C., Liu, S., and Yuan, Y. (2014). A Bayesian design for phase II clinical trials with delayed responses based on multiple imputation. *Statistics in Medicine*, 33(23), 4017–4028.

Capen, C., Christopher, D., Forenzo, P., Ireland, C., Liu, O., Lyapustina, S., O'Neill, J., Patterson, N., Quinlan, M., Sandell, D., Schwenke, J., Stroup, W., and Tougas, T. (2012). On the shelf life of pharmaceutical products. *AAPS PharmSciTech*, 13(3), 911–918.

Carpenter, B., Gelman, A., Hoffman, M.D., Lee, D., Goodrich, B., Betancourt, M., Brubaker, M., Guo, J., Li, P., and Riddell, A. (2017). Stan: A probabilistic programming language. *Journal of Statistical Software*, 76(1), 1–32.

Carstensen, J.T., and Nelson, E. (1976). Terminology regarding labeled and contained amounts in dosage forms. *Journal of Pharmaceutical Sciences*, 65(2), 311–312.

Casella, G., and George, E.I. (1992). Explaining the Gibbs sampler. *The American Statistician*, 46(3), 167–174.

Chang, M. (2008). *Adaptive Decision Theory and Implementation Using ASA and R.* Chapman & Hall/CRC Press, Boca Raton, FL.

Chevret, S. (1993). The continual reassessment method in cancer phase I clinical trials: A simulation study. *Statistics in Medicine*, 12, 1093–1108.

Chevret, S. (2006). *Statistical Methods for Dose-Finding Experiments*. Wiley, Chichester, UK.

Chow, S.C. (2007). *Statistical Design and Analysis of Stability Studies*. Chapman & Hall/CRC, Boca Raton, FL.

Chow, S.-C., and Chang, M. (2007). *Adaptive Design Methods in Clinical Trials*. Hall/CRC Press, Boca Raton, FL.

Chow, S.-C., and Liu, J.-P. (1998). *Design and Analysis of Animal Studies in Pharmaceutical Development*. 1st ed. CRC Press, Boca Raton, FL.

Chuang-Stein, C. (1993). An application of the beta-binomial model to combine and monitor medical event rates in clinical trials. *Drug Information Journal*, 27, 515–523.

Chuang-Stein, C., McDermott, S., Meyerson, L., and Hoffman, J. (1998). Report of the adverse event working group: Analysis and presentation. Unpublished report.

Clopper, C., and Pearson, E. S. (1934). The use of confidence or fiducial limits illustrated in the case of the binomial. *Biometrika*. 26, 404–413.

CMC Biotech Working Group (2009). *A-Mab: A Case Study in Bioprocess Development*. www.casss.org/associations/9165/.../A-Mab_Case_Study_Version_2-1.pdf. Accessed on January 9, 2019.

CMC Vaccine Working Group (2012). *A-VAX: Applying Quality by Design to Vaccines*. www.ispe.org. Accessed on April 15, 2016.

Colosimo, B.M., and del Castillo, E. (2007). *Bayesian Process Monitoring, Control and Optimization*. Chapman & Hall/CRC, Boca Raton, FL.

Delaney, M. (2006). History of HAART – The true story of how effective multi-drug therapy was developed for treatment of HIV disease. *Retrovirology*, 3(Suppl 1), S6. . International Meeting of The Institute of Human Virology, Baltimore, MD, 17–21 November 2006.

DeMets, D.L., and Lan, K.K.G. (1994). Interim analysis – The alpha spending function approach. *Statistics in Medicine*, 13, 1341–1352.

Denwood, M.J. (2016). Runjags: An R package providing interface utilities, model templates, parallel computing methods, and additional distributions for MCMC models in JAGS. *Journal of Statistical Software*, 71(9), 1–25.

Derringer, G., and Suich, R. (1980). Simultaneous optimization of several response variables. *Journal of Quality Technology*, 12, 214–219.

De Santis, F. (2006). Sample size determination for robust Bayesian analysis. *Journal of the American Statistical Association*, 101(473), 278–291.

De Santis, F. (2007). Using historical data for Bayesian sample size determination. *Journal of the Royal Statistical Society, Series A*, 170(1), 95–113.

DeSilva, B., Smith, W., Weiner, R. et al. (2003). Recommendations for the bioanalytical method validation of ligand-binding assays to support pharmacokinetic assessments of macromolecules. *Pharmaceutical Research*, 20, 1885–1900.

DeWoody, K., and Raghavarao, D. (1997). Some optimal matrix designs in stability studies. *Journal of Biopharmaceutical Statistics*, 7, 205–213.

Dortant, P.M., Claassen, I.J.T.M., van Kreyl, C.F., van Steenis, G., and Wester, P.W. (1997). Risk assessment on the carcinogenic potential of hybridoma cell DNA: Implications for residual contaminating cellular DNA in biological products. *Biologicals*, 25, 381–390.

EMA (1995). ICH Topic Q 2 (R1) Validation of Analytical Procedures: Text and Methodology. http://www.ema.europa.eu/docs/en_GB/document_library/Sc ientific_guideline/2009/09/WC500002662.pdf. Accessed on May 18, 2019.

EMA (2007). Guideline on clinical trials in small populations. https://www.ema. europa.eu/documents/scientific-guideline/guideline-clinical-trials-small-populations_en.pdf. Accessed on December 25, 2018.

EMA (2014). Guideline on similar biological medicinal products containing biotechnology-derived proteins as active substance: non-clinical and clinical issues. http://www.ema.europa.eu/docs/en_GB/document_library/Scientific_guidel ine/2015/01/WC500180219.pdf. Accessed on May 18, 2019.

EMA (2017). Reflection paper on statistical methodology for the 5 comparative assessment of quality attributes in drug development. http://www.ema.europa.eu/docs/en_GB/document_library/Scientific_guideline/2017/03/WC500224995.pdf. Accessed on May 18, 2019.

Ermer, J. and Nethercote, P. (2015). *Method Validation in Pharmaceutical Analysis*. Wiley-VCH, Weinheim, Germany.

Etzioni, R. and Kadance, J.B. (1995). Bayesian statistical methods in public health and medicine. *Annual Review of Public Health*, 16, 23–41.

FDA (1987a). *FDA guideline on General Principles of Process Validation*. https://variation.com/wp-content/uploads/guidance/FDA-Process-Validation-Guidance-1987.pdf. Accessed on May 3, 2019.

FDA (1987b). *Guideline for Submitting Documentation for the Stability of Human Drugs and Biologics*. Center for Drugs and Biologics, Office of Drug Research and Review. Food and Drug Administration, Rockville, MD. https://www.fda.gov/drugs/guidancecomplianceregulatoryinformation/guidances/ucm149499.htm. Accessed on January 6, 2019.

FDA (1995). Current good manufacturing practice in manufacturing, processing, packing, or holding of drug: Amendment of certain requirements for finished pharmaceuticals. *Federal Registry*, 60(13), 4087–4091.

FDA (1998). Guidance for industry: E9 statistical principles for clinical trials. https://www.fda.gov/downloads/drugs/guidancecomplianceregulatoryinformation/guidances/ucm073137.pdf. Accessed on January 29, 2018.

FDA (1999). Guidance for Industry: Providing Regulatory Submissions to the Center for Biologics Evaluation and Research (CBER) in Electronic Format – Biologics Marketing Applications [Biologics License Application (BLA), Product License Application (PLA)/Establishment License Application (ELA) and New Drug Applications (NDA)]. https://www.fda.gov/downloads/BiologicsBloodVaccines/GuidanceComplianceRegulatoryInformation/Guidances/General/UCM192413.pdf. Accessed on January 1, 2019.

FDA (2001). *Guidance for Industry: Statistical Approaches to Establishing Bioequivalence*. https://www.fda.gov/media/70958/download. Accessed on May 3, 2019.

FDA (2004a). *Pharmaceutical cGMPs for the 21st Century: A Risk-Based Approach: Final Report*. https://www.fda.gov/media/77391/download. Accessed on May 3, 2019.

FDA (2004b). *Guidance for Industry: PAT – A Framework for Innovative Pharmaceutical Development, Manufacturing and Quality Assurance*. http://snowdonpharma.com/wp-content/uploads/2014/08/UCM070305.pdf. Accessed on May 3, 2019.

FDA (2004c). *FDA Guidance for Industry: Sterile Drug Products Produced by Aseptic Processing – Current Good Manufacturing Practice*. file:///C:/Users/kvcg781/Downloads/fda_cgmp_pharma%20(3).pdf. Accessed on May 3, 2019.

FDA (2006). Guidance for Industry: Investigating Out-of-Specification (OOS) Test Results for Pharmaceutical Production. https://www.gmp-compliance.org/guidelines/gmp-guideline/fda-guidance-for-industry-investigating-out-of-specification-oos-results-for-pharmaceutical-production. Accessed on May 18, 2019.

FDA (2007). *Guidance for Industry: Good Laboratory Practices: Questions and Answers*. https://www.fda.gov/downloads/iceci/enforcementactions/bioresearchmonitoring/ucm133748.pdf, assessed on 1 January 2019.

FDA (2010a). *The Use of Bayesian Statistics in Medical Device Clinical Trials: Guidance for Industry and Food and Drug Administration Staff*. https://www.fda.gov/media/71512/download. Accessed on May 3, 2019.

FDA (2010b). *Guidance for Industry: Characterization and Qualification of Cell Substrates and Other Biological Materials Used in the Production of Viral Vaccines for Infectious Disease Indications.* https://www.fda.gov/downloads/biologicsbloodvaccines/guidancecomplianceregulatoryinformation/guidances/vaccines/ucm202439.pdf. Accessed on January 10, 2019.

FDA (2011a). *Guidance for Industry on Process Validation: General Principles and Practices.* https://www.fda.gov/downloads/drugs/guidances/ucm070336.pdf. Accessed on January 10, 2019.

FDA (2011b). *Guidance for Industry: Clinical Considerations for Therapeutic Cancer Vaccines.* https://www.fda.gov/downloads/biologicsbloodvaccines/guidancecomplianceregulatoryinformation/guidances/vaccines/ucm278673.pdf. Accessed on December 25, 2018.

FDA (2012). *Kefauver-Harris Amendments Revolutionized Drug Development.* https://www.fda.gov/ForConsumers/ConsumerUpdates/ucm322856.htm. Accessed on January 1, 2019.

FDA (2015). *Guidance for Industry: Analytical Procedures and Methods Validation for Drugs and Biologics.* http://www.fda.gov/downloads/drugs/guidancecomplianceregulatoryinformation/guidances/ucm386366.pdf. Accessed on January 1, 2019.

FDA (2015). Guidance for industry: Scientific considerations in demonstrating biosimilarity to a reference product. Silver Spring, MD: The United States Food and Drug Administration. https://www.fda.gov/downloads/drugs/guidances/ucm291128.pdf. Accessed on May 18, 2019.

FDA (2016a). *ISO 17025 ORA Laboratory Procedures Volume II – Assuring the Quality of Test Results ORA-LAB.5.9.* http://www.fda.gov/ScienceResearch/FieldScience/LaboratoryManual/ucm171889.htm. Accessed on January 17, 2019.

FDA (2016b). *Adaptive designs for medical device clinical studies: Guidance for Industry and Food and Drug Administration Staff.* https://www.fda.gov/media/92671/download. Accessed on May 3, 2019.

FDA (2016c). *Leveraging existing clinical data for extrapolation to pediatric uses of medical devices: Guidance for Industry and Food and Drug Administration staff.* http://www.fda.gov/downloads/MedicalDevices/DeviceRegulationand Guidance/GuidanceDocuments/UCM444591. Accessed on January 29, 2018.

FDA (2017). *Draft Guidance to industry: Statistical approach to evaluate analytical similarity.* https://www.fda.gov/downloads/Drugs/GuidanceCompliance RegulatoryInformation/Guidances/UCM576786.pdf. (Link is no longer available).

Fieller, E. C. (1944). A fundamental formula in the statistics of biological assay and some applications. *Journal of Pharmacy and Pharmacoloy,* 17, 117–123.

Findlay, J. W. A., Smith, W. C., Lee, J. W. et al. (2000). Validation of immunoassays for bioanalysis: a pharmaceutical industry perspective. *Journal of Pharmaceutical and Biomedical Analysis,* 21, 1249–1273.

Flaherty, K.T., Puzanov, I., Kim, K.B., Ribas, A., McArthur, G.A., Sosman, J.A., O'Dwyer, P.J., Lee, R.J., Grippo, J.F., Nolop, K., and Chapman, P.B. (2010). Inhibition of mutated, activated BRAF in metastatic melanoma. *The New England Journal of Medicine,* 363(9), 809–819.

Fleming, T.R. (1982). One-sample multiple testing procedure for phase II clinical trials. *Biometrics,* 38(1), 143–151.

Gehan, E.A. (1961). The determination of the number of patients required in a preliminary and a follow-up trial of a new chemotherapeutic agent. *Journal of Chronic Diseases*, 13, 346–353.

(comment on article by Browne and Draper). *Bayesian Analysis*, 1(3), 515–534.

Gelman, A. (2008). Objections to Bayesian statistics. *Bayesian Analysis*, 3(3), 445–449.

Gelman, A., Carlin, J., Stern, H., Dunson, D., Vetari, A., and Rubin, D. (2013). *Bayesian Data Analysis*. 3rd ed. CRC Press, Boca Raton, FL.

Gelman, A., and Hill, J. (2007). *Data Analysis Using Regression and Multilevel Hierarchical Models*. Cambridge University Press, New York.

Ghosh, S.K., Mukhopadhyay, P., and Lu, J.-C.J. (2006). Bayesian analysis of zero-inflated regression models. *Journal of Statistical Planning and Inference*, 136(4), 1360–1375.

Goldman, B., LeBlanc, M., and Crowley, J. (2008). Interim futility analysis with intermediate endpoints. *Clinical Trials*, 5(1):14–22.

Goodman, S., Zahurak, M.L., and Piantadosi, S. (1995). Some practical improvements in the continual reassessment method for phase I studies. *Statistics in Medicine*, 14, 1149–1161.

Govaerts, B., Dewe, W., Maumy, M. and Boulanger, B. (2008). Pre-study analytical method validation: comparison of four alternative approaches based on quality-level estimation and tolerance intervals. *Quality and Reliability Engineering International*, 24, 557–680.

Greco, W., Unkelbach, H.-D., Pöch, G., Sühnel, J., Kundi, M., and Bödeker, W. (1992). Consensus on concepts and terminology for combined-action assessment: The Saariselkä agreement. *Archives of Complex Environmental Studies*, 4, 65–69.

Greco, W.R., Bravo, G., and Parsons, J.C. (1995). The search for synergy: A critical review from a response surface perspective. *Pharmacological Reviews*, 47, 331–385.

Green, S., Benedetti, J., and Crowley, J. (2002). *Clinical Trials in Oncology*. 2nd ed. Chapman & Hall/CRC Press, Boca Raton, FL.

Green, S.J., and Dahlberg, S. (1992). Planned versus attained design in phase II clinical trials. *Statistics in Medicine*, 11, 853–862.

Hahn, G.J. and Meeker, W.Q. (1991). *Statistical Interval: A Guide for Practitioners*. Wiley, Hoboken, NJ.

Harrington, E.C., Jr (1965). The desirability function. *Industrial Quality Controlled*, 21, 494–498.

Hather, G., Liu, R., Bandi, S., Mettetal, J., Manfredi, M., Shyu, W.C., Donelan, J., and Chakravarty, A. (2014). Growth rate analysis and efficient experimental design for tumor xenograft studies. *Cancer Informatics*, 13(Suppl 4), 65–72.

He, W., Liu, J., Binkowitz, B., and Quan, H. (2006). A model-based approach in the estimation of the maximum tolerated dose in phase I cancer clinical trials. *Statistics in Medicine*, 25(12), 2027–2042.

Heitjan, D.F. (1997). Bayesian interim analysis of phase II cancer clinical trials. *Statistics in Medicine*, 16, 1791–1802.

Heyd, J.M., and Carlin, B.P. (1999). Adaptive design improvements in continual reassessment method for phase I studies. *Statistics in Medicine*, 18(11), 1307–1321.

Hobbs, B.P., and Carlin, B.P. (2008). Practical Bayesian design and analysis for drug and device clinical trials. *Journal of Biopharmaceutical Statistics*, 18(1), 54–80.

Hofer, J. (2009). Discussion. *Journal of Quality Technology*, 41(2), 137–139.

Hoffman, D. (2004). Negative binomial control limits for count data with extra-Poisson variation. *Pharmaceutical Statistics*, 2, 127–132.

Hoffman, D. and Kringle, R. (2007). A total error approach for the validation of quantitative analytical methods. *Pharmaceutical Research*, 24, 1157–1164.

Hubert, Ph., Nguyen-Huu, J. J., Boulanger, B., et al. (2004). Harmonization of strategies for the validation of quantitative analytical procedures: a SFSTP proposal—part I. *Journal of Pharmaceutical and Biomedical Analysis*, 36, 579–586.

Hubert, Ph., Nguyen-Huu, J. J., Boulanger B., et al. (2007a). Harmonization of strategies for the validation of quantitative analytical procedures: a SFSTP proposal—part II. *Journal of Pharmaceutical and Biomedical Analysis*, 45, 70–81.

Hubert, Ph., Nguyen-Huu, J. J., Boulanger B., et al. (2007b). Harmonization of strategies for the validation of quantitative analytical procedures: a SFSTP proposal—part III. *Journal of Pharmaceutical and Biomedical Analysis*, 45, 82–96.

Hung, H.M.J. (1993). Two stage tests for studying monotherapy and combination therapy in two by two factorial trials. *Statistics in Medicine*, 12, 645–660.

ICH (1993). Q1A Stability Testing of New Drug Substances and Products. http://www.pharma.gally.ch/ich/q1a038095en.pdf. Accessed on January 6, 2019.

ICH (1995). Q2A Validation of Analytical Methods: Definitions and Terminlology. http://www.pharma.gally.ch/ich/q2a038195en.pdf. Accessed on May 18, 2019.

ICH (1995b). Q5C Quality of Biotechnological Products: Stability Testing of Biotechnological/Biological Products. https://www.ich.org/fileadmin/Public_Web_Site/ICH_Products/Guidelines/Quality/Q5C/Step4/Q5C_Guideline.pdf. Accessed on January 6, 2019.

ICH (2002). Q1D Bracketing & Matrixing Designs for Stability Testing of New Drug Substances and Drug Products. https://www.ema.europa.eu/en/documents/scientific-guideline/ich-q-1-d-bracketing-matrixing-designs-stability-testing-drug-substances-drug-products-step-5_en.pdf. Accessed on May 3, 2019.

ICH (2003a). Q1A (R2) Stability Testing of New Drug Substances and Products. https://www.ich.org/fileadmin/Public_Web_Site/ICH_Products/Guidelines/Quality/Q1A_R2/Step4/Q1A_R2_Guideline.pdf. Accessed on January 6, 2019.

ICH (2003b). Q1E Evaluation of Stability Data. https://www.ich.org/fileadmin/Public_Web_Site/ICH_Products/Guidelines/Quality/Q1E/Step4/Q1E_Guideline.pdf. Accessed on January 6, 2019.

ICH (2005). Q2(R1) Validation of Analytical Procedures: Text and Methodology – International Conference on Harminisation of Technical Requirements for Registration of Pharmaceuticals for Human Use. http://www.ich.org/fileadmin/Public_Web_Site/ICH_Products/Guidelines/ Quality/Q2_R1/Step4/Q2_R1__Guideline.pdf. Accessed on May 18, 2019.

ICH (2005a). International Conference on Harmonisation Safety Guideline S7B – Therapeutic Non-Clinical Evaluation of the Potential for Delayed Ventricular Repolarization (QT Interval Prolongation) by Human Pharmaceuticals. http://www.ich.org/products/guidelines/safety/article/safetyguidelines.html. Accessed on January 3, 2019.

ICH (2005b). International Conference on Harmonisation Safety Guideline S8 – Immunotoxicitystudies for Human Pharmaceuticals. http://www.ich.org/products/guidelines/safety/article/safety-guidelines.html. Accessed on January 3, 2019.

ICH (2006). Q8(R2) Pharmaceutical Development. http://www.fda.gov/downloads/Drugs/.../Guidances/ucm073507.pdf. Accessed on May, 3 2019.

ICH (2007a). Q9 Quality Risk Management. http://www.ich.org/fileadmin/Public_ Web_Site/ICH_Products/Guidelines/Quality/Q9/Step4/Q9_Guideline.pdf. Accessed on May, 3 2019.

ICH (2007b). Q10 Pharmaceutical Quality Systems. http://www.fda.gov/downloads/ Drugs/.../Guidances/ucm073517.pdf. Accessed on May, 3 2019.

Irwin, M. (2005). Prior choice, summarizing the posterior. http://www.markirwin. net/stat220/Lecture/Lecture3.pdf. Accessed on January 2, 2019.

Ishii, K.J., Gursel, I., Gursel, M., and Klinman, D.M. (2004). Immunotherapeutic utility of stimulatory and suppressive oligodeoxynucleotides. *Current Opinion in Molecular Therapeutics*, 6, 166–174.

Jeffreys, H. (1961). *Theory of Probability*. 3rd ed. Oxford University Press, London.

Ji, Y., Li, Y., and Bekele, B.N. (2007). Bayesian dose-finding in oncology clinical trials based on toxicity probability intervals. *Clinical Trials*, 4, 235–244.

Joseph, L., and Belisle, P. (1997). Bayesian sample size determination for normal means and difference between normal means. *Journal of the Royal Statistical Society*, 46, 209–226.

Joseph, L., du Berger, R., and Bélisle, P. (1997). Bayesian and mixed Bayesian/likelihood criteria for sample size determination. *Statistics in Medicine*, 16, 769–781.

Jung, S.H., Lee, T., Kim, K.M., and George, S.L. (2004). Admissible two-stage designs for phase II cancer clinical trials. *Statistics in Medicine*, 23, 561–569.

Kay, R. (2015). *Statistical Thinking for Non-Statisticians in Drug Regulations*. John Wiley & Sons, Ltd, Hoboken, NJ.

Kiermeier, A., Jarrett, R.G., and Verbyla, A.P. (2004). A new approach to estimating shelf-life. *Pharmaceutical Statistics*, 3, 3–11.

Kola, I., and Landis, J. (2004). Can the pharmaceutical industry reduce attrition rates? *Nature Reviews Drug Discovery*, 3(8), 711–715.

Komka, K., Kemény, S., and Bánfai, B. (2010). Novel tolerance interval model for the estimation of the shelf life of pharmaceutical products. *Journal of Chemometrics*, 24(3–4), 131–139.

Korn, E.L., Midthune, D., Chen, T.T., Rubinstein, L.V., Christian, M.C., and Simon, R.M. (1994). A comparison of two phase I trial designs. *Statistics in Medicine*, 13, 1799–1806.

Kozlowski, S., and Swann, P. (2009). Considerations for biotechnology product quality by design. In: *Quality by Design for Biopharmaceuticals: Principles and Case Studies*, edited by Rathore, A.S., and Mhatre, R. Wiley & Sons, Inc, Somerset, UK.

Krause, P. R. and Lewis, Jr., A. M. (1998). Safety of viral DNA in biological products. *Biologicals*, 36(3), 184–197.

Kringle, R. O. and Khan-Malek, R. C. (1994). A statistical assessment of the recommendations from a conference on analytical methods validation in bioavailability, bioequivalence, and pharmacokinetic studies. *Proceedings of the Biopharmaceutical Section of the American Statistical Association*, Alexandria, VA, 510–514.

Krishnamoorthy, K. and Mathew, T. (2009). *Statistical Tolerance Regions: Theory, Applications, and Computation*. Wiley, Hoboken, NJ.

Lakatos, E. (2016). Sample size for survival trials in cancer. In: *Cancer Clinical Trials*, edited by George, S.L., Wang, X., and Pang, H. CRC Press, Boca Raton, FL.

Laska, E.M., and Meisner, M.J. (1989). Testing whether an identified treatment is best. *Biometrics*, 45, 1139–1151.

LeBlond, D., Tan, C. and Yang, H. (2013). Confirmation of analytical method calibration linearity. *Pharmacopeial Forum*, May–June Issue, 39(3).

LeBlond, D. (2015). Applied non-clinical Bayesian statistics. Presented at 2015 Nonclinical Biostatistics Conference, Villanova, PA, 13 October 2015.

LeBrun, P. (2012). Bayesian Design Space Applied to Pharmaceutical. Unpublished dissertation, University de Liege. https://www.google.com/url?sa=t&rct=j&q=&esrc=s&frm=1&source=web&cd=3&ved=0ahUKEwijkrXoq8HKAhXI1x4KHXjoDEYQFggoMAI&url=https%3A%2F%2Forbi.ulg.ac.be%2Fbitstream%2F2268%2F126503%2F1%2Fthesis.pdf&usg=AFQjCNG-IxFztbhvUfL_3qMwMqKXH4LvZw&bvm=bv.112454388,d.dmo. Accessed on January 8, 2019.

Lebrun, P., Sondag, P., Lories, X., Michiels, J.-F., Rozet, E., and Boulanger, B. (2018). Quality by design applied in formulation development and robustness. In: *Statistics for Biotechnology Process Development*, edited by Coffey, Yang. Chapman & Hall/CRC Press, Boca Raton, FL.

Ledolter, J., and Burrill, C. (1999). *Statistical Quality Control: Strategies and Tools for Continual Improvement*. Wiley.

Lee, J.J., and Liu, D.D. (2008). A predictive probability design for phase II cancer trials. *Clinical Trials*, 5, 93–106.

Lee, J., Devanarayan V., Barrett Y., Weiner R., Allinson J., Fountain S., Keller S., Weinryb I., Green M., Duan L., Rogers J., Millham R., O'Brien P., Sailstad J., Khan M., Ray C. and Wagner J. (2006). Fit-for-purpose method development and validation for successful biomarker measurement. *Pharmaceutical Research*, 23(2), 312–28

Lehmann, E.L. (1952). Testing multiparameter hypotheses. *The Annals of Mathematical Statistics*, 23, 541–552.

Lin, T.Y.D., and Fairweather, W.R. (1997). Statistical design (bracketing and matrixing) and analysis of stability data for the US market. In *Proceedings of IBC Bracketing and Matrixing*, London.

Lin, Y., and Shih, W.J. (2001). Statistical properties of the traditional algorithm-based designs for phase I cancer clinical trials. *Biostatistics*, 2(2), 203–215.

Lin, Y., and Shih, W.J. (2004). Statistical properties of the modified algorithm-based designs for phase I cancer clinical trials. Technical report, Department of Biostatistics, University of Medicine and Dentistry of New Jersey.

Little, R.J. (2006). Calibrated Bayes: A Bayes/frequentist roadmap. *The American Statistician*, 60, 213–223.

Little, T.A. (2014). Design of experiments for analytical method development and validation. *BioPharm International*, 4(3). http://www.biopharminternational.com/design-experiments-analytical-method-development-and-validation. Assessed on May 18, 2019.

Loewe, S. (1928). Die quantitativen probleme der pharmakologie. *Ergebnisse Der Physiologie*, 27, 47–187.

Lunn, D., Spiegelhalter, D., Thomas, A., and Best, N. (2009). The BUGS project: Evolution, critique and future directions (with discussion). *Statistics in Medicine*, 28, 3049–3067.

Manola, A. (2012). Assessing release limits and manufacturing risk from a Bayesian perspective. Mid-West Biopharmaceutical Statistics Workshop, May 2012, Muncie, ID.

Martin, A.D., Quinn, K.M., and Park, J. (2011). MCMCpack: Markov Chain Monte Carlo in R. *Journal of Statistical Software* 42(9): 1–21. http://www.jstatsoft.org/v42/i09/.

Martin, G.P., Barnett, K.L., Burgess, C., Curry, P.D., Ermer, J., Gratzl, G.S., Hammond, J.P., Herrmann, J., Kovacs, E., LeBlond, D.J., LoBrutto, R., McCasland-Keller, A.K., McGregor, P.L., Nethercote, P., Templeton, A.C., Thomas, D.P., and Weitzel, J. (2013). Stimuli to the revision process: lifecycle managmement of analytical procedures: method development, procedure performance quantification,and procedure performance verification. *Phamacopeial Forum*, 39(5), http:/www.usp.org/uspnf/stimuli-article-lifecycle-management-analytical-procedures-posted-comment. Accessed on May 18, 2019.

Miller, K. and Bowsher, R., Celniker, A. et al. (2001). Workshop on bioanalytical methods validation for macromolecules: summary report. *Pharmaceutical Research*, 18, 1373–1383.

Møller, S. (1995). An extension of the continual reassessment methods using a preliminary up-and-down design in a dose finding study in cancer patients, in order to investigate a greater range of doses. *Statistics in Medicine*, 14, 911–922; discussion 923.

Montgomery, D.C. (2013). *Introduction to Statistical Quality Control*. 7th ed. Wiley, New York.

Morita, S., Thall, P.F., and Müller, P. (2008). Determining the effective sample size of a parametric prior. *Biometrics*, 64, 595–602.

Moyé, L.A. (2008). Bayesians in clinical trials: Asleep at the switch. *Statistics in Medicine*, 27, 469–482; discussion 483.

Murphy, J.R. (1996). Uniform matrix stability study designs. *Journal of Biopharmaceutical Statistics*, 6, 477–494.

Natanegara, F., Neuenschwander, B., Seaman, J.W., Kinnersley,N., Heilmann, C.R., Ohlssen, D., and Rochester, G. (2014). The current state of Bayesian methods in medical product development: Survey results and recommendations from the DIA Bayesian Scientific Working Group. *Pharmaceutical Statistics*, 13(1), 3–12.

Nelson, L.S. (1984). Technical aids. *Journal of Quality Technology*, 16(4), 238–239.

Nethrcote, P., Borman, P., Bennett, T., Martin, G., and McGregor, P. (2010). QbD for better method validation and transfer. *Pharmaceutical Manufacturing*, http://www.pharmamanufacturing.com/articles/2010/060/. Accessed on April 17, 2016.

Netherote, P. and Ermer, J. (2012). Quality by design for analytical methods: implications for method validation and transfer. *Pharmaceutical Technology*, 36(10), 74–79.

Ng, K., and Rajagopalan, N. (2009). Application of quality by design and risk assessment principles for the development of formulation design space. In: *Quality by Design for Biopharmaceuticals: Principles and Case Studies*, edited by Rathore, A.S., and Mhatre, R. Wiley & Sons, Inc, Somerset, UK.

Nordbrock, E. (1992). Statistical comparison of stability designs. *Journal of Biopharmaceutical Statistics*, 2, 91–113.

Nordbrock, E., and Valvani, S. (1995). PhRMA Stability Working Group. In: *Guideline for Matrix Designs of Drug Product Stability Protocols*, January, 1995.

Novick, S., Ho, S., and Best, N. (2018a). Data-driven prior distribution for a Bayesian phase-2 COPD dose-finding clinical trial. *Statistics in Biopharmaceutical Research*, 10(3), 166–175.

Novick, S. and Yang, H. (2013). Directly testing the linearity assumption for assay validation. *Journal of Chemometrics*, 27(5):117–123.

Novick, S., and Peterson, J. (2015). Drug combination design strategies. In: *Statistical Methods in Drug Combination Studies*, edited by Zhao, W., and Yang, H. CRC Press, Boca Raton, FL.

Novick, S.J. (2013). A simple test for synergy for a small number of combinations. *Statistics in Medicine*, 32(29), 5145–5155.

Novick, S., Yang, H. and Peterson, J. (2012). A Bayesian approach to parallelism testing. *Statistics in Biopharmaceutical Research*. 4(4), 357–374.

Novick, S.J., Sachsenmeier, K., Leow, C.C., Roskos, L., and Yang, H. (2018b). A novel Bayesian method for efficacy assessment in animal oncology studies. *Statistics in Pharmaceutical Research*, 10(3), 151–157.

O'Brian, P.C., and Fleming, T.R. (1979). A multiple testing procedure for clinical trials. *Biometrics*, 35, 549–556.

O'Hagan, A., Stevens, J.W., and Campbell, M.J. (2005). Assurance in clinical trial design. *Pharmaceutical Statistics*, 4, 187–201.

Ohlssen, D. (2016). An industry perspective of the value of Bayesian methods. American course on drug development and regulatory sciences (ACDRS) special workshop: Substantial evidence in 21st century of regulatory sciences – Borrowing strength from accumulating data, April 21st 2016. https://pharm.ucsf.edu/sites/pharm.ucsf.edu/files/ohlssen.pdf. Accessed on January 20, 2019.

O'Quigley, J. (1992). Estimating the probability of toxicity at the recommended dose following a phase I clinical trial in cancer. *Biometrics*, 48, 885–893.

O'Quigley, J., and Chevret, S. (1991). Methods for dose-finding studies in cancer clinical trials: A review and results of a Monte Carlo study. *Statistics in Medicine*, 10, 1647–1664.

O'Quigley, J., Pepe, M., and Fisher, L. (1990). Continual reassessment method: A practical design for phase I clinical trials in cancer. *Biometrics*, 46(2), 203–2015.

O'Quigley, J., and Zhen, L.Z. (1995). Continual reassessment methods: A likelihood approach. *Biometrics*, 52, 673–684.

Oron, A.P., and Flournoy, N. (2017). Centered isotonic regression: Point and interval estimation for dose-response studies. *Statistics in Biopharmaceutical Research*, 9(3), 258–267.

Page, E.S. (1954). Continuous inspection schemes. *Biometrika*, 41 (1/2), 100–115.

Peden, K., Sheng, L., Pal, A., and Lewis, A. (2006). Biological activity of residual cell substrate DNA. *Developmental Biology (Basel)* 123, 45–56; discussion 55–73.

Peltzman, S. (1973). An evaluation of consumer protection legislation: The 1962 drug amendments. *Journal of Political Economy*, 81(5):1049–1091.

Peterson, J.J. (2007). A review of Bayesian reliability approaches to multiple response surface optimization. In: *Bayesian Statistics for Process Monitoring, Control, and Optimization*, edited by Colosimo, B.M., and del Castillo, E. Chapman and Hall/CRC Press, Boca Raton, FL.

Peterson, J.J. (2008). A Bayesian approach to the ICH Q8 definition of design space. *Journal of Biopharmaceutical Statistics*, 18, 959–975.

Peterson, J.J. (2009). What your ICH Q8 design space needs: A multivariate predictive distribution. *Pharmaceutical Manufacturing*, 8(10), 23–28.

Peterson, J.J., and Lief, K. (2010). The ICH Q8 definition of design space: A comparison of the overlapping means and the Bayesian predictive approaches. *Statistics in Biopharmaceutical Research*, 2, 249–259.

Peterson, J.J., Snee, R.D., McAllister, P.R., Schofield, T.L., and Carella, A.J. (2009). Statistics in pharmaceutical development and manufacturing (with discussion). *Journal of Quality Technology*, 41, 111–134.

Peterson, J. J. and Yahyah, M. (2009). A Bayesian design space approach to robustness and system suitability for pharmaceutical assays and other processes. *Statistics in Biopharmaceutical Research*, 1(4), 441–449.

Petricciani, J., and Loewer, J. (2001). An overview of cell DNA issues. *Developments in Biologicals*, 106, 275–282; discussion 317.

Petrova, R.D. (2012). New scientific approaches to cancer treatment: Can medicinal mushrooms defeat the curse of the century? *International Journal of Medicinal Mushrooms*, 14(1), 1–20.

PhRMA (2015). Biopharmaceutical research & development: The process behind new medicines. http://phrma-docs.phrma.org/sites/default/files/pdf/rd_brochure_022307.pdf. Accessed on January 1, 2019.

Piantadosi, S., and Liu, G. (1996). Improved design for dose escalation studies using pharmacokinetic measurements. *Statistics in Medicine*, 15, 1605–1618.

Plummer, M. (2003). JAGS: A program for analysis of Bayesian graphical models using Gibbs sampling. In: Proceedings of the 3rd International Workshop on Distributed Statistical Computing (DSC 2003), March 20–22, Vienna, Austria. ISSN 1609-395X.

Pocock, S.J. (1977). Group sequential methods in the design and analysis of clinical trials. *Biometrika*, 64, 191–199.

Pocock, S.J. (1982). Interim analyses for randomized clinical trials: The group sequential approach. *Biometrics*, 38, 153–162.

Pong, A., and Raghavarao, D. (2000). Comparison of bracketing and matrixing designs for a two-year stability study. *Journal of Biopharmaceutical Statistics*, 10, 217–228.

Pourkavoos, N. (2012). Unique risks, benefits, and challenges of developing drug–drug combination products in a pharmaceutical industry setting. *Combination Products in Therapy*, 2(2), 1–31.

Press, S.J. (1972). *Applied Multivariate Analysis: Using Bayesian and Frequentist Methods of Inference*. R.E. Krieger Pub. Co., Malabar, FL.

Qian, J., Stangl, D.K., and George, S. (1996). A Weibull model for survival data: Using prediction to decide when to stop a clinical trial. In: *Bayesian Biostatistics*, edited by Berry, D.A., and Stangl, D.K. CRC, Boca Raton, FL.

Quinlan, M., Stroup, W., Christopher, D., and Schwenke, J. (2013). On the distribution of batch shelf lives. *Journal of Biopharmaceutical Statistics*, 23, 897–920.

R Core Team (2018). *R: A Language and Environment for Statistical Computing*. R Foundation for Statistical Computing, Vienna, Austria. https://www.R-project.org/.

Ramaswamy, S. (2007). Rational design of cancer-drug combinations. *The New England Journal of Medicine*, 357, 299–300.

Ratain, M.J., Mick, R., Schilsky, R.L., and Siegler, M. (1993). Statistical and ethical issues in the design and conduct of phase I and II clinical trials of new anticancer agents. *Journal of the National Cancer Institute*, 85, 1637–1643.

Rathore, A.S., and Mhatre (2009). *Quality by Design for Biopharmaceuticals: Principles and Case Studies*. Wiley & Sons, Inc, Somerset, UK.

Richmond, A., and Su, Y. (2008). Mouse xenograft models vs. GEM models for human cancer therapeutics. *Disease Models and Mechanisms*, 1, 78–82.

Riley, C.M., and Yang, H. (2019). General principles and regulatory considerations: Specifications and shelf life setting. In: *Specification of Drug Substances and Products: Development and Validation of Analytical Methods.* 2nd ed., edited by Riley, C.M., Rosanke, T.W., and Riley, S.R.R. Elsevier, Amsterdam, the Netherlands.

Robert, C., and Casella, G. (2004). *Monte Carlo Statistical Methods.* Springer, New York.

Robert, C.P. (2013). Bayesian Computational Tools. https://arxiv.org/pdf/1304.2048.pdf. Accessed on January 20, 2019.

Roberts, S. W. (1959). Control chart tests based on geometric moving averages. *Technometrics*, 1, 239–250.

Robertson, A., Wright, F.T., and Dykstra, R. (1988). *Order Restricted Statistical Inference.* John Wiley, New York.

Rodriguez, G. (2010). Survival models. https://data.princeton.edu/wws509/notes/c7.pdf. Accessed on January 20, 2019.

Rogatko, A., Schoeneck, D., Jonas, W., Tighiouart, M., Khuri, F.R., and Porter, A. (2007). Translation of innovative designs into phase I trials. *Journal of Clinical Oncology*, 25(31), 4982–4986.

Rothenfusser, S., Tuma, E., Wagner, M., Endres, S., and Hartmann, G. (2003). Recent advance in immunostimulatory CpG oligonucleotides. *Current Opinion in Molecular Therapeutics*, 5, 98–106.

Rozet, E., Govaertsb, B., Lebruna, P., Michail, K., Ziemons, E., Wintersteigerc R., Rudaz, S., Boulanger, B., and Hubert, P. (2011). Evaluating the reliability of analytical results using a probability criterion: A Bayesian perspective. *Analytica Chimica Acta*, 705, 193–206.

Saffaj, T. and Ihsane, B. (2012). A Bayesian approach for application to method validation and measurement uncertainty. *Talanta*, 92, 15–25.

Sahu, S.K., and Smith, T.M.F. (2006). A Bayesian method of sample size determination with practical applications. *Journal of the Royal Statistical Society, Series A*, 169, 235–253.

Sambucini, V. (2008). A Bayesian predictive two-stage design for phase II clinical trials. *Statistics in Medicine*, 27, 1199–1224.

Satterthwaite FW. (1946). An approximate distribution of estimates of variance components. *Biometrics Bulletin*, 2, 110.

Schenerman, M.A., Axley, M.J., Oliver, C.N., Ram, K., and Wasserman, G.F. (2009). Using a risk assessment process to determine criticality of product quality attributes. In: *Quality by Design for Biopharmaceuticals: Principles and Case Studies*, edited by Rathore, A.S., and Mhatre, R. Wiley & Sons, Inc., Somerset, UK.

Schoot, R., Kaplan, D., Denissen, J., Asendorpf, J.B., Neyer, F.J., and Aken, M.A.G. (2013). A gentle introduction to Bayesian analysis: Applications to developmental research. *Children Development*, 85(3), 842–860.

Seber, G. F., and Wild, C.J. (2003). *Nonlinear Regression.* Wiley, Hoboken, NJ.

Shao, J., and Chow, S.-C. (1991). Constructing release targets for drug products: A Bayesian decision theory approach. *Journal of Applied Statistics*, 40(3), 381–391.

Shao, J., and Chow, S.-C. (2001). Drug shelf life estimation. *Statistica Sinica*, 11, 737–745.

Sheng, L., Cai, F., Zhu, Y., Pal, A., Athanasiou, M., Orrison, B., Blair, D.G., Hughes, S.H., Coffin, J.M., Lewis, A.M., and Peden, K. (2008). Oncogenicity of DNA in vivo: Tumor induction with expression plasmids for activated H-ras and c-myc. *Biologicals*, 36, 184–197.

Sheng-Fowler, L., Cai, F., Fu, H., Zhu, Y., Orrison, B., Foseh, G., Blair, D.G., Hughes, S.H., Coffin, J.M., Lewis, A.M. Jr, and Peden, K. (2010). Tumors induced in mice by direct inoculation of plasmid DNA expressing both activated H-ras and c-myc. *International Journal of Biological Sciences*, 6, 151–162.

Sheng-Fowler, L., Lewis, A.M. Jr, and Peden, K. (2009a). Issues associated with residual cell-substrate DNA in viral vaccines. *Biologicals*, 37, 190–195.

Sheng-Fowler, L., Lewis, A.M. Jr, and Peden, K. (2009b). Quantitative determination of the infectivity of the proviral DNA of a retrovirus in vitro: Evaluation of methods for DNA inactivation. *Biologicals*, 37, 259–269.

Shewhart , W. A. (1931). *Economic Control of Manufactured Product*. D. Van Nostrand Co., Inc., New York.

Simon, R. (1989). Optimal two-stage designs for phase II clinical trials. *Controlled Clinical Trials*, 10, 1–10.

Singh, K., Kirchhoff, C.F., and Banerjee, A. (2009). Application of QbD principles to biologics product: Formulation and process development. In: *Quality by Design for Biopharmaceuticals: Principles and Case Studies*, edited by Rathore, A.S., and Mhatre, R. Wiley & Sons, Inc., Somerset, UK.

Smith, M.K., and Marshall, S. (2006). A Bayesian design and analysis for dose-response using informative prior information. *Journal of Biopharmaceutical Statistics*, 16, 695–709.

Snapinn, S., Chen, M.G., Jiang, Q., and Koutsoukos, T. (2006). Assessment of futility in clinical trials. *Pharmaceutical Statistics*, 5(4):273–281.

Snapinn, S.M. (1987). Evaluating the efficacy of a combination therapy. *Statistics in Medicine*, 6, 657–665.

Sondag, P., Lebrun, P., Rozet, E., and Boulanger, B. (2016). Assay validation. In: *Nonclinical Statistics for Pharmaceutical and Biotechnology Industries*, edited by Zhang, L., Kuhn, M., Peers, I., and Altan, S. Springer, Cham, Switzerland.

Spiegelhalter, D.J., Abrams, K.R., and Myles, J.P. (2004). *Bayesian Approaches to Clinical Trials and Health-Care Evaluation*. Wiley, Chichester, UK.

Spiegelhalter, D.J. and Freedman, L.S. (1986). A predicative approach to selecting the size of a clinical trials, based on subjective clinical opinion. *Statistics in Medicine*, 5, 1–13.

Stan Development Team (2018). *Stan Modeling Language Users Guide and Reference Manual*, Version 2.18.0. http://mc-stan.org.

Stand, A., and Strickland, H. (2016). Process capability and statistical control. In: *Nonclinical Biostatistics for Pharmaceutical and Biotechnology*, edited by Zhang, L. et al. Springer, Cham, Switzerland.

Stein, W.D., Figg, W.D., Dahut, W., Stein, A.D., Hoshen, M.B., Price, D., Bates, S.E., and Fojo, T. (2008). Tumor growth rates derived from data for patients in a clinical trial correlate strongly with patient survival: A novel strategy for evaluation of clinical trial data. *The Oncologist*, 13, 1046–1054.

Stein, W.D., Gulley, J.L., Schlom, J., Madan, R.A., Dahut,W., Figg, W.D., Ning, Y.M., Arlen, P.M., Price, D., Bates, S.E., and Fojo, T. (2011). Tumor regression and growth rates determined in five intramural NCI prostate cancer trials: The growth rate constants as an indicator of therapeutic effect. *Clinical Cancer Research*, 17, 907–917.

Stein, W.D., Huang, H., Menefee, M., Edgerly, M., Kotz, H., Dwyer, A., Yang, J., and Bates, S.E. (2009). Other paradigms: Growth rate constants and tumor burden determined using computed tomography data correlate strongly with the overall survival of patients with renal cell carcinoma. *Cancer Journal*, 15, 441–447.

Stigler, S.M. (1986). *The History of Statistics: The Measurement of Uncertainty before 1900.* Harvard University Press, Cambridge, MA.

Stockdale, G.W., and Cheng, A. (2009). Finding design space and a reliable operating region using a multivariate Bayesian approach with experimental design. *Quality Technology and Quantitative Management*, 6(4), 391–408.

Storer, B.E. (1989). Design and analysis of phase I clinical Trials. *Biometrics*, 45, 925–937.

Stroup, W., and Quinlan, M. (2010). Alternative shelf life estimation methodologies. In: Proceedings of 2010 Joint Statistical Meeting. American Statistical Association, Alexandria, VA, 2056–2066.

Stroup, W., and Quinlan, M. (2016). Statistical considerations for stability and estimation of shelf life. In: *Nonclinical Statistics for Pharmaceutical and Biotechnology Industries*, edited by Zhang, L., Kuhn, M., Peers, I., and Altan, S. Springer, Cham, Switzerland.

Thall, P.F., and Lee, S.J. (2003). Practical model-based dose-finding in phase I clinical trials: Methods based on toxicity. *International Journal of Gynecological Cancer*, 13(3), 251–261.

Thall, P.F., and Simon, R. (1994a). Practical Bayesian guidelines for phase IIB clinical trials. *Biometrics*, 50, 337–349.

Thall, P.F., and Simon, R. (1994b). A Bayesian approach to establishing sample size and monitoring criteria for phase II clinical trials. *Controlled Clinical Trials*, 15, 463–481.

Thall, P.F., and Simon, R.M. (1995). Recent developments in the design of phase II clinical trials. *Cancer Treatment and Research*, 75, 49–71.

Thall, P.F., Simon, R.M., and Estey, E.H. (1995). Bayesian sequential monitoring designs for single-arm clinical trials with multiple outcomes. *Statistics in Medicine*, 14, 357–379.

Thomas, N., and Roy, D. (2017). Analysis of clinical dose–response in small-molecule drug development: 2009–2014. *Statistics in Biopharmaceutical Research*, 9(2), 137–146.

Thomas, N., Sweeney, K., and Somayaji, V. (2014). Meta-analysis of clinical dose–response in a large drug development portfolio. *Statistics in Biopharmaceutical Research*, 6(4), 302–317.

Tsong, Y. (1992). False alarm rates of statistical methods used in determining increased frequency of reports on adverse drug reaction. *Journal of Biopharmaceutical Statistics*, 2(1), 9–30.

Tsong, Y. (1999). Statistical considerations in the analysis of postmarketing adverse event report. Presented at the 1999 Midwest Biopharmaceutical Statistics Workshop. Ball University, Muncie, IN, 24–25 May.

Tsutakawa, R.K. (1972). Design of experiment for bioassay. *Journal of the American Statistical Association*, 67(339), 584–590.

USP (1989). General information <1225> validation of compendial methods. *United States Pharmacopeia*, XXVI, 2439–2442.

USP (2013). General information <1210> statistical tools for analytical procedure validation. *Pharmacopeial Forum*, 40(5).

USP (2015). USP <1010> analytical data—Interpretation and treatment. *USP 38–NF* 33, 19–34. http://www.usp.org/sites/default/files/usp/document/our-work/DS/2015-dsc-chapters-561-616-1010-1092.pdf. Accessed on January 21, 2019.

Vardi, Y., Ying, Z., and Zhang, C.-H. (2001). Two-sample tests for growth curves under dependent right censoring. *Biometrika*, 88, 949–960.

Wang, F., and Gelfand, A.E. (2002). A simulation-based approach to Bayesian sample size determination for performance under a given model and for separating models. *Statistical Science*, 17(2), 193–208.

Wang, S.K., and Tsiatis, A.A. (1987). Approximately optimal one-parameter boundaries for a sequential trial. *Biometrics*, 43, 605–611.

Wei, G.C.G. (1998). Simple methods for determination of the release limits for drug products. *Journal of Biopharmaceutical Statistics*, 8(1), 103–114.

Wei, G.C.G. (2003). Release targets. In: *Encyclopedia of Biopharmaceutical Statistics*, edited by Chow, S.-C. Marcel Dekker, New York.

Whitehead, J., Valdés-Márquez, E., Johnson, P., and Graham, G. (2008). Bayesian sample size for exploratory clinical trials incorporating historical data. *Statistics in Medicine*, 27, 2307–2327.

WHO (2006). WHO Guidelines on Stability Evaluation of Vaccines. http://www.who.int/biologicals/publications/trs/areas/vaccines/stability/Microsoft%20Word%20-%20BS%202049.Stability.final.09_Nov_06.pdf. Accessed on January 6, 2019.

WHO (World Health Organization) (2007). Meeting Report (11–12 June, 2007) Study Group on Cell Substrates for Production of Biological, 1–30. https://www.who.int/biologicals/publications/meetings/areas/vaccines/cells/Cells.FINAL.MtgRep.IK.26_Sep_07.pdf?ua=1. Accessed on May 3, 2019.

WHO (2009). Handbook for Good Laboratory Practice (GLP). https://www.who.int/tdr/publications/documents/glp-handbook.pdf. Accessed on January 1, 2019.

Winkler, R.L. (2001). Why Bayesian analysis hasn't caught on in healthcare decision making. *International Journal of Technology Assessment in Health Care*, 17, 56–66.

Woodcock, J. (2012). Reliable drug quality: An unresolved problem. *PDA Journal of Pharmaceutical Science and Technology*, 66, 270–272.

Wolfinger, R.D. (1998). Tolerance intervals for variance component models using Bayesian simulation. *Journal of Quality Technology*, 30, 18–32.

Wu, J., Banerjee, A., Jin, B., Menon, S.M., Martin, S.W., and Heatherington, A.C. (2018). Clinical dose–response for a broad set of biological products: A model-based meta-analysis. *Statistical Methods in Medical Research*, 27(9), 2694–2721.

Yang, H. (2012). Ensure product quality and regulatory compliance through novel stability design and analysis. *The Journal of Validation Technology*, 18(3), 52–59.

Yang, H. (2013a). Setting specifications of correlated quality attributes. *PDA Journal of Pharmaceutical Science and Technology*, 67, 533–543.

Yang, H. (2013b). Establishing acceptable limits of residual DNA (2013). *PDA Journal of Pharmaceutical Science and Technology*, 67(March–April Issue), 155–163.

Yang, H. (2017). *Emerging Non-Clinical Biostatistics for Biopharmaceutical Development and Manufacturing*. Chapman & Hall/CRC, Boca Raton, FL.

Yang, H., Wei, Z., and Schenerman, M. (2015). A statistical approach to determining criticality of residual host cell DNA. *Journal of Biopharmaceutical Statistics*, 25(2), 234–246.

Yang, H., and Zhang, J. (2016). A Bayesian approach to residual host cell DNA safety assessment. *PDA Journal of Pharmaceutical Science and Technology*, 70, 157–162.

Yang, H., and Zhang, L. (2012). Evaluation of statistical methods for estimating shelf life of drug products: A unified and risk-based approach. *The Journal of Validation Technology*, http://www.ivtnetwork.com/sites/default/files/IVTJVT0512_067-074_Yang-%7B1237440%7D.pdf. Accessed on January 8, 2019.

Yang, H., Zhang, J., Yu, B., and Zhao, W. (2016). *Statistical Methods for Immunogenicity Assessment*. Chapman & Hall/CRC Press, Boca Raton, FL.

Yang, H., Zhang, L., and Cho, I. (2007). Statistical modeling in detecting safety signals for product quality issue. In: Proceedings of 2007 JSM. American Statistical Association, Alexandria, VA.

Yang, H. and Zhang, L. (2015). A generalized pivotal quantity approach to analytical method validation based on total error. *PDA Journal of Pharmaceutical Science and Technology*, 69, 725–735

Yang, H., Zhang, L., and Galinski, M. (2010). A probabilistic model for risk assessment of residual host cell DNA in biological products. *Vaccine*, 28(19), 3308–3311.

Yang, H., Novick, S., and LeBlond, D. (2015). Testing analytical method linearity within a pre-specified range. *Journal of Biopharmaceutical Statistics*, 25(2), 334–350.

Yang, H. and Schofield, T. (2014). Statistical considerations in design and analysis of analytical method bridging studies. *Journal of Validation Technology*. Spring Issue. http://www.ivtnetwork.com/article/statistical-considerations-design-and-analysis-bridging-studies. Accessed on May 18, 2019.

Yang, R., and Berger, J.O. (1998). A catalog of noninformative priors. http://www.stats.org.uk/priors/noninformative/YangBerger1998.pdf. Accessed on January 2, 2019.

Yu, B., Zeng, L., Ren, P., and Yang, H. (2017). Evaluation of different estimation methods for accuracy and precision in biological assay validation. *PDA Journal of Pharmaceutical Science and Technology*, 71(4), 297–305.

Yu, B., Zeng, L., and Yang, H. (2017). Determination of acceptance criteria and sample sizes for accelerated stability comparability studies for biologics. *Biologicals*, 49, 46–50.

Yu, B., Zeng, L., and Yang, H. (2018). A Bayesian Approach to setting the release limits for critical quality attributes. *Statistics in Biopharmaceutical Research*, 10(3), 158–165.

Yu, L.X., Amidon, G., Khan, M.A., Hoag, S.W., Polli, J., Raju, J.K., and Woodcock, J. (2015). Understanding pharmaceutical quality by design. *The AAPS Journal*, 16(4), 71–783.

Zeng, L., Novick, S., Yu, B., and Yang, H. (2018). A general framework for equivalence testing over a range of linear outcomes with CMC applications. *Statistics in Biopharmaceutical Research*. DOI: 10.1080/19466315.2018.1470029.

Zacks, S., Rogatko, A., and Babb, J. (1998). Optimal Bayesian feasible dose escalation for cancer phase I trials. *Statistics in Medicine*, 25, 2365–2383.

Zhao, W., and Yang, H. (2015). *Statistical Methods in Drug Combination Studies*. CRC Press, Boca Raton, FL.

Zhang, J. and Yang, H. (2018). Multivariate Analysis for Process Understanding and Troubleshooting. In *Statistics for Biotechnology Process Development*, edited by Coffey, T. and Yang, H. CRC Press, Boca Raton, FL.

Index

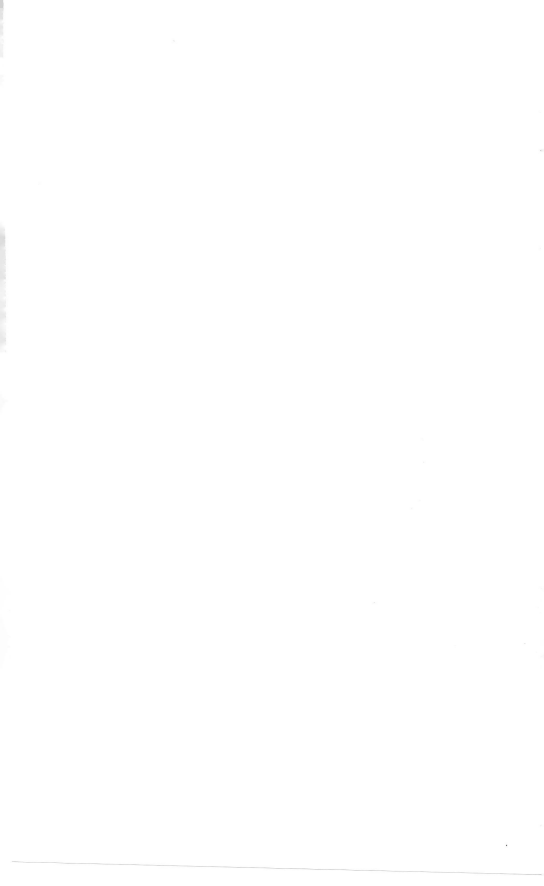